# Forensic Medicine

## for the Police

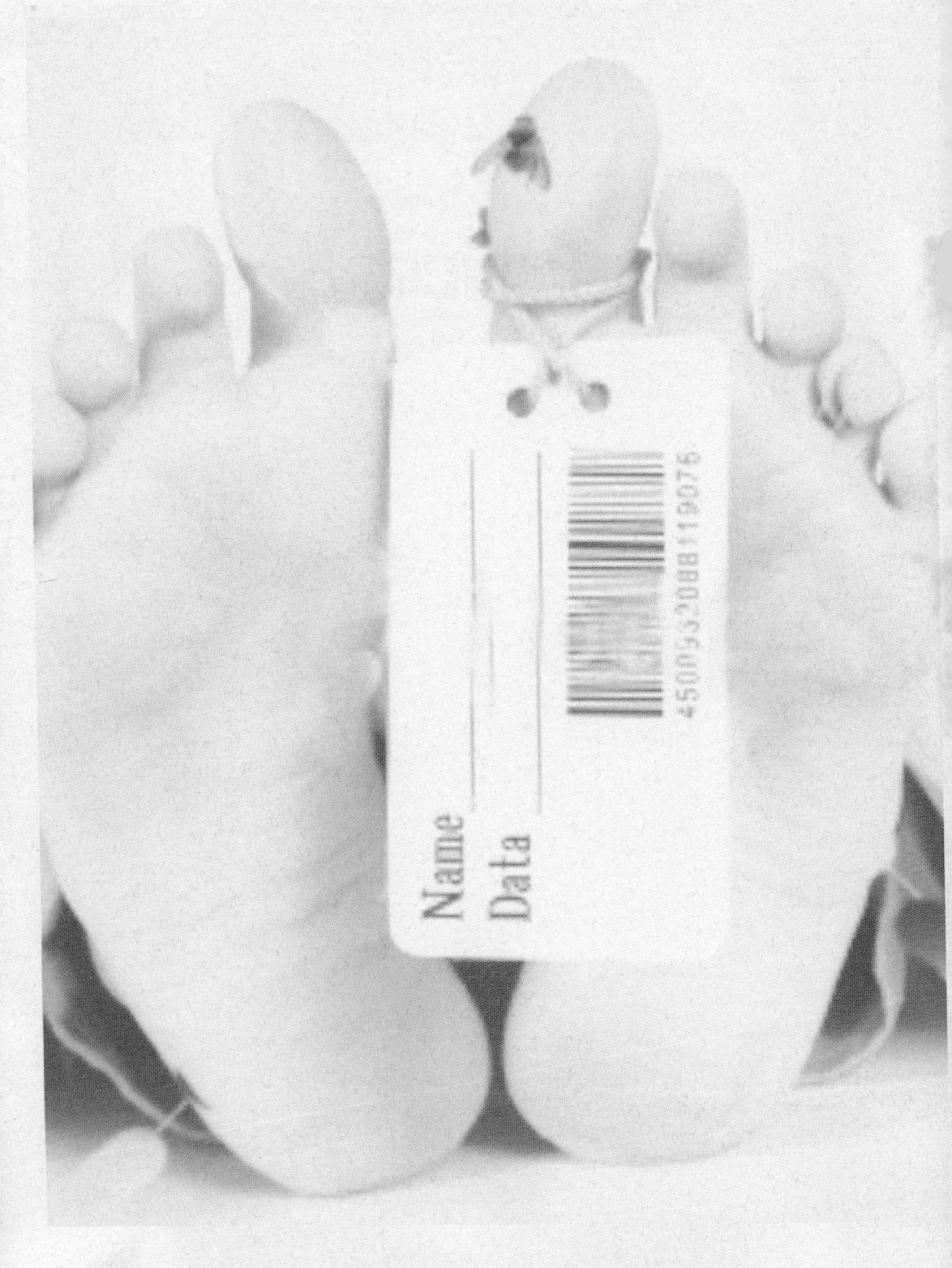

Name _____

Data _____

450093208811907b

# Forensic Medicine

## for the Police

### B. Umadethan MD

Professor and Head, Department of Forensic Medicine
Professor in charge and Coordinator
Department of Medical Education, College of Medicine
Amrita Institute of Medical Sciences, Kochi, Kerala

Formerly Professor and Head, Department of Forensic Medicine, and Police Surgeon
Medical Colleges of Thiruvananthapuram, Alappuzha and Thrissur

Director, State Medicolegal Institute
State Medicolegal Expert and Consultant
Medicolegal Adviser to Kerala Police

Principal, Medical College, Thiruvananthapuram

Director of Medical Education, Kerala, and

Medicolegal Consultant, Libyan Arab Republic

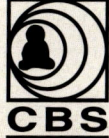

CBS

## CBS PUBLISHERS & DISTRIBUTORS Pvt Ltd

New Delhi • Bengaluru • Pune • Kochi • Chennai

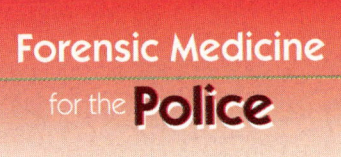

Forensic Medicine for the **Police**

ISBN: 978-81-239-1976-8 (Hard cover)
ISBN: 978-81-239-1905-8 (Soft cover)

Copyright © Author and Publishers

**First Edition:** 2011

Published by Satish Kumar Jain and produced by Vinod K. Jain for

**CBS Publishers & Distributors** Pvt Ltd

4819/XI Prahlad Street, 24 Ansari Road, Daryaganj,
New Delhi 110 002, India.
Ph: 23289259, 23266861/67          Fax: +91-011-23243014

Website: www.cbspd.com
e-mail:   delhi@cbspd.com;
          cbspubs@vsnl.com;
          cbspubs@airtelmail.in.

**Branches**

- Bengaluru: Seema House 2975, 17th Cross, K.R. Road,
  Banasankari 2nd Stage, Bengaluru 560 070, Karnataka
  Ph: +91-80-26771678/79          Fax: +91-80-26771680          e-mail:  bangalore@cbspd.com

- Pune: Bhuruk Prestige, Sr. No. 52/12/2+1+3/2 Narhe, Haveli
  (Near Katraj-Dehu Road Bypass), Pune 411 051, Maharashtra
  Ph: 020-32404169          e-mail:  pune@cbspd.com

- Kochi: 36/14 Kalluvilakam, Lissie Hospital Road, Kochi 682 018, Kerala
  Ph: +91-484-4059061-65          Fax: +91-484-4059065          e-mail:  cochin@cbspd.com

- Chennai: 20, West Park Road, Shenoy Nagar, Chennai 600 030, Tamil Nadu
  Ph: +91-44-26260666, 26208620          Fax: +91-44-45530020          email:  chennai@cbspd.com

*Printed at* Magic International Private Limited, Greater Noida, UP

*to*

*The officers and men of the police forces who
relentlessly work to enforce law and order
and toil in the pursuit of truth in
the investigation of crimes*

# Foreword

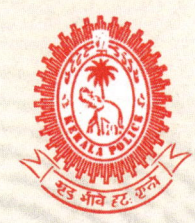

**Jacob Punnoose** IPS
Director General of Police

Police Headquarters, Trivandrum-695 010
Phone : (0) 0471 2721601
(M) 0944 6111221
*e-mail:* jacobpunnoose@gmail.com

Every year Police in Kerala conduct almost 15,000 inquests over dead bodies. In each, the police officer has to answer the question "accident, suicide or homicide?" The answer has to be supported by sound reasoning and convincing evidence. Additionally, there are thousands of cases of hurt, injury, drunkenness, etc. where the forensic medical expert can help the policeman in arriving at a correct decision in evaluating clues and in judging the authenticity of conflicting versions of witnesses.

Knowledge of forensic medicine comes to the help of the professional policeman who is trying to answer such questions. Such knowledge will enable him to look for clues and circumstances which can later help the forensic medical expert give a decisive opinion on examining the body or the injury. Ignorance of forensic medicine may cause disregard for such vital clues.

Usually books on forensic medicine are written for the medical expert and some medical knowledge is assumed on the part of the reader. Therefore the policeman who reads such books is left with doubts. Therefore a book which answers the needs of the policeman, the lawyer and the doctor alike was long overdue.

At long last Prof. (Dr.) Umadethan has taken the trouble to enrich his profession by writing such a book. From first to last, it is a book written for the practical police officer, the professional doctor and the practicing lawyer. The structure of the book, the style of presentation, the explanatory annexures, the details given about procedural nuances, the pragmatic hints governing practical situations — all these make this book an essential volume in the library of every policeman, doctor and lawyer. This book will be an invaluable tool in guiding them to a better observation for clues which can yield decisive forensic evidence and to a better understanding of the intricacies of forensic interpretation of observed conditions.

I have known Dr. Umadethan for nearly a quarter of a century. I have been associated with him in solving and seeking solutions to many a forensic mystery. He combines unparalleled knowledge of the nuances of forensic medicine with rare investigative perception, enabling him not only to divine the cause of death or injury, but also to reconstruct, with great accuracy, the process which led to the causation of death or injury. I am happy that he has written this book which will be the best possible practical guide to the practitioners and beneficiaries of forensic sciences.

**Jacob Punnoose** IPS

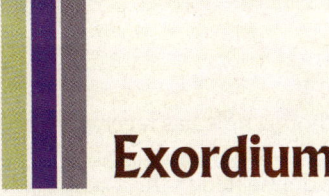

# Exordium

## Justice K.T. Thomas
Former Judge, Supreme Court of India
('Padma Bhushan' awardee President of India)

I have great pleasure in introducing this monumental work to the readers. I have two reasons, mainly, to feel so happy about it. First is that my own experience (as counsel practised actively for seventeen years and thereafter as judge at three different levels: Sessions Court, High Court and the Supreme Court) showed that proper awareness on medical aspects has wholesome usefulness in unfurling the truth in criminal cases. Second is the impression I formed about the author for over a period of three decades that he is a connoisseur in the field of forensic medicine.

I recollect with all vividness the evidence given by Dr Umadethan on photographic superimposition technique, which was then only in its nascent stage. Though the advantage of the evidence based on that technique is not conclusive in establishing the identity of the *corpus delicti* (dead body), it has a salutary impact on the process of reaching conclusions in sensitive areas. The testimony given by him including his answers in grilling cross-examination conducted by a seasoned criminal lawyer instilled great impression in my mind. Ultimately I acted on that testimony which was a fillip in unraveling the mystery which surrounded the dispute regarding the identity of a skeleton disinterred from a pit. This does not mean that photographic superimposition technique is flawless. Apart from the possibility of human error, there is the possibility of technicians and doctors leaning in favour of positive finding actuated by predisposition of mind developed from police versions submitted to them. It is, therefore, advisable not to accept the result of the technique as conclusive proof for identity of the *corpus delicti*. The Supreme Court of India, in its wisdom, repeatedly held that evidence-based on this technique has only corroborative value.

I had the occasion to know Dr Umadethan at closer quarters during later years. The opinion given by him in a number of cases gave me the impression that he is not only an expert in the subject but one who dauntlessly gives his opinion unmindful of public opinion built up by any media publication. He would dare to face any consequence for steadfastly adhering to his conviction formed from the data available. I am much relieved to learn that the High Court of Kerala had, in its majesty, exercised inherent powers on two occasions to erase some unsavoury remarks injudiciously and imprudently passed against him by the lower judiciary and thereby restored his probity. Thus his credibility remains unsullied.

During my early stages of practice as trial lawyer, the subject Forensic Medicine became attracted to me because a proper understanding of the nature of wounds, duration of time for different putrefactive changes, and time for digestion of different kinds of food articles and a lot more can have great influence on choreographing the defence strategy. After I became judge, my interest in that subject became doubled as it helped to arrive at judicial conclusions in a variety of cases.

I realised that frontiers of medical jurisprudence as a subject have widened, thanks to the dedicated researches conducted by the studious members of the faculty of medicolegal science in different medical colleges. During the first half of the constitutional history of India, books available for legal fraternity were only handful but in the second half the number of books multiplied as newer areas on the subject have been surveyed by connoisseurs of this topic. It is heartening to note that the list of new authors includes doctors in India.

A cursory perusal of this book provided me the perception that the author's angle has reached many new areas. He has taken pains to collect important decisions of the Supreme Court of India which dealt with medical jurisprudence and he has cited them at appropriate contexts delineated in this book. Such references will give a fair idea to the students as well as members of the faculty, apart from their utility to the members of legal profession, regarding the contours of the subject being developed now. In due course of time this book will become an oft quoted work in criminal courts and the extracts therefrom will become oft quoted passages in judgments also.

I wish this endeavour Godspeed to reap beneficial results.

**Justice K. T. Thomas**

Muttambalam
Kottayam 686 004
Kerala (India)

# Preface

Forensic medicine, otherwise known as legal medicine, is a broad medical specialty concerned with the application of the principles of medicine for the purpose of law. The relevance of this branch of medicine has considerably increased in the past few decades. Investigation of offences against human body and unnatural deaths are the two main important functions of the police. Basic knowledge of forensic medicine and forensic sciences is absolutely essential for the effective investigation of these cases. Apart from this, a police officer should be aware of the modern trends and recent advances in the field of criminal investigation, such as polygraph, DNA fingerprinting, brain fingerprinting, toxicology, drug abuse, etc.

Medical evidence often plays a crucial role in the investigation of offences against human body. Statements of witnesses and circumstantial evidence can be analysed and corroborated with the findings of the medical examination of the victim as well as the accused. Proper interpretation and evaluation of the medical evidence is necessary to arrive at definite conclusions. This is all the more important in the investigation of unnatural deaths.

Investigation starts from the examination of the scene and the dead body. Valuable clues can be obtained by proper scientific examination of the crime scene and dead body. A crime scene can be preserved for continued scrutiny, but a dead body will be available for a few hours for examination during the police inquest. Therefore the investigating officer should be able to collect as much evidence as possible within the short period. This requires knowledge, skill and attitude.

I have been teaching the police trainees relevant aspects of forensic medicine, scientific methods of investigation and first aid since 1970 in the Police Training College, Thiruvananthapuram. I was also closely associated with criminal investigation for more than thirty years as Police Surgeon and Medicolegal Adviser to Kerala Police. This has helped me very much to understand the strength and weakness of the investigating officer in tackling medicolegal problems. This experience has been very helpful in writing this book.

There are innumerable textbooks on the subject but hardly any of them caters to the needs of a novice in the police profession. This book is written with the objective of imparting basic knowledge to the police trainees and officers so that they will develop fine skills and attitude in scientific criminal investigation. Stress is given to the practical aspects of forensic medicine and scientific methods of investigation. The formats of common medicolegal forms and requisitions are also appended wherever necessary for the ready reference of the investigating officers. The points to be observed and materials to be collected in all types of unnatural deaths are also included.

I hope this publication will be helpful for the police trainees as well as officers in service to achieve the educational objectives mentioned at the outset and inspire them to acquire more knowledge and skills in their career.

B. Umadethan

# Acknowledgements

I am extremely grateful to Honourable Justice KT Thomas, former Justice of Supreme Court, who has written the Foreword to this book. My association with that great personality dates back to the early seventies when he was the most popular and charming criminal lawyer in the Kottayam Bar. When he was the Justice of Kerala High Court in 1995, he had baptised my earlier work *Practical Forensic Medicine*. I consider it as a privilege to receive commendations and encouragement from an eminent jurist and authority on criminal law like Hon. Justice Thomas.

I am very grateful to my respected friend Sri Jacob Punnoose, IPS, Director General of Police, Kerala, for writing an excellent review of this work. As the helmsman of Kerala Police, Sri Punnoose is a man of admirable qualities and I have been associated with him professionally and personally for more than two decades.

I worked as Medicolegal Adviser to Kerala Police for twelve years. The former Director Generals of Police Sri MK Joseph, Sri Sathar Kunju and Sri MGA Raman were instrumental in appointing me to that unique post. I am thankful to those stalwarts for providing me an opportunity to learn the intricacies of criminal investigation by associating and interacting with so many investigating officers. It was a golden period in my professional life. The impetus to write this book came from many of the great officers in the Police Department. I acknowledge with gratitude their zeal with which they spurred me into action.

I express my sincere thanks to my colleagues in the fraternity of forensic medicine, learned members of the legal profession and law enforcement agencies for their love and concern towards me.

I am indebted to my sister Prof. Lalithabhai formerly Professor of English at SN College for helping me with the semantics of the book. I am thankful to Prof. Ambika, Professor of Physiology at Trivandrum Medical College who edited the annexations of this book containing elements of human anatomy and physiology. I express my sincere gratitude to Prof. Sheela Pavithran who took the painstaking task of correcting the draft and rectifying the mistakes.

I am very much thankful to my wife Smt Padmakumari for all the help and support.

I thank Mr TC Nandakumar, my Secretary, for assisting me in the preparation and editing of the text and photographs.

I am thankful to CBS Publishers & Distributors and their Regional Manager Mr PD Damodaran Namboodiri for bringing out the book in an attractive form.

**B. Umadethan**

# Contents

# Introduction

Forensic medicine is a broad medical speciality in which the principles of medicine are applied for the purpose of law. The word **forensic** is derived from the Latin word *Forum* which means court. The synonyms are court medicine, legal medicine, etc. **Medical jurisprudence** is a set of legal principles which govern the medical practice.

**Toxicology** deals with the chemistry, signs and symptoms of various types of poisons. **Forensic Science** is concerned with the application of the principles of physics, chemistry, biology and other basic sciences for the purpose of law. Forensic medicine and science form an integral part of the scientific criminal investigation.

Forensic medicine is mainly concerned with the offences against human body. Principles of other branches of medicine such as anatomy, pathology, Radiology, obstetrics, etc. are applied in the methods of examination of the victim and the accused, the living and the dead. The forensic expert is really a medical detective. He examines the victims and the accused and records his findings. His scientific observations and inferences are highly essential for the investigator and the judiciary for the proper dispensation of justice.

Legal medicine dates back to 4000 BC. There are references about medicolegal problems in the ancient Codes of India, China, Egypt and Babylon. Code of Manu, *Manusmriti* and *Bhrigusamhita* narrate various medicolegal principles. Codes of the King Hammurabi of Babylon contains principles of legal medicine. Hippocrates of Greece, the Father of Medicine, has mentioned about the fatality of various types of injuries and ethical principles involved in the practice of medicine.

By the turn of 16th century, legal medicine gained importance in many countries. The penal code of the Bishop of Bamberg, Caroline Code, etc. highlight the importance of medical evidence in criminal trials. The first medicolegal autopsy was conducted in the year 1762 in Paris. By the beginning of 17th century, medicolegal autopsies were routinely conducted in suspicious deaths. The first textbook on Forensic Medicine was written by an Italian doctor named Fortunato Fedele. In the 18th century, Departments of forensic medicine were started in many universities of Germany, Italy and England.

In India, legal medicine, in the present form emerged during the British rule. Medical jurists were appointed in many medical institutions. British doctors like Norman Chevers and Grewal had written books on forensic medicine in accordance with the legal and social conditions prevailing in the country. The first Indian book on forensic medicine was written by Dr. Jaisingh Modi (1875–1954). His book *Medical Jurisprudence and Toxicology* is even today accepted as a standard reference book by the members of the medical and legal profession.

At present, there are full fledged Departments of Forensic Medicine in all the medical colleges of the country. The professors of forensic medicine are appointed as police surgeons having jurisdiction in one or more districts. Important and sensational medicolegal cases are handled by these experts. Routine medicolegal cases are conducted by the government medical officers. Forensic medicine is an important subject in the medical curriculum. This subject is taught in law schools also.

All the police training academies have included forensic medicine in their training modules. The relevance and status of the speciality has increased during the past years. Society, judiciary, police and other law enforcement agencies are benefited by the services of this field of medicine in the administration of justice.

*"The search for truth is the essence of forensic medicine. This truth forms an essential link between the enforcement of law and protection of the public in the administration of justice"— Caption of a sculpture by Una Hanbury, situated in the lobby of Maryland Medical Examiner-Coroner's Office at Baltimore.*

# Learning Objectives

At the end of the training programme, the learner should be able to:

- Recognise the scope and role of forensic medicine in criminal investigation.
- Enumerate various offences against the human body as described in the Indian Penal Code.
- Identify situations where physical examination of the accused/victim by a doctor for the purpose of investigation and collection of evidence is required.
- Prepare requisitions to the medical officers in accordance with the legal provisions.
- Identify different types of injuries, their causation, medicolegal classification and importance.
- Prepare inquest report under Section 174 of the Cr. P. C incorporating the relevant details of the dead body and the scene of occurrence.
- Identify various changes seen in a dead body in relation to the postmortem interval.
- Identify various postmortem features seen in different types of unnatural deaths.
- Assess approximate time since death, apparent cause and manner of death.
- Conduct a systematic and thorough examination of the scene of crime.
- Collect, preserve and despatch the evidentiary materials to the appropriate laboratories.
- Interpret the results of laboratory analysis correctly.
- Recognise situations where the services of other experts would be required.
- Prepare a proper requisition containing all relevant details to the medical officer requesting him to conduct a medicolegal autopsy.
- Interpret the various medicolegal certificates/ reports, question the doctor and record the statement.
- Investigate hospital deaths alleged to have been caused by negligence on the part of medical personnel.
- Elucidate the medicolegal aspects of unsoundness of mind with regard to civil and criminal responsibility, restraint of persons in accordance with the provisions of law.
- Be aware of the modern trends and recent advances in scientific criminal investigation.
- Maintain good interpersonal relation with medical experts and establish rapport with them.
- Realise the limitations of knowledge and skills and seek help from appropriate sources in different medicolegal situations.

## INSTRUCTIONAL OBJECTIVES

### General

At the end of the training program, the learner should be able to conduct scientific investigation in the common medicolegal situations, adopting modern techniques and recent advances in forensic medicine and forensic sciences. He should be able to take appropriate steps in the collection/ preservation/despatch of material objects to the laboratories concerned and interpret the certificates and results of the experts.

3

For achieving these objectives, he should acquire knowledge and skills in the following subject areas.

## Curricular Elements
### Introduction
- Definition of the terms such as forensic medicine, medical jurisprudence, forensic sciences, toxicology.
- Historical development of the specialities of forensic medicine and forensic sciences.
- Scope and role of forensic medicine in the scientific criminal investigation.
- Modern trends and recent advances in forensic medicine.
- Medicolegal system in the country, departments of forensic medicine, police surgeons.
- Different types of medicolegal cases—scope of medical examination-investigation and collection of trace evidence.

### Death
- Diagnosis — brain death, criteria of death.
- Excerpts from Transplantation of Human Organs Act.
- Duties of a police officer — cardiopulmonary resuscitation.
- Classification, mechanism and manner of death.
- Disposal of unclaimed dead bodies for anatomical dissection.
- Death certification, death intimation and death report.

### Police Inquest
- Unnatural deaths — Section 174 of Criminal Procedure Code.
- Inquiry by the Magistrate — Section 176 of the Criminal Procedure Code.
- Inquest procedure — sketch and photograph of the scene.
- Examination of the dead body — columns 7 and 8 of the inquest report.
- Collection of evidentiary materials from the scene and dead body.
- Preparation of the inquest report.
- Duties, responsibilities and jurisdiction of the police surgeons.
- Forwarding dead body for autopsy-preparation of requisition in KPF 102 Form.

### Trace Evidence
- Survey of crime scene
- Collection of trace evidence
- Collection and preservation of different types of exhibits
- Biological stains, hair and fibres
- Role of experts in the scene of occurrence.

### Medicolegal Autopsy
- Objectives of an autopsy.
- Autopsy technique, interpretation of findings, theory and demonstration
- Collection of body fluids and viscera for laboratory analysis
- Cause of death, time of death and manner of death.
- Interpretation of postmortem certificate
- Questioning the medical witness.

### Forensic Taphonomy
- Changes in the buried dead body
- Locating graves
- Objectives of disinterring a dead body
- Relevance of Section — 176 of Cr. P. C
- Demonstration of the procedure of exhumation by slide/video show.

### Human Skeletal Remains
- Examination of decomposed dead body and skeletal remains
- Determination of sex, age, stature and features of identity
- Methods of identification — photographic and computerised superimposition
- Reconstruction of face-plastic and computer methods.

### Mechanical Injuries
- Mechanism of wounding
- Different types of injuries — abrasion, contusion, laceration, incised wound, punctured wound.
- Fractures
- Dismemberment.

### Firearm and Explosion Injuries
- Basic ballistics.
- Firearms, ammunition, mechanism of firing, fire effects.
- Autopsy on victims of gunshot injury.

- Examination of gunshot residues
- Explosion wounds.

## Regional Injuries
- Head injuries—skull fractures, injuries to brain
- Injuries to the neck, vertebral column and spinal cord
- Injuries to chest, abdomen and limbs.

## Traffic Accidents
- Injuries to pedestrian — primary, secondary and tertiary impacts
- Injuries to occupants
- Injuries sustained to cyclists/motor cyclists
- Effects of alcohol on driving
- Railway/aviation accidents.

## Medicolegal Aspects of Injuries
- Antemortem/postmortem injuries
- Cause of death from injuries
- Manner of causation of injuries
- Wound certification
- Referring an injury case.

## Asphyxial Deaths
- General features of asphyxia
- Different types of asphyxial deaths — hanging, strangulation, drowning, suffocation
- Irrespirable gases — carbon dioxide, carbon monoxide
- Diving hazards — barotrauma
- Laboratory tests — cellophane test, Diatom test
- Choking — first aid – Heimlich maneuver
- Traumatic asphyxia.

## Death due to Electric Shock and Lightning
- Electric burns
- Lightning injuries.

## Burns
- Effects of burns on the body
- Antemortem and postmortem burns
- Chemical burns.

## Virginity
- Signs of virginity
- Hymen/vagina.

## Sexual Offences
- Rape–definition–legal aspects.

- Examination of victim
- Investigation of a case of alleged rape
- Accused–examination and certification.
- Collection, preservation and despatch of trace evidence from the accused and victim
- Unnatural sexual offences and sexual perversions.
- Sexual harassment of working women
- Trial of child sex abuse.

## Pregnancy
- Presumptive, probable and conclusive signs of pregnancy
- Preconception and prenatal diagnostic techniques —prohibition of sex selection Act.

## Delivery
- Medicolegal aspects
- Signs of recent delivery in the living and dead
- Signs of parity in a woman.

## Abortion
- Types of abortion
- Deaths due to abortion.

## Medical Termination of Pregnancy Act
- MTP Act—provisions
- Maintenance of records
- Different proformas.

## Neonaticide and Infanticide
- Legal aspects
- Investigation of infanticide
- Foetal autopsy—signs of live birth
- Battered baby, cot deaths, shaken baby syndrome.

## Impotence
- Medicolegal aspects
- Physiology of erection
- Causes of impotence
- Female sexual dysfunction.

## Drunkenness
- Alcohol and its effects on humans
- Drunkenness and crime
- Drunken driving
- Drunken and disorderly behaviour
- Examination and certification of a drunken person—Sec: 53 Cr.PC.

- Laboratory analysis of blood, urine—breath analyser.
- Interpretation of clinical and laboratory findings.
- Drunkenness and criminal/civil responsibility
- Methyl alcohol—liquor tragedies.

## *Poisoning*

- Signs of poisoning
- First aid in poisoning
- Inquest in death due to poisoning
- Different types of poisons
- Common poisons — symptoms, signs, death, postmortem findings
- Collection, preservation and despatch of viscera for chemical analysis
- Miscellaneous examination — material objects other than viscera
- Detection of poison—chemicolegal rules—chemical analysis.

## *Narcotic Drugs and Psychotropic Substances*

- NDPS Act, Narcotics Control Bureau, Central Bureau of Narcotics
- Drug addiction, drug abuse, drug dependence
- Drug trafficking
- Narcotic drugs — opium alkaloids, synthetic and semisynthetic narcotics
- Psychotropic substances — depressants, stimulants, hallucinogens
- Identification of a drug addict — medical examination
- List of narcotic drugs and psychotropic substances — small quantity/commercial quantity.

## *Sudden Natural Death*

- Sudden death — medicolegal aspects
- Sudden death due to heart disease

- Miscellaneous conditions causing sudden death.

## *Investigation of Hospital Deaths*

- Anesthetic deaths
- Operative deaths
- Maternal deaths
- Medical negligence — criminal negligence
- Investigation of hospital deaths.

## *Recent Advances in Forensic Medicine and Forensic Sciences*

- DNA fingerprinting
- Brain fingerprinting
- Polygraph examination
- Narcoanalysis
- Forensic radiology
- Forensic odontology.

## *Violation of Human Rights*

- Human rights — National Human Rights Commission
- Torture —investigation
- Child rape — directives
- Human rights and policing — rape, custodial deaths, polygraph, interrogation.

## *Biological and Chemical Terrorism*

- Biological agents
- Chemical agents.

## *Annexations*

- Anatomical planes and terms
- Basic human anatomy and physiology
- Skeletal, muscular, respiratory, circulatory, gastrointestinal, endocrine, nervous, excretory, reproductive, integumentary, lymphatic systems and blood.

# Scope and Role of Forensic Medicine

Some years ago, in a remote village in Egypt, the inhabitants were attempting to clean a disused well. They recovered three pieces of bones from the bottom of the well. The bones were handed over to the police, who in turn sent them to Prof. Sir. Sydney Smith, the Head of Forensic Medicine of Cairo University. Police wanted to know whether the bones were human or not. After examining the bones, Prof. Smith gave the following opinion.

"The bones belonged to a woman aged about 18–22 years; she had a limp on her right leg; she might have delivered once or perhaps more; cause of death was a gun shot injury of the abdomen; the gun was a country gun; the woman was standing three yards in front of the assailant who was sitting; she did not die immediately; died only after a week due to infection; the incident might have occurred one year ago."

Needless to say that the Police officials were astonished when they received so many clues from the examination of three pieces of bones. Their subsequent investigations proved that the deductions of Prof. Smith were correct. Police found out that a 20-year-old woman, who was staying with her father and only son was missing since one year. She had a limp on her right leg too. Soon, her father was interrogated by the police and he confessed to having committed the crime. One day he was sitting on a door step, cleaning his muscle loading country gun. The gun was discharged accidentally and the daughter, standing in front of him was hit. The old man was scared and kept the incident secret. He nursed his daughter keeping her in the house. When she died after a week, he dumped her body into the disused well near his house. After one year, the old man came to know that the villagers are going to renovate the well. He got into the well one night, collected all the already skeletonised body remains in a gunny bag and threw them into the river Nile. At that time he did not know that he had left behind three pieces of bones which could provide incriminating evidence later.

This anecdote illustrates the role of forensic medicine in the detection of crimes. It is possible to make deductions based on scientific facts. The three pieces of bones were the hip bones. Sex can be easily determined from the characteristics of bones, especially hip bone of a human being. Similarly, age can be determined from the developmental changes seen in the bones. In the particular case, severe arthritic changes were present in right hip joint. It is only probable that such a person would have severe limitations of movement of the limb on that side. Presence of small pits which appear on the inner aspect of the hip bone due to pregnancy and delivery provided the clue for parity.

Prof. Smith had detected small irregular lead pellets embedded in the hip bone. These pellets were similar to those used in a country gun. It is possible to calculate the range of firing from the dispersion of the pellets. From the position of the embedded pellets in the pelvic bone, relative positions of the accused and victim can be found out. Prof. Smith could notice new bone formation over the pellets embedded in the bone. This finding meant that the victim survived after sustaining the injury. He examined the new bone formation microscopically to determine the age of the new bone formed and this tallied with the time of survival. Based on the stage of putrefaction and skeletonisation, time since death could also be found out.

Medicolegal work consists of examination of the dead and the living in civil and criminal cases. Conducting autopsies on persons who die an unnatural or suspicious death forms the major part of the work. The main objective of an autopsy is to find out the cause of death, time of death and to establish the identity of unknown dead bodies. Examination of human remains such as tissues and bones also form part of the medicolegal work. The doctor can also help the investigating officer to arrive at a conclusion regarding the manner of death also.

Accused and victims of sexual offences, victims of assault, etc. are examined by the doctor for recording the physical findings as well as for collecting trace evidence. These examinations help to prove the offence if any committed by the accused. The medicolegal expert also conducts examination of drunken persons and insane persons. Determination of the age of the juvenile offenders are also done by the doctor. In civil cases like disputed paternity and nullity of marriage, both parties are examined for signs of potency, pregnancy, virginity, delivery, etc.

In all these examinations, the doctor acts as a common witness as well as an expert. When he describes the findings of his examination, he acts as a common witness. When he interprets his findings and furnishes his opinion, he acts as an expert witness. He is the person who can give an opinion about the severity and fatality of various types of injuries. His opinion is very essential for the police to conduct a successful investigation. The judiciary also relies on the evidence of the medical witness in deciding the case.

When a medical officer or forensic specialist is conducting a medicolegal case, the relevant history of the case should be furnished prior to the examination. The doctor should be taken to the scene of the crime if it is necessary to arrive at an opinion. The investigating officer should elicit all possibilities and probabilities from the doctor.

Be that as it may, the investigating officer should never rely heavily on medical evidence. Forensic medicine is not an exact science. No opinion can be formed with hundred percent certainty. In all cases, there can be biological variations and hence absolute proof may be a rarity. The officer should give due importance to the evidence collected during investigation and see whether the medical evidence corroborates and supports. Opinion of experts has to be appreciated and evaluated in conjunction with all the other forms of evidence collected through field verification. There are several instances when the entire investigation has gone astray due to wrong medical opinion. This, of course, will result in either an unjust conviction or unworthy acquittal. Therefore, it is the duty of every investigating officer not to leave any stone unturned to find out the truth of the case.

*"Truth is incontrovertible, panic may resent it, ignorance may deviate it, malice may distort it; but there it is"*— *Sir Winston Churchill*

# 4

# Death

Death is defined as the complete and permanent cessation of circulation, respiration and functions of the brain. Survival of a person depends on the integrity and proper functioning of the heart, lungs and brain, called the **tripod of life**. If any one of these fail, the other two will also fail. Of these three organs, brain is the most vulnerable as it will be irrevocably damaged if it does not get oxygen for more than five minutes. Lungs are concerned with the intake of oxygen through the respiratory process and its diffusion into the blood. Heart is concerned with the circulation of blood and transport of oxygen and nutrients to all tissues of the body.

## BRAIN DEATH

Functions of the brain can be divided into two categories; vegetative and cognitive. **Brainstem** is that part of the brain which connects the higher centres to the periphery. It controls the vegetative functions such as circulation and respiration. **Cerebral cortex** is concerned with cognitive functions like perception, memory, awareness, etc. When the supply of the oxygenated blood stops, the cerebral cortex is affected first. Brainstem is more resistant to anoxia. By resuscitative measures, it is possible to revive a person whose heart and lungs have stopped functioning. If there is delay in reviving a person for a few minutes, his cognitive functions will be lost due to the anoxic damage of the cerebral cortex; but he will have spontaneous respiration and circulation. In other words, he will live like a vegetable. This is called **cerebral death**.

The person will not show any awareness of self or environment; but the sleep-wake cycles may be present. This state is known as **persistent vegetative state** (PVS).

If there is further delay in resuscitation, the brainstem will also be affected and there will be irreversible loss of all functions of the brain. There will not be any spontaneous circulation and respiration. Corneal and pupillary reflexes will be absent. This is the real death and is termed "brain stem death".

## Criteria of Death

1. Cessation of the functions of heart.
2. Cessation of spontaneous respiration.
3. Bilateral dilatation and fixation of pupils.
4. Absence of brainstem reflexes.
5. Completely flat brain waves in the EEG tracings.

The moment of death became a material point in the case of resuscitation and organ transplantation. For transplanting organs, they have to be removed immediately after death; otherwise the cells of the organs will die. Due to many reasons, it may not possible to do so. Circulation and respiration of a brain-dead person can be maintained with the help of life support systems like ventilators and organs can be removed for transplantation. In such instances, a team of doctors shall confirm and certify brain death before removal of the organs. Similarly brain death certification is necessary before stopping the life support systems while treating a patient in irreversible coma before stopping the life support systems while treating a patient in irreversible coma. Under Sub-section 6 of Section 3 of the "Transplantation of Human Organs Act", a Board of medical experts should certify brain death.

The Board shall consist of:
1. The medical officer in charge of the hospital.
2. The doctor who treated the person.
3. A neurologist or neurosurgeon.
4. An independent specialist nominated by the hospital (approved by the appropriate authority).

## Excerpts from the Transplantation of Human Organs Act 1994

**The purpose of this Act is to:**
1. Provide for the regulation of removal, storage and transplant of human organs for therapeutic purposes.
2. Prevent commercial dealings in human organs.
   - Any person can authorise the removal, before his death of any organ of his body for therapeutic purposes.
   - Any person in writing, in the presence of two witnesses (one of them, a near relative) can authorise the removal of his organs after his death. After his death, the person lawfully in possession of the dead body can authorise the removal of organs.
   - The person lawfully in possession of the dead body can authorise the removal of organs for therapeutic purposes with the permission of the near relatives, provided the deceased before his death, had not objected for such removal.
   - If the brain dead person is less than 18 years of age, any of the parents of the deceased can authorise the removal of organs.
   - Organs can be removed from an unclaimed dead body with the authorisation of the person in charge of the dead body provided the relatives do not claim the body.
   - Organs cannot be removed if any police or judicial inquest on the dead body is to be conducted or if the body is given for burial or cremation.
   - In the case of a living donor, organs cannot be removed and transplanted to a recipient, unless the donor is a near relative of the recipient.
   - Prior approval of the authorisation committee is essential if the recipient is not a relative. For this purpose, every state has constituted authorisation committee. This is to prevent commercial dealing of organs. Transplantation operations can be conducted only in well-equipped hospitals authorised by the Government.

## First Duty of a Police Officer at a Scene of Accident/Crime

A police officer on reaching a scene of accident or crime shall ascertain whether the victim is alive or not. If life is not extinct, he has to provide resuscitation measures and necessary first aid to save the life of the person. If there are no signs of circulation or respiration, if the pupils are dilated and fixed, if muscles of the body have started stiffening (**rigor mortis**) the person can be considered dead. These can be confirmed by the following tests.

1. To check for breathing look, listen and feel. Place the ear next to the victims mouth and nose and listen for breath sounds. Look at the chest and abdomen to rise and fall due to respiration.
2. Check for arterial pulse (Figs 4.1 and 4.2). This requires some practice. Pulse is the rhythmic expansile pulsation of arteries caused by the heart pumping of blood into the aorta. Pulse can be felt by palpating an artery like carotid or radial. Pulsations of the radial artery can be felt on the inner aspect of wrist near the root of thumb. Place two or three fingers on the artery applying slight pressure. To locate the carotid artery, firstly tilt the head and lift the chin (lift up with two fingers on the chin while pushing down on the forehead with the other hand). Place two or three fingers on the Adam's apple. Slide the fingers into the groove between the Adam's apple and the muscle (sternomastoid). Pulsations will be felt when the fingers are pressed lightly and pulled outwards (Fig. 4.2).
3. Pupil is an aperture in the iris of the eye. It acts like a shutter in a camera. It dilates in dim light and constricts in bright light. When a person is brain dead, the pupils will be dilated and fixed. This is tested by shining a torch light into the eye.

procedure is called cardiopulmonary resuscitation (CPR).

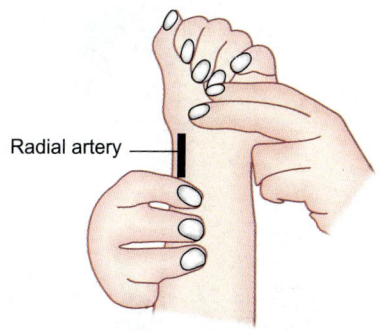

Radial artery

**Fig. 4.1:** Feeling the radial pulse

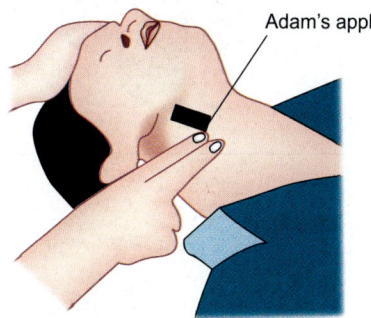

Adam's apple

**Fig. 4.2:** Feeling the carotid pulse

### Steps of Cardiopulmonary Resuscitation (CPR)

a. First, check to see whether the victim is responsive by tapping or gently shaking the victim and shouting "Are you OK ?" If there is no response keep the victim lie on his back.

b. The next step is to check for breathing as described above. If the victim is not breathing, open the airway by the head-tilt chin-lift maneuver. Place the mouth around the victims mouth and pinch the nose. Give two slow breaths into the victim's mouth. A piece of cloth can be used as a barrier to avoid direct mouth-to-mouth contact. Make sure that the chest of the victim rises when rescue breath is given. Continue till the victim starts breathing (Figs 4.3 A and B).

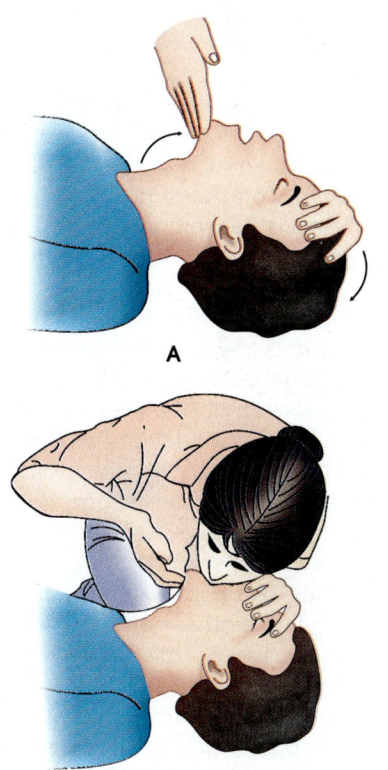

A

B

**Figs 4. 3A and B:** Head-tilt chin-lift maneuver, B. Mouth-to-mouth breathing

4. After death, the muscles of the body will become stiff. The stiffness, known as rigor mortis develops first in the head, and neck and spread to the entire body. If the jaw, neck and limb muscles are stiff, it can be inferred that the person has been dead for some time.

Consciousness is the awareness of oneself and the environment. In unconsciousness, the person is unaware of the external stimuli. This state is different from sleep. A sleeping person can be aroused, while an unconscious person cannot be aroused. The level of unconsciousness (coma) varies depending upon the causative factor. Coma may be due to brain injury, poisoning, intoxication, epilepsy, metabolic disorders, etc. Stoppage of the heart (cardiac arrest) or respiration can render a person unconscious immediately. The police officer should attempt to rescue the person by giving artificial respiration and cardiac massage to revive the heart. The

c. The next step is to check for the pulse as described above. If the victim has a pulse, and he has started breathing, place the victim in the recovery position (Fig. 4.4).

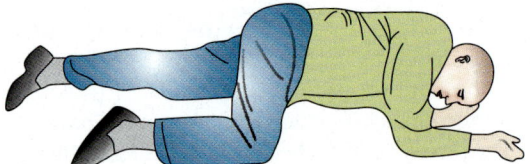

**Fig. 4.4:** Recovery position. All unconscious persons should be placed in this position

d. If there is no pulse, start chest compressions. The victim should lie on his back with the head-tilt-chin lift position. The rescuer should kneel by the side of the victim (Fig. 4.5 A).

e. Find a position on the lower half of the breast bone—sternum (Fig. 4.5 B).

f. Place the heel of one hand on this location.

g. Place the heal of the second hand on the top of the first hand.

h. The rescuer should position his body over his hands. His shoulders should be above his hands and he should look down on his hands.

i. Provide 15 compressions at the rate of 100 compressions per minute. Count the compressions by saying "a, b ,c, d, e, f, g, h, i, j, k, l, m, n, off and again a, b, c, d....(Fig. 4. 5 C).

j. Continue one rescuer CPR with chest compressions and two slow breaths.

k. After one minute of CPR (four cycles of 15 compressions and two breaths), check the pulse to see whether circulation has been restored. Check the pulse every few minutes. If the pulse returns, stop the chest compressions and continue providing rescue breaths if needed (one breath every five seconds).

If there are two rescuers, one can give rescue breaths, while the other can give chest compressions. Give necessary first aid such as arresting bleeding, prevention of shock, etc. along with CPR and transport the victim to the nearest hospital. Alert the hospital casualty before transporting the victim. CPR should continue till the victim regains pulse and respiration. It can be stopped when obvious signs of death are apparent.

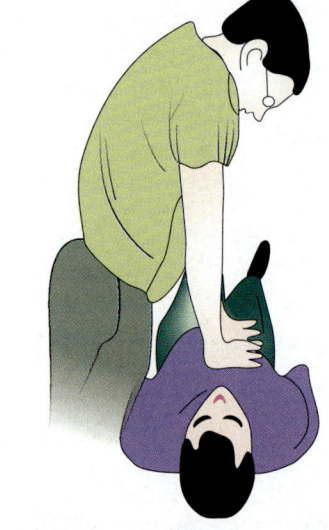

A

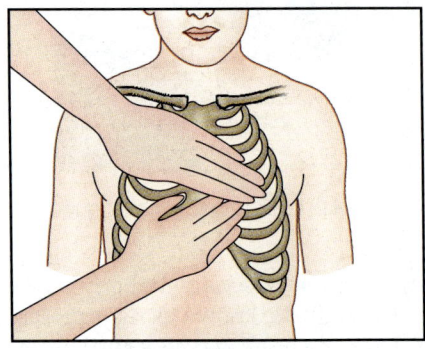

B

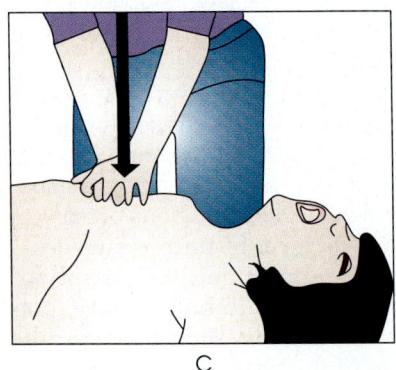

C

**Figs 4.5 A to C:** Cardiopulmonary resuscitation: A. Position of the rescuer, B. Position on the lower half of breast bone, C. Position of hands while compressing the chest

## Cause of Death

For every death, there will be a cause. It may be a natural cause like disease or old age. Death due to natural cause is called natural death. Death due to accident, suicide or homicide is called unnatural death. A natural death may also be considered unnatural, if it occurs unexpectedly and suddenly under suspicious circumstances.

When a person is admitted in the hospital for certain complaints, a clinical diagnosis is made based on the signs, symptoms and investigations. If that patient dies due to the natural consequences of that condition, the attending doctor can certify death. This is an inference based on scientific reasoning and it will satisfy the legal requirements in our country. The actual cause of death can only be found out by a detailed autopsy.

The death certificate (Proforma 4.1) is issued only if the cause of death is known beyond any doubt. Family physicians have also to observe certain formalities and take precautions in certifying death. If a patient dies while under treatment at his or her residence, the doctor can certify death, provided he has seen the patient within 24 hours preceding death and he has no suspicion of any foul play. A doctor will not certify death in the following instances:

1. Persons brought dead to the casualty
2. Persons dying in the casualty
3. Persons dying after admission, but before making a diagnosis
4. All cases of unnatural deaths-accidents, suicide and homicides
5. Deaths caused by animals, snakebites, etc.
6. Anaesthetic deaths
7. Suspicious death of a married woman within 7 years of her marriage.
8. When there is suspicion that death is due to the commission of an offence by some person

All the above mentioned types of death are intimated to the nearest police station (Proforma 4.2).

## Manner of Death

Manner of death is the way in which death has occurred. This is an important issue in the case of all unnatural deaths. The manner can be accident,

---

**Proforma 4 .1:** Death certificate

Name of the deceased................................................................................................................ .Sex...............................

Occupation.....................................................................................Religion ...............................................................

Date of death ................................Age in years........................... If under one year,................months............days

If under  24 hours, .............................hours ...................minutes

Cause of death...........................................................................................................................................

Disease or condition (a) .........................................................................................................................

directly leading to death (due to or as a consequence of)

(This does not mean the mode of dying, e.g.. heart failure, asthma, etc., it means disease, injury or complications)

Antecedent cause (b) .............................................................................................................

Morbid condition, if any giving rise to (due to or consequence of)

above cause stating the underlying condition

Other significant conditions (c) ............................................................................................................

contributory to death, but not related to the disease or condition causing it.

If the deceased was a female, was the death associated with pregnancy/delivery?.......................

Signature...........................................

Designation.......................................

Date:......................                    Reg. No...........................................

**Proforma 4.2:** Death Intimation

Hospital............................................................................    Date.........................
No.........................

From

Dr.........................................................................
................................................................ .(Designation)

To
The Sub Inspector, ........................................ Police station

Sir,

This is to inform you that  Sri/Smt..................................................................................................................
aged................years  admitted on ...........................with history of........................................................................
and referred from ................................... expired on.....................at........... hours.
Body is kept in the mortuary. Please do the needful.

Yours faithfully,
Signature..............................

---

suicide or homicide. For example, when a dead body is recovered from a well, the cause of death could be drowning. If the deceased had fallen accidentally into the well, it is considered as an accidental drowning. If he had jumped into the well to end his life, it is a suicidal drowning. If somebody had pushed him into the well, it is a case of homicidal drowning. Manner of death can be ascertained only by an investigation into the circumstances of death.

### Mechanism of Death

Mechanism of death is the exact physiological change or changes which produced death. In a particular case, there may be more than one mechanisms of death. For example, when a person sustains a stab in the heart, death may be due to neurogenic shock, bleeding, secondary shock, cardiac tamponade, etc. Some times it may not be possible to detect the exact mechanism of death. For instance: A stabbed B with a sharp knife on the chest and B died immediately. Autopsy revealed that the knife had penetrated the chest wall covering of the heart and its wall. There was 500 ml of blood and clots in the sac (pericardium) covering the heart. Actual mechanism of death could have been compression of the heart by the blood and clots collected within the pericardial sac (cardiac tamponade). But the cause of death is expressed in the autopsy certificate in morbid anatomical terms as "stab injury involving the heart". This will satisfy the legal requirement.

### Reporting Deaths

The doctor has to notify all deaths occurring in his hospital to the local administration (Registrar of births and deaths) within three days in urban areas and within seven days in rural areas. The Police Officer has also to notify all deaths which he investigate to the local authority. The proforma of the Death report is given in Proforma 4.3.

### DEALING WITH UNCLAIMED DEAD BODIES (Sec. 4 of the Anatomy Act)

If a person dies in a hospital or in a prison and his body is not claimed by any of his near relatives

**Proforma 4.3:** Death Report

Ward .................No ............. Municipality .......................... Taluk ...................................

Panchayat ...............................District............................Corporation........................................

Full name of the deceased ........................................................................................................

Sex:  Male/Female

Age at death........years.......months....days.......

Nationality and caste .......................................

Occupation  of the deceased............................

Marital status ................................................

Normal residence ...........................................

Place of death .................Door No..................

Street ..........................Ward No....................

Cause of death (if death certificate is issued) ...............................................................

Date of death ...............................................

Name of father/husband ............................................................................

Name of burial or burning ground..........................................................................................

Informant's name ......................................................... Relationship ...............................

Designation and address .............................................................................................

Name  of medical attendant ...............................................................................................

Date:.............                                           Signature of Medical Officer.........................................

within 24 hours, if he is resident of the same district, or within 72 hours if he is a resident outside the district, the authority in charge of such hospital or prison shall, without delay, report the fact to the authorised officer. Government has authorised the health officers of corporations and municipalities as authorised officers for the purpose of this Act. In other areas, the local Sub Inspector of police will be the authorised officer. The said officer shall take possession of the unclaimed body and hand it over to the authority in charge of a teaching medical institution if it is required by that authority, for the purpose of conducting anatomical examination and dissection except in the following circumstances:

1. When a near relative of the deceased person is known to be alive and he has failed to claim the body within the prescribed time for reasons beyond his control.
2. When the deceased person has prior to his death declared that his body shall not be subjected to anatomical examination or dissection or both

(in that case the body has to be handed over to such religious or public institutions belonging to the religion of the deceased).

3. When there is any doubt regarding the cause of death (in that case, he shall forward the unclaimed body to the police officer as per Section 174 of the Code of Criminal Procedure).
4. When the unclaimed body taken possession of by the authorised officer is not required by the authority in charge of a teaching medical institution (in that case the body shall be disposed off as per the rules of the local administration).

## Donation of Dead Body (Living Will)

If any person, either in writing at any time or orally in the presence of two or more persons during his last illness has expressed an unequivocal request that his body be used for the purpose of conducting anatomical examination and dissection after his death, the party lawfully in possession of his body after his death, may, unless, the said party has reason to believe that the request was subsequently withdrawn, report the fact to the authorised officer and permit the said officer to take possession of the body and hand it over to the authority in charge of a teaching medical institution, if it is required by that authority.

The party lawfully in possession of the body of a deceased person may permit the authorised officer to take over possession of the body for the purposes aforesaid unless that party has reason to believe: (a) That the deceased had expressed an objection to his body being so dealt with after his death, and had not withdrawn it: or (b) that the surviving spouse or any near relative of the deceased objects to the body of the deceased being so dealt with.

If any person who has been entrusted with a dead body solely for the purpose of its interment, burial, cremation or disposal otherwise shall not give permission to the authorised officer to take over possession of the body. If there is any doubt or dispute as to the near relative, the matter is to be referred to a Magistrate of the first class, who will conduct a summary enquiry. The decision of such Magistrate shall be final and conclusive. Pending such decision, the body of the deceased person shall be preserved from decay by keeping in a mortuary.

Whoever disposes of, or abets the disposal of, an unclaimed body or obstructs any authority in charge of a teaching medical institution or an authorised officer from handing over, taking possession of, removing or using, such dead body to the medical institution shall be punishable with fine which may extend to five hundred rupees.

No suit, prosecution or other legal proceeding shall be against any person for anything which is in good faith done or intended to be done in pursuance of this Act.

## Duty of Police and Other Officers

All officers and servants of the police, medical and public health departments, all officers and servants in the service of a local authority and all village officers and servants who come to know of the death of any person in any public place in an area in which he had no permanent place of residence, shall report the fact to the authorised officer with the least practicable delay. The responsibility for immediately reporting the fact to the authorised

officer and also arranging the removal of the dead body to the hospital for preservation from decay shall be that of the officer in charge of the police station having jurisdiction over the area or the health inspector of the area or the executive officer of the Panchayath as the case may be.

If the body of such person is not claimed by any of his near relative within a period of 24 hours, the Authorised Officer shall proceed to deal with the body in the manner laid down in Section 4 of the Act (except in the circumstances mentioned).

Dead bodies which are received shall be kept temporarily in the cold storage of the mortuary until they are removed to the anatomy department. In the anatomy department, they shall be washed and preserved by means of formalin or glycerine solution. Those which are not required for immediate use, shall be kept in a tank containing preservative solution.

**Nothing contained in these rules shall apply to cases where death has taken place under suspicious circumstances and the body is required for medicolegal examination. In such cases, if the Police have not taken possession of by themselves the body shall be handed over to the police.**

## DIRECTIONS TO THE INVESTIGATING OFFICER

- On reaching the scene of occurrence, examine the victim for signs of life.
- Examine the carotid or radial pulse for signs of circulation.
- Look for breath sounds and respiratory movements.
- Open the eyelids and examine the pupils for reaction to light.
- If life is not extinct, attempt cardiopulmonary resuscitation.
- In the meanwhile, make arrangements for transportation to the nearest hospital.
- Give necessary first aid like arresting bleeding, splinting fractures, etc.
- Removal of the victim from the scene should be done carefully to prevent further injury.
- Preserve the scene of occurrence by cordoning the area.
- If death is certain, proceed under section 174 of Criminal Procedure Code.

# 5

# Inquest

Inquest is an enquiry into the cause and circumstances of death when death is unnatural or has occurred under suspicious circumstances. Different inquest systems are existing in different countries of the world. In the United Kingdom, a coroner and jury holds inquest. Coroner is an officer appointed from amongst the legal profession. In United States, a Medical Examiner who is a doctor specialised in Forensic Medicine conducts inquest. In Italy, a public prosecutor known as Procurator-Fiscal holds inquest. In India, inquests are held by police officers not below the rank of a Station House Officer. Coroner's system existed in Mumbai city and Kolkata, but now it is abolished.

## Section 174 of Criminal Procedure Code

1. "When an officer in charge of a police station, or some other police officer, specially empowered by the State Government in that behalf receives information that a person has committed suicide or has been killed by another or by an animal or by machinery or by an accident or has died under circumstances raising a reasonable suspicion that some other person has committed an offence, he shall immediately give intimation thereof to the Executive Magistrate concerned and shall proceed to the place where the dead body of such deceased person is and therein the presence of two or more respectable inhabitants of the neighbourhood, shall make an investigation U/S Section 174 draw up a report of the apparent cause of death, describing such wounds, fractures, bruises and other marks of injury as may be found on the body and stating in what manner, or by what weapon or instrument (if any) such marks appear to have been inflicted."

2. The report shall be signed by such police officer and other persons and shall be forwarded to the Magistrate concerned.

3. When:
   i.   The case involves suicide by a woman within seven years of her marriage; or
   ii.  The case relates to the death of a woman within seven years of her marriage in any circumstance raising a reasonable suspicion that some other person committed an offence in relation to such woman; or
   iii. The case relates to the death of a woman within seven years of her marriage and any relative of the woman has made a request in this behalf; or
   iv.  There is any doubt regarding the cause of death; or
   v.   The police officer for any other reason considers it expedient to do so, he shall, subject to such rules as the State Government may prescribe in this behalf, forward the body, with a view to it being examined to the nearest Civil Surgeon, or other qualified medical man appointed in this behalf by the State Government, if the state of the weather and the distance admit of it being so forwarded without the risk of such putrefaction on the road render such examination useless.

4. The following Magistrates are empowered to hold inquests, namely any District Magistrate or

Subdivisional Magistrate and any other Executive magistrate specially empowered in this behalf by the State Government or the District Magistrate.

According to this section, when the police officer in charge of a police station receives intimation of death from a medical officer or any citizen, he registers a case of unnatural death and prepares a first information report (**FIR**). The FIR is forwarded to the Executive Magistrate concerned. If the intimation is about a cognizable offence like murder, as per Sec 154 Cr. P.C, the case is registered and the FIR is forwarded to the judicial magistrate concerned.

The Police Officer then proceeds to the spot and conducts the inquest and prepares a report. If there is inevitable delay, he should send police men to guard the scene of occurrence to prevent trespass by the people and loss of evidence. The object of the inquest is to ascertain whether a person had died under the circumstances which were doubtful or an unnatural death and if so what is the cause of death. The details such as how the deceased was assaulted or who assaulted him are beyond the scope of this enquiry under this section.

Sub-section 3 of Section 174 was added in 1983. The purpose was to deal with the increasing incidence of dowry deaths or cases of cruelty to married women by the husbands and in laws which will attract Section 498 A of the Indian Penal Code.

## INQUIRY BY MAGISTRATE INTO CAUSE OF DEATH

In certain circumstances, Magistrates have to conduct inquiry into the cause of death as per **Section 176 of Criminal Procedure Code** (amended in 2005) which states as follows:

1. When the case is of the nature referred to in clause (i) or clause, (ii) of subsection (3) of Section 174, the nearest Magistrate empowered to hold inquests shall, and in any other case mentioned in sub-section (1) of Section 174, any magistrate so empowered may hold an inquiry into the cause of death either instead of, or in addition to, the investigation held by the police officer; and if he does so, he shall have all the powers in conducting in which he would have in holdingan inquiry into an offence.

2. Where (a) any person dies or disappears or (b) rape is alleged to have been committed on any woman while such person or woman is in the custody of the police or in any other custody authorised by the Magistrate or the court, under this code in addition to the inquiry or investigation held by the police, an inquiry shall be held by the Judicial Magistrate or the Metropolitan Magistrate as the case may be, within whose local jurisdiction the offence has been committed.

3. The Magistrate holding such an inquiry shall record the evidence taken by him in connection therewith in any manner hereinafter prescribed according to the circumstances of the case.

4. Whenever the Magistrate considers it expedient to make an examination of the dead body of any person who has been already interred, in order to discover the cause of death, the Magistrate may cause the body to be disinterred and examined.

5. Where an inquiry is to be held under this section, the Magistrate shall wherever practicable, inform the relatives of the deceased whose names and addresses are known, and shall allow them to remain present at the inquiry.

6. The Judicial Magistrate or the Metropolitan Magistrate or Executive Magistrate or police officer holding an inquiry or investigation, as the case may be under subsection (1A) shall, within 24 hours of the death of the person, forward the body with a view to its being examined to the nearest Civil Surgeon or other qualified medical man appointed in this behalf by the state government, unless it is possible to do so for reasons to be recorded in writing. Explanation: In this section, the expression 'relative' means parents, children, brothers, sisters and spouse.

Section 176 was amended in the year 2005. In the case of a custodial death or custodial rape or disappearance of a person, the Judicial Magistrate is empowered to conduct enquiry in addition to the enquiry or investigation conducted by the police. If the dead body is buried, such Magistrate can order the body to be disinterred and examined. The dead body in these cases shall be forwarded to the nearest Civil Surgeon or other qualified medical man within 24 hours of the death of the person.

## INQUEST PROCEDURE

Investigation of an unnatural death begins with the inquest. It should be held carefully in a systematic manner adopting all scientific methods. Much evidence can be collected from the examination of a dead body and the scene of occurrence. A scene can be preserved for continued examination at a later stage. But the investigating officer gets very little time for examining the dead body. It has to be sent for autopsy at the earliest after completing the inquest; otherwise it will putrefy. Therefore, the IO has to collect as much evidences as possible from the scene and dead body. Useful inferences can be drawn from the scientific observations made at the scene which will help to solve the case. As per the Police Standing Orders, except in emergent situations, inquests are to be conducted during day time.

### General Directions
### Sketch of the Scene of Occurrence

Detailed description of the scene and the dead body are to be recorded in the inquest report (Columns 7 and 8). The descriptions should be supported by measurements wherever needed. The measurements should be taken in metric scale. A rough sketch of the scene (Fig. 5.1) and the position of the dead body in relation to various objects in the scene should be prepared with measurements shown. The dead body and the articles present in the scene may be numbered and a legend may be appended to it. The preparation of a sketch in the beginning will be helpful in preparing the inquest report accurately.

### Photographs of the Scene

Description of the dead body and the scene entered under columns 7 and 8 of the inquest report can be better understood if a number of good photographs are taken. A descriptive

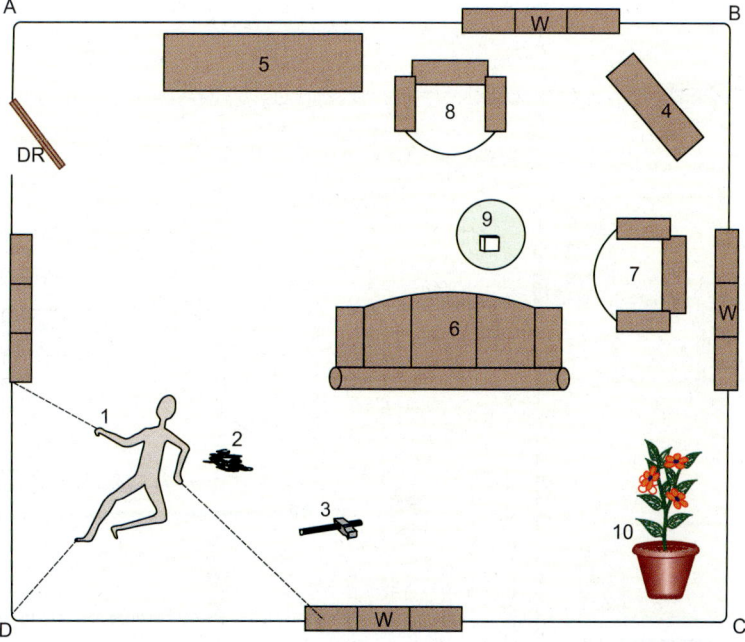

**Fig. 5.1:** Rough sketch of the crime scene— Door (DR), window (W) relative measurements (--------interrupted line), dead body (1), blood stain (2), blood stained hammer (3), television set (4), diwan (5), sofa 3 seater (6), single seaters (7 and 8), round table (9) flower vase (10), AB and CD—5 meters each, BC and DA—4 meters each

photograph is better than a few pages of description. The photographer should be given proper guidance and direction when he takes the photographs. If the police photographer is not available, a local photographer can be summoned to take the photographs. The negative should be obtained from him after taking the pictures for taking prints and preservation.

Photographs of the dead body and the scene are to be taken in conformity with the description given in the inquest report. The pictures must be taken sequentially. The pictures should be self-explanatory. For example, if a dead body is found inside a room in a house, the first picture should be that of the road leading to the house. The next photograph should be that of the house viewed from the road. Subsequent photographs should be in the same order of entry into the room (Figs 5.3 to 5.10). It will be better if a floor plan of the house is also included (Fig. 5.2).

Photographs of the dead body should be taken from various angles to show its relative position to various articles in the room. Close up photographs of the injuries, marks of violence, foreign bodies and other material objects should be taken. When injuries are photographed, a cloth tape scale should be placed nearby, so that the actual size can be easily understood from the photograph. A detailed inquest report with descriptive photographs will be helpful for reconstructing the crime in future. This will also be helpful for another agency who may take up the investigation of the case at a later stage.

Ordinarily, black and white photographs need be taken. But to highlight blood stains, injuries, etc. colour pictures have to be taken. At present, high resolution digital cameras are available for taking excellent photographs. The photographs can be stored as a permanent record in a compact disc (CD) and any number of prints can be taken. As digital images can be manipulated using suitable software, there can be problems in the admissibility of evidence. The photographs can be attached to the case diary file as shown in Fig. 5.11.

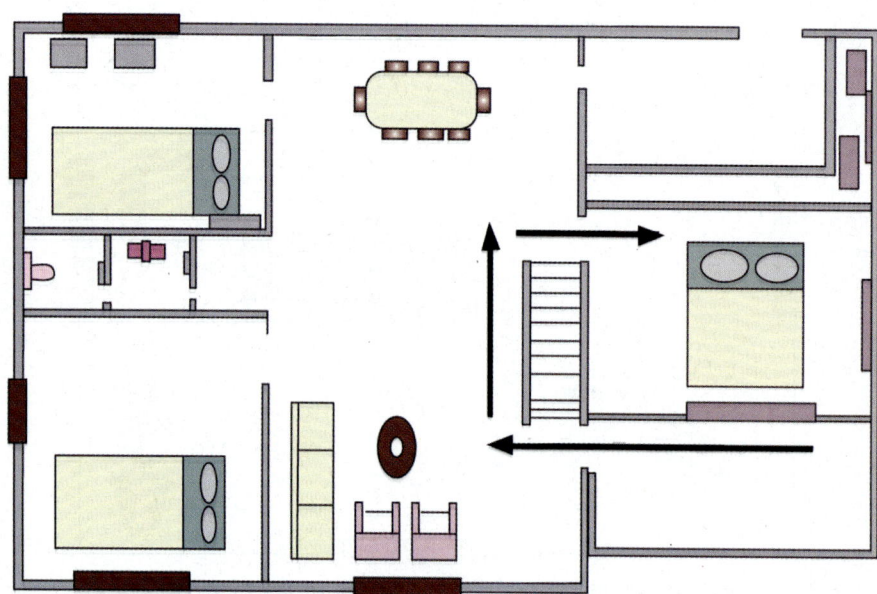

**Fig. 5.2:** Scene of occurrence — Floor plan of the house —Arrows indicate the location of the crime scene

## Photographs of the Scene of Occurrence taken in a Sequential Manner

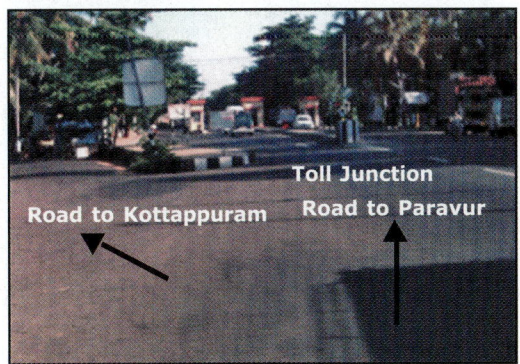

Fig. 5.3: Kottappuram toll junction road on the left goes to Kottappuram

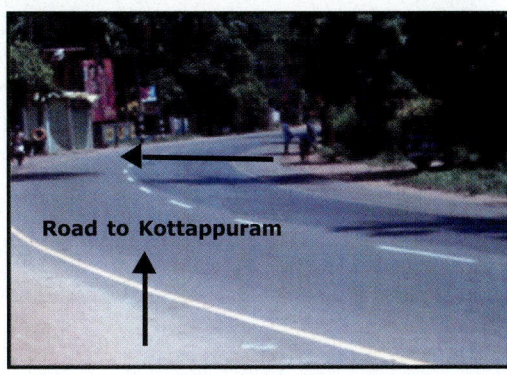

Fig. 5.4: Two hundred meters from toll junction, the road curves — arrow points to the scene

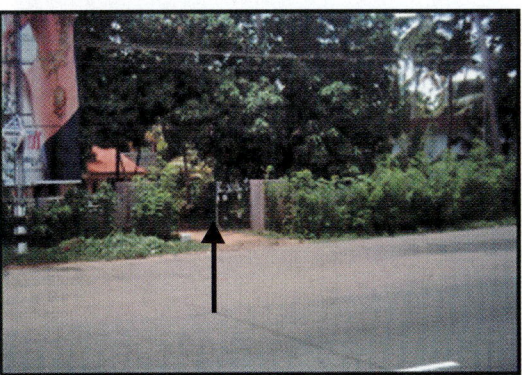

Fig. 5.5: View of the house from the road

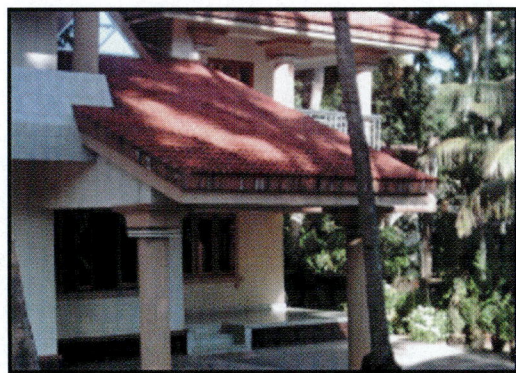

Fig. 5.6: Crime scene—the front of the house

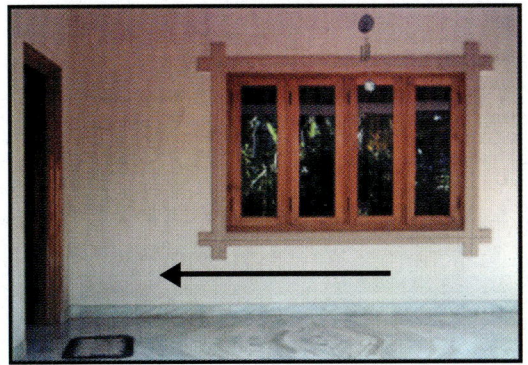

Fig. 5.7: The veranda of the house —the door on the left opens to the living room

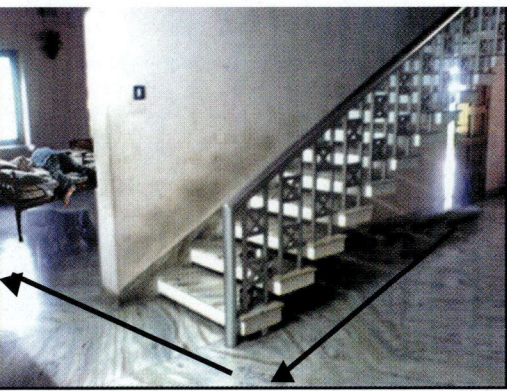

Fig. 5.8: Living room—the room on the right is the crime scene

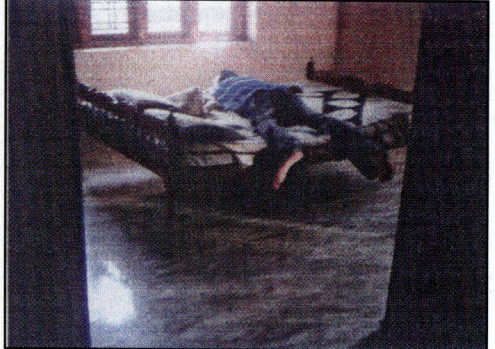

**Fig. 5.9:** Body of the victim is found lying in a prone position on a cot

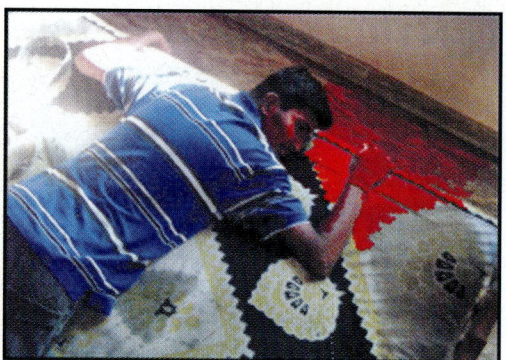

**Fig. 5.10:** Victim lying in a pool of blood

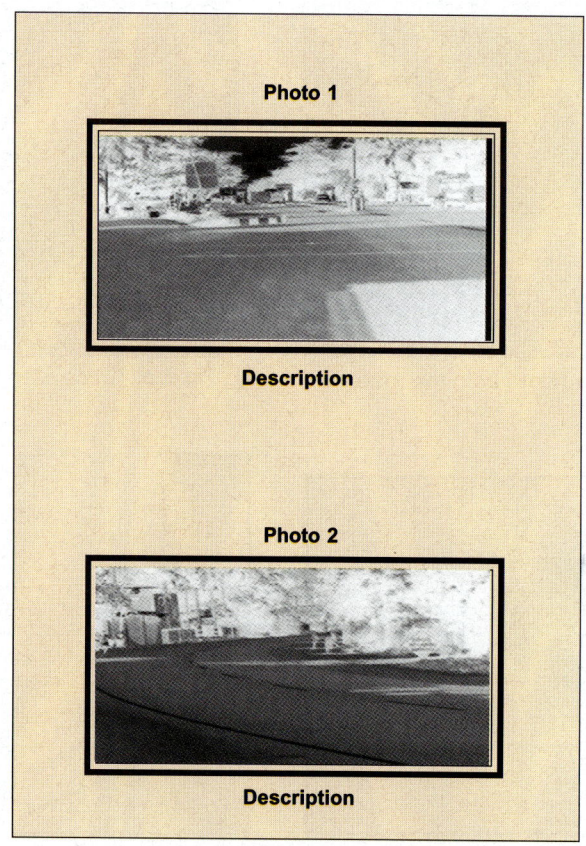

**Fig. 5.11:** Method of filing photographs in the Crime Diary File. Photographs can be pasted on a thick black/white card paper. Photos have to be numbered. The description is noted beneath each photo

## EXAMINATION OF THE DEAD BODY

Under column 7 of the inquest report, a detailed description of the dead body should be entered. Measurements of the dead body and its relative position to the nearby articles and landmarks should be noted. Description of the external body orifices, position of the limbs, appearance of external genitalia are to be noted. The investigating officer, being the first person to examine the dead body, can observe the salient postmortem changes which will be helpful in estimating the time of death. As per the directives of the Human Rights Commission, it is mandatory to note the **temperature of the dead body** and state of **rigor mortis** in death due to torture, sexual assault, etc. If the forensic pathologist is not available during inquest, the investigating officer should note down the temperature of the dead body, postmortem rigidity of muscles and postmortem staining.

### Cooling of Dead Body (Algor Mortis)

After death, temperature of the body will progressively fall and reach the temperature of the surroundings by conduction, convection and radiation. Some time after death, the body will be cold to touch, but the inner core of the body may not have attained the temperature of the environment. The best method of finding out the cadaver's temperature is by noting the rectal temperature using a 25 cm long thermometer having a range of 0 to 50°C (Fig. 5.12A). Bulb of the thermometer is introduced into the rectum and kept there for 2 minutes. It is taken out and note the temperature (Fig. 5.13). Digital thermometer will be a better choice (Fig. 5.12B). The temperature of the environment should also be noted. Roughly the hours after death can be calculated as follows:

$$\frac{\text{Normal body temperature } (37° +/-0.5) - \text{Rectal temperature}}{\text{Rate of fall of temperature/hour (approximately 0.5 °C/hour)}}$$

Cooling depends upon so many factors like clothing of the body, environmental conditions, physique, etc. However, a dead body will attain the room temperature in 12 – 18 hours after death. Owing to so many variable factors, estimation of the time of death based on cooling of the body is not reliable.

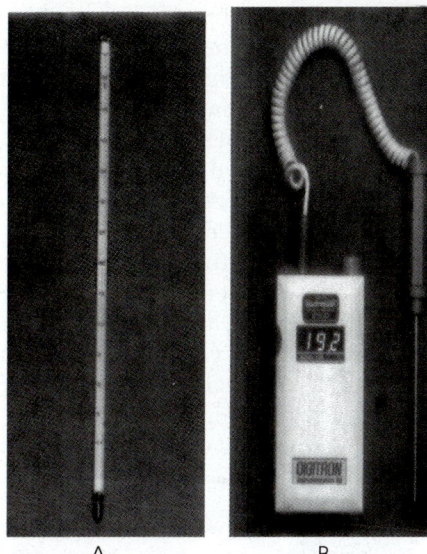

**Figs 5.12A and B:** Rectal thermometers, A. Mercury analog, B. Digital

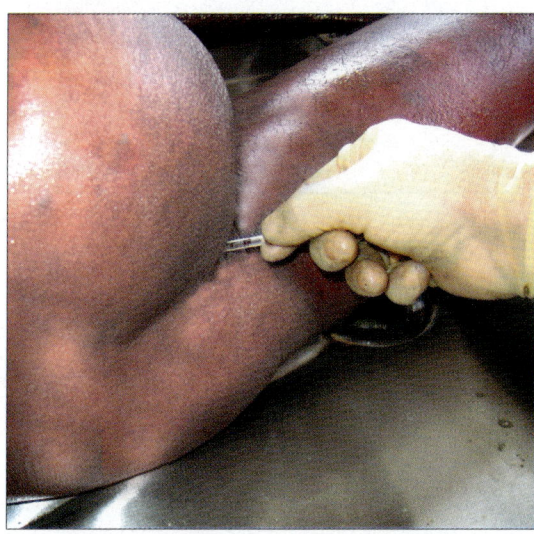

**Fig. 5.13:** Taking rectal temperature

### Postmortem Lividity (Suggillation, Livor Mortis, Hypostasis, Postmortem Staining)

This is a bluish or reddish blue discolouration occurring on the dependent parts of a dead body. After death, the blood vessels will lose the tone and blood will gravitate into them, imparting a discolouration of the subjacent skin. In a body lying on its back, the staining will be on the back aspect and vice versa (Figs 5.14 and 5.15). In a hanging body, postmortem staining is seen on the limbs. The staining, at first appears in patches, but by about 3 hours after death, it spreads. The postmortem staining becomes permanent and fixed by 6 to 12 hours after death.

The exact reason for fixation of postmortem staining is not known. But it is believed that when the muscles become stiff after death, the muscle fibres compress the blood vessels and prevents the flow of blood. Therefore even if the position of the body is changed, postmortem lividity does not change. But if the position of the body is changed

before 6 – 12 hours, the staining will disappear from the original area and reappear in the new dependent parts. So in a hanging body, if staining is noted in any area other than the limbs, the assumption is that the body was suspended after death. If a hanging body is cut down and laid on its back, the postmortem staining can develop slightly on the back; even if it was fixed on the limbs already.

Examine the dependent parts in good light. Staining is easily distinguished in fair complexioned bodies and cannot be distinguished in dark bodies or in those which have lost large quantities of blood. If blanching of the stained area occurs on pressing with the thumb, it is assumed that the staining is not fixed (Figs 5.16 and 5.17).

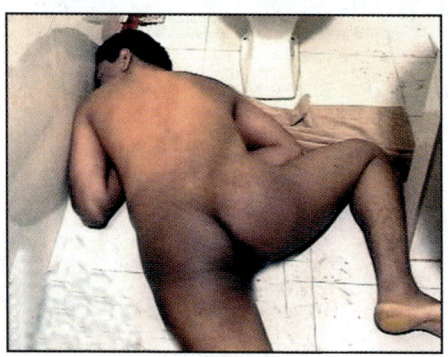

**Fig. 5.14:** Dead body lying prone in a bathroom. Death was due to inhalation of carbon monoxide from a faulty water heater

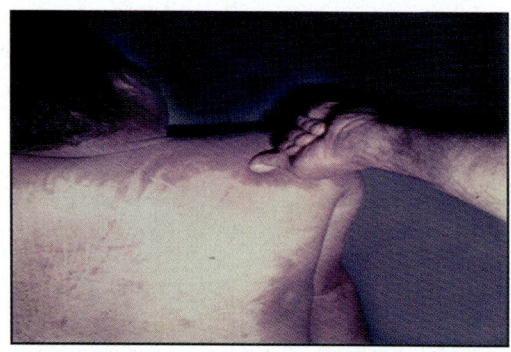

**Fig. 5.16:** To find out whether the lividity is fixed or not, press area with thumb

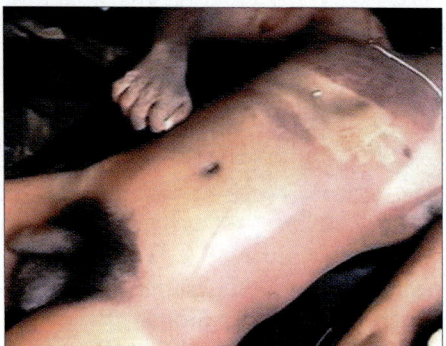

**Fig. 5.15:** Postmortem lividity on the front. The cherry pink colour is due to carboxyhemoglobin. Note the contact pallor in the areas on the chest which were in close contact with the folded hands

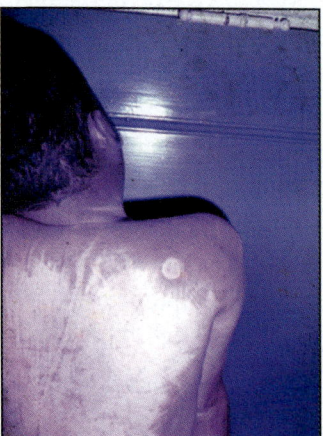

**Fig. 5.17:** Blanching indicates that the lividity is not fixed

Staining may be absent on those areas which are in close contact with the surface, e.g. shoulder blades and buttocks in the case of a supine body (contact pallor). Loss of muscle tone in those areas will make them flattened in appearance (contact flattening). In some case of poisoning, postmortem staining will have distinctive colour. Carbon monoxide will impart a cherry red colour, cyanides will give a bright red colour and nitrate poisoning can cause brown staining. Postmortem staining is sometimes mistaken for contusions. There will be swelling and abrasions around a contusion. It can be confirmed during autopsy by incising and examining the suspected livid area. On incision, extravasated dark clotted blood is seen in the tissues in the case of a contusion. But only droplets of blood are seen in the cut vessels when an area of hypostasis is incised. Microscopical examination of the tissue can also be done in doubtful cases.

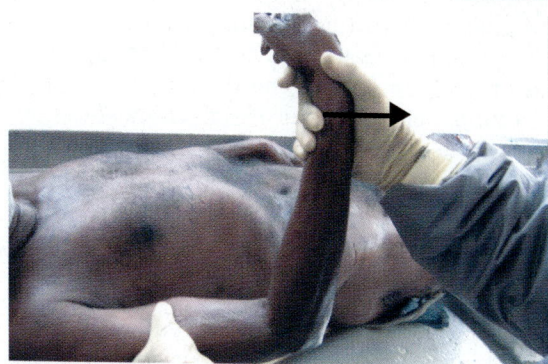

**Fig. 5.18:** Testing for rigor mortis—Try to extend a bent limb

## Postmortem Rigidity (Rigor Mortis)

Stiffening of muscles after death is called rigor mortis. Soon after death, all the muscles of the body become flaccid **(primary relaxation)**. Muscles are composed of bundles of muscle fibres, made up of interdigitating protein filaments, viz. actin and myosin. When a nerve impulse reaches the muscle, the muscle fibres contract. After death, muscles lose their plasticity and elasticity. The actin and myosin filaments combine to form a rigid compound of actomyosin and the muscles become stiff. This is the reason for the development of rigor mortis.

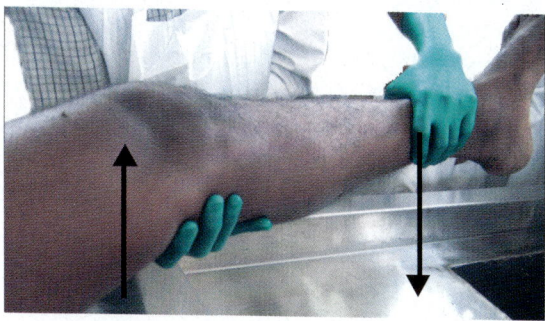

**Fig. 5.19:** Testing for rigor mortis—Try to bend an extended limb

Smaller muscles are affected first and hence apparently, rigor starts first in the eyelids, face, neck and apparently establishes in a proximo-distal fashion. In tropical climate, rigor establishes in the muscles of face and neck in 1-2 hours, in the upper limbs by 2 –4 hours and in lower limbs by 4 –6 hours. The whole body becomes stiff in 6 hours. By trying to open the jaw or flexing an extended limb or extending a flexed limb, one can find out whether rigor has set in or not (Figs 5.18 and 5.19). Once the rigor is broken by force or during transportation, it will not reappear.

The rigor will start disappearing by 18 –24 hours after death. Many factors affect the onset and duration of rigor. Muscular activity prior to death, diseases, etc. hasten the onset; while cold weather may retard the onset and prolong the duration. Rigor will also occur in the internal muscular organs like heart, uterus, etc. It can develop in paralysed limbs. When a dead body is kept in a cold storage, the development of rigor mortis will be arrested. When the body is subsequently taken out and thawed, rigor mortis will progress further. Estimation of time of death based on rigor mortis in the case of a dead body kept in the cold chamber will be erroneous. The body has to be examined and the extent of rigor should be noted at the time of inquest or before placing it in the cold chamber. Time of death can be ascertained from the establishment and retaining of rigor mortis.

Many conditions simulate rigor mortis. **Cadaveric spasm** or instantaneous rigor is a condition where muscles which were contracting at the time of death may become stiff just after death without undergoing the stage of primary flaccidity. The cause for its development is not known. In deaths due to drowning, the deceased may catch hold of weeds/water plants as a last act of life and the materials will be found firmly clasped in the hands of the dead body. This is a good evidence to indicate that death was due to drowning. In suicidal gunshot/cut throat cases, sometimes the weapon may be found held firmly by the person due to cadaveric spasm (Fig. 5.20). This appearance cannot be fabricated easily.

Extreme heat will coagulate the muscle proteins and the body will become stiff **(heat stiffening)**. When a dead body is subjected to intense heat, stiffening of the muscles will result in the flexion of neck, elbows, thighs and knees. The body assumes the posture of a boxer. This is called **pugilistic attitude**. Likewise, extreme cold can also cause stiffening of muscles and solidification of subcutaneous fat **(cold stiffening)**. Putrefactive gases can also produce rigidity in the muscles **(gas rigidity)**.

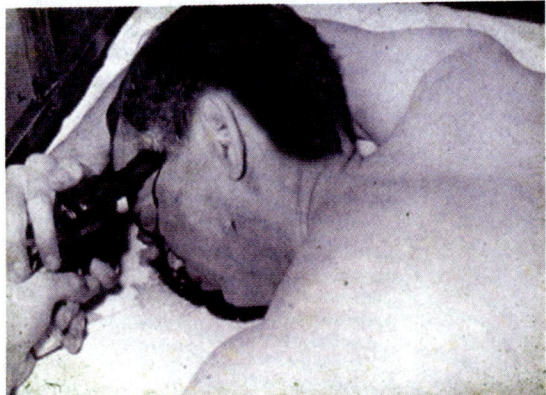

**Fig. 5.20:** Cadaveric spasm. Suicide by revolver shot. The gun is firmly clasped in the hands

## Putrefaction

Putrefactive changes appear after the disappearance of rigor mortis. Even though the process of decomposition starts at cellular level much earlier,

appearance of different shades of colour in the skin, formation of gases and liquefaction of tissues are the main presenting features. Bacteria, fungi and various enzymes are responsible for these changes. Putrefaction is optimum at temperatures of 20°C to 40°C. That is why bodies exposed to the sun, especially in summer, decompose faster. Decomposition will be arrested below 0°C. Bodies can be kept in cold chambers or covered with ice and salt to prevent decomposition. If the body has to be preserved for weeks, it has to be deep frozen or embalmed.

### Colour Changes

Appearance of a greenish discolouration on the right side of lower abdomen is the first change, indicating putrefaction (Fig. 5.21). Usually, it appears after rigor has started to disappear. The colour changes are due to the hemolysis and subsequent disintegration of haemoglobin and its combination with the gases of putrefaction such as hydrogen sulphide. The green colour will spread to all regions; but will be marked in areas where there is postmortem staining. The colour will change to greenish yellow, blue or black. Later the skin of the whole body will assume a dark colour. The walls of veins, stained by the haemoglobin derivatives will stand out prominently. This

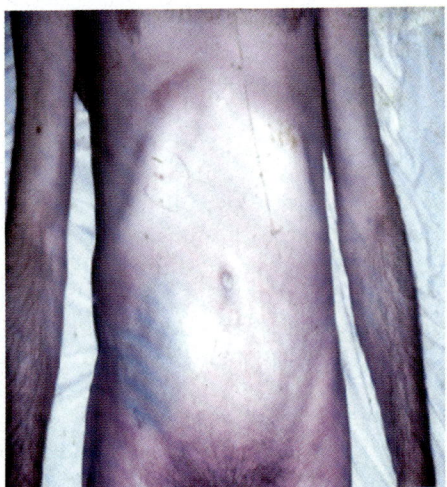

**Fig. 5.21:** Onset of putrefaction—greenish discolouration on the right side of lower abdomen

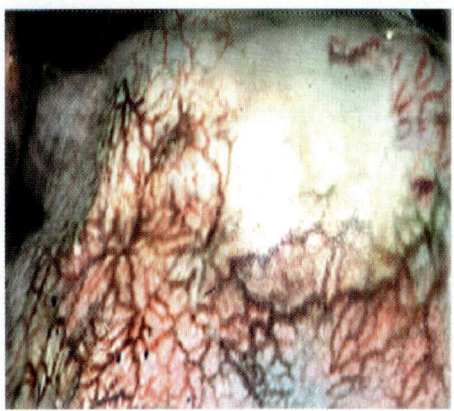

**Fig. 5.22:** Marbling

appearance is called **marbling** (Fig. 5.22). The above mentioned changes will be complete within 36 – 48 hours.

In putrefied bodies, skin of the hand may peel off like a glove (Fig. 5.23). This glove-like skin is to be dried, spread out and prints can be taken. Doctors can help the investigating officer and fingerprint expert. If there are no facilities for taking prints during inquest, the tips of fingers can be amputated and preserved in 10% formalin in separate labelled bottles for fingerprinting later.

## Gas Formation

The bacteria present in the body liberate gases during the putrefactive process. The foul smelling gases collect in the intestine and the abdomen is distended. Because of increased pressure in the tissues and body cavities, the eyeballs and the tongue will be protruded; rectum and uterus will be prolapsed. If the uterus is gravid, the foetus may be expelled **(postmortem delivery)**. The protrusion of tongue may simulate strangulation or hanging. If so, find out whether the tongue is bitten to exclude an asphyxial death. The face and genitalia will be bloated up. Gases collecting under the skin will form blebs. These blebs may be similar to the blebs in burns (Fig. 5.24). But when the skin of the bleb is punctured; the floor will be white without any vital reaction and there will not be any fluid as in the case of a bleb of burns. These changes will take place in 36 to 72 hours. After 72 hours, the skin peels off, hairs and nails become loose, and tissues become soft.

Floatation of a submerged body is due to the formation of gases of decomposition. In tropics, this can occur in 24 hours after submersion.

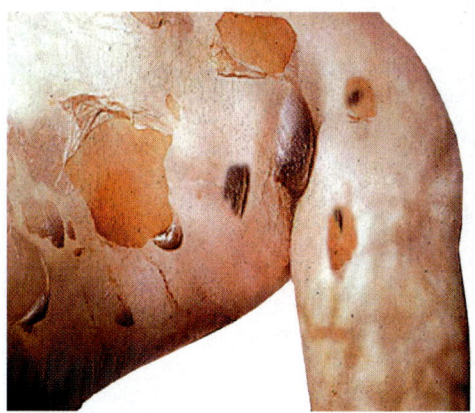

**Fig. 5.24:** Postmotem blebs and peeling of skin

## Skeletonisation

If a dead body is lying in the open, it may take 1 – 2 months for complete skeletonisation. If the body is buried without a coffin, skeletonisation may take place in 2–6 months. If the body is encased in a coffin, more time is required for skeletonisation. Many factors such as temperature, humidity, etc. are responsible for these changes. Hence a definite opinion as to the time since death

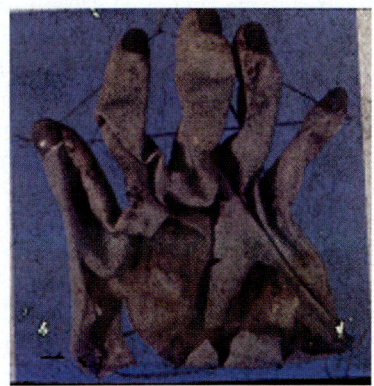

**Fig. 5.23:** Peeling of skin of hands like a glove (degloving)

cannot be given based on the changes of putrefaction alone.

Sometimes if the body is buried in a marshy area, the fatty tissues of the body are converted to higher fatty acids like stearic, palmitic, etc. A soap like substance is formed in the subcutaneous areas. This is called **adipocere** (Fig. 5.25). Minimum time required for the development of adipocere is 3 to 7 days. Similarly bodies buried in warm, sandy areas, become shrunken and shrivelled; the change is called **mummification** (Fig. 5.26). It may take 3 months to one year for this change to develop. In both these states, the features will be preserved and identity of the deceased can be established. Injuries if any, can also be recognised.

Putrefaction is delayed if a dead body remains in water. But if it is taken out, the putrefactive processes are hastened due to the imbibition of water. That is why when a drowned body is taken out of water for inquest, it appears fresh.

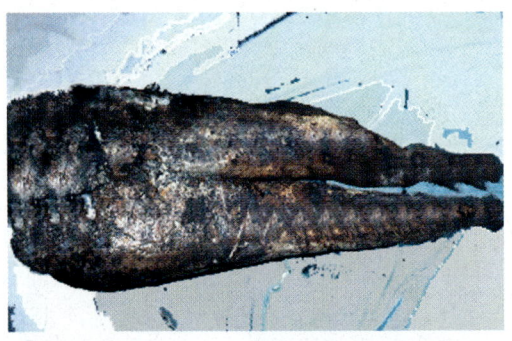

**Fig. 5.25:** Adipocere formation of lower limbs of dead body

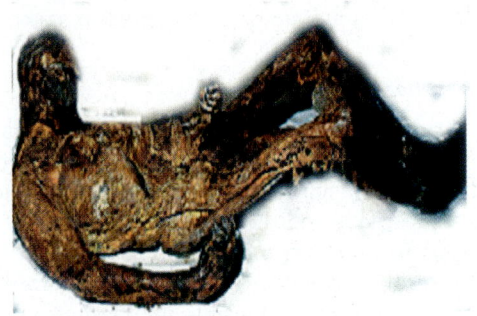

**Fig. 5.26:** Mummified body

By the time the inquest is finished, the features will be grossly altered due to putrefaction. Rate of decomposition of a dead body in air is twice as quickly as in water and eight times as quickly as in earth **(Casper's dictum)**.

### Internal Changes

Internal organs also undergo various putrefactive changes. Discolouration appears first in the intestine. This is often mistaken as contusion. Brain becomes soft in 24 hours and will liquefy in 72 to 96 hours. Lungs, liver, spleen, kidneys, etc. become pulpy in 72 to 96 hours. Putrefactive gases in the liver will give it a foamy appearance **(foamy liver)**. Histological examination is useless at this stage, but toxicological analysis is possible even if the organs are highly putrefied.

### Putrefaction and Injuries

When the skin is peeled off, superficial injuries like abrasions cannot be made out. But contusions may be distinguished even after many days. All the suspected discoloured areas should be incised. The extravasated blood in a contusion will be present even though it might have started to disintegrate. In doubtful cases, the tissues may be subjected to microscopical examination. As long as the tissues surrounding the wound are not destroyed, incised and lacerated wounds can also be discernible.

### Entomological Evidence

When the dead bodies start decaying, house flies lay eggs on them. The eggs hatch out in 10–12 hours into larvae called maggots. The innumerable maggots will destroy the soft tissues of the body. After 6 to 7 days, maggots crawl out to become pupae. These maggots may be preserved in rectified spirit and sent for examination to an entomologist to assess their age. From this, time of death can be calculated (Figs 5.27 and 5.28).

### Unknown, Unidentified Dead Bodies

All possible efforts should be taken to the identify the unknown dead bodies. Without establishing the identity of the corpse, it may not be even possible to proceed with the investigation of the case. Every day a number of person-missing cases

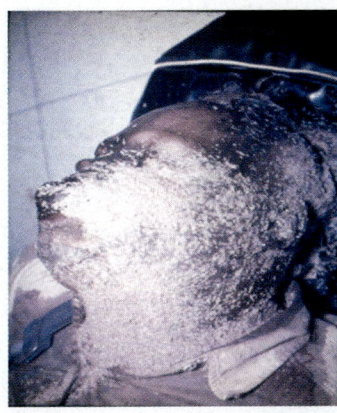

**Fig. 5.27:** Putrefied dead body infested with maggots

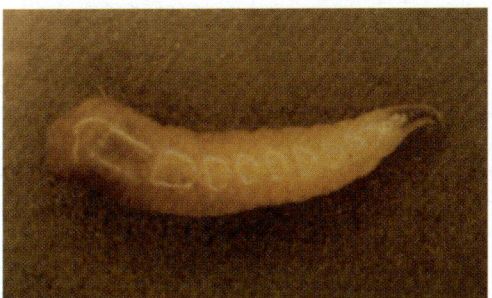

**Fig. 5.28:** Maggot

are registered in the police stations. The physical details of the missing person should be compared and correlated with the physical features of unidentified dead bodies. Usually, the investigating officers note two identification marks such as moles or scars. This will not help to identify the body.

## Photographs

Photographs of the dead body including close up pictures of the face are to be taken. Dead bodies lack animation and hence difficulty will be experienced in identifying the deceased from a photograph taken at the crime scene or mortuary. Postmortem changes of skin, rigor mortis, injuries, putrefactive changes, etc. can alter the facial appearance. So photographs should be taken after the disappearance of rigor. The body should be propped up or the photo can be taken with a digital camera with a variangle LCD screen. Postmortem

drawing can be applied by 'lifting' the facial structures and giving an 'expression' to the face (Figs 5.29A and B).

## Determination of Sex

Determining the sex is usually not difficult. Examination of the external genital organs will help in distinguishing the sex except in cases of intersex. Intersex is the intermingling of both sexes in one individual. In some individuals, there will be total failure of development of sex organs (gonadal agenesis). In some others, there will be undeveloped sex organs (gonadal dysgenesis). Chromosomal studies may be required to determine the genetic sex in these cases.

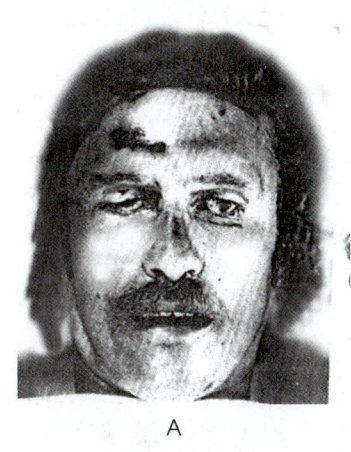

A

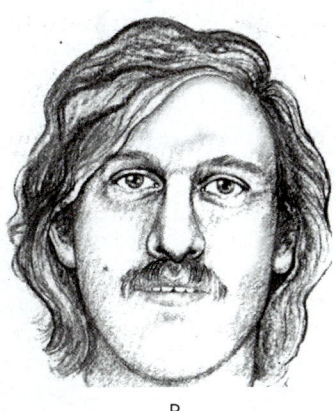

B

**Figs 5.29 A and B:** A. Postmortem photograph of face, B. Modified by drawing the artist (*Courtesy:* Karen Taylor)

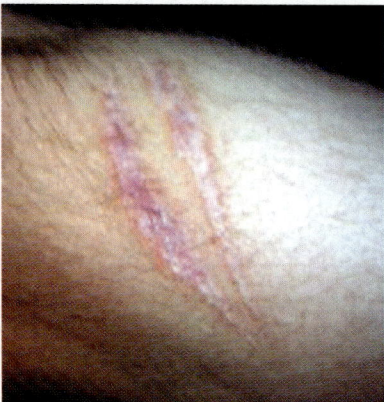

**Fig. 5.30:** Scars

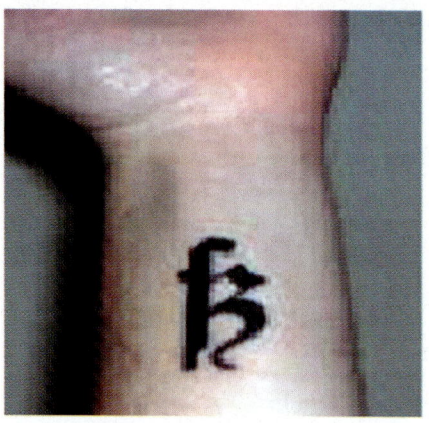

**Fig. 5.32:** Tattoo mark

## Scars, Moles and Tattoo Marks

A scar is formed as a result of healing of an injury and is composed of fibrous tissue (Fig. 5.30). Only if the injury has involved dermis and deeper tissues, a scar is formed. A clean incised wound, without sepsis will heal in 6–7 days and a vascular scar appears. By about 14 days, the scar becomes pale. In about 2–6 months, the scar becomes white, tough and remains permanent. A scar being a permanent one, is often taken as an identification mark.

Mole is a pigmented spot either flat or raised; hairy or hairless (Fig. 5.31). Medically it is called intradermal naevus. These are permanent marks; usually noted as an identification mark.

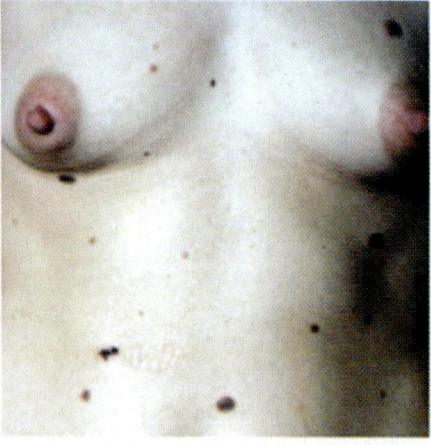

**Fig. 5.31:** Multiple black moles

Tattoos are designs imprinted in the skin, using tattoo machines or needles dipped in dyes (Fig. 5.32). They are seen in areas like arms, chest, etc. and will depict names, diagrams of deities, flowers and symbols. They are permanent and can be made out even in putrefied dead bodies where the epidermis has peeled off. The local lymph gland will also contain the pigment.

## Other Features

Bony deformities, occupational marks, circumcised penis, pierced ear lobules, callosities on the forehead, etc. are features which will help to identify the caste, occupation, etc. Circumcision is performed by Muslims and Jews. It is also performed in children and adults when the foreskin of the penis is tight and cannot be retracted. Callosities are seen in the hands of manual labourers. Persons engaged in climbing trees will have callosities in their legs, chest and abdomen. Coal miners will have deposits of coal particles in the wound scars. Soft callosities are seen in the fingers, especially on the outer aspect of right middle finger in those who write for long time using pens. Personal habits of a person are reflected in his teeth. Smoker's teeth will be stained yellow or blackish brown with nicotine. The stain found adjacent to the gingival margin on the lingual aspect will be blackish brown in colour. On the labial aspect, the colour of the stain will be yellow. Pipe smokers and those who use cigarette holders will develop irregular gaps in the anterior teeth of both jaws. Teeth of persons who chew betel leaves will be stained black.

Other dental peculiarities like extractions, fillings, dental works, mal alignment, staining due to chewing or smoking, etc. will help to establish the identity. Artificial dentures and other dental work will also help in establishing identity. The forensic surgeon or a forensic odontologist may be requested to make a detailed examination to provide clues regarding age and identity.

## Determination of Age

Age can be estimated from the examination of teeth more or less accurately up to 14 years as they erupt in a chronological order. A detailed description of the teeth will help very much to establish the identity. Age can also be assessed from a single tooth by noting the secondary changes occurring in the dental tissues as age advances. The method is known as **Gustafson's technique** named after a Sweedish dentist. For this, one of the incisor teeth is removed, ground; and a thin section made is examined microscopically. The tooth can be sent to the forensic odontology section of the oral pathology department of dental colleges or the department of forensic medicine in the medical colleges of the state for estimating the age by Gustafson's method.

Forensic surgeon may be able to assess the age by observing the closure of cranial sutures. During autopsy, when the skull cap is removed, the sutures are inspected. The estimation is not very accurate. There could a difference of +/- 10 years.

## Hair

Detailed description of scalp hair, moustache, beard, axillary hair, chest hair, and pubic hair should be recorded; length, colour and texture are to be noted. Microscopical comparison of the morphology of the hair samples is possible. In the neutron activation analysis method (NAA), hairs are made radioactive and quantitative analysis of the elements contained in the hairs is done for comparison and identification of the samples. The unique method of DNA typing is possible from the cells attached to the hair roots. For this, entire hairs with roots are necessary. DNA typing provides absolute proof of identity.

Chemical examination of the hair samples can reveal the presence of hair dyes or bleaching agents applied to the hair for cosmetic purpose. Poisoning with heavy metals like arsenic can also be detected by chemical analysis. Samples may be collected.

## Fingerprints

Skin of the fingers, palms of hands and soles of feet contain 'friction ridges'. These are characterised by a complicated pattern of ridges and furrows. On the pulps of fingers, the friction ridges form a number of basic patterns (Figs 5.33 A to D). The four basic patterns are 'arches, loops, whorls and composites'. Within these basic patterns, many other variations are also seen. These ridge patterns are formed in the humans in the foetal stage and remain constant throughout life. Within the fingerprint pattern, a number of features like islands, bifurcations, deltas, dots, etc. are seen. These are called minutiae, the basis of fingerprint comparison.

Statistical probability of two individuals (even in twins of same sex) having the same fingerprint pattern is almost nil. In unidentified bodies, fingerprints from the dead body have to be taken for establishing identity by comparison with fingerprints from documents or crime records.

In murder cases, suspicious deaths and unknown dead bodies, it may be necessary to take

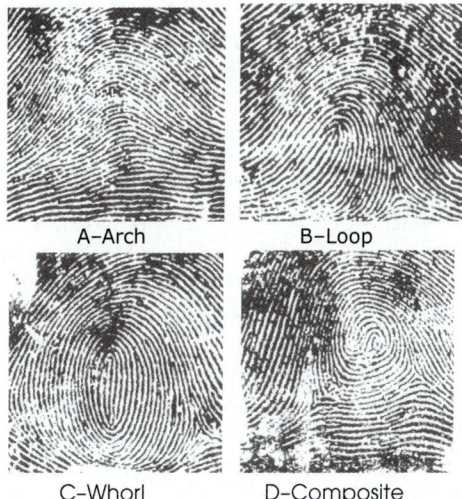

A–Arch  B–Loop

C–Whorl  D–Composite

**Figs 5.33A to D:** Different patterns of fingerprints, A–Arch, B–Loop, C–Whorl, D–Composite

the fingerprints of the deceased. It is not an easy task to take fingerprints from a dead body. Therefore, services of a fingerprint expert may be made available for this work. A special fingerprint kit with specially designed spatulas is available for taking fingerprints from dead bodies. If the fingers are stiff due to rigor mortis, it should be broken by manipulating the fingers.

If the fingerprint expert is not available, the forensic surgeon may be requested to amputate the finger tips (in unclaimed bodies). The fingers may be put in individual bottles, preserved in 10% formalin, labelled and sealed. The fingers are later taken out of formalin, cleaned and dried. Glycerine is injected under the skin of the pulp of the finger if the skin is shrivelled before taking the fingerprints by the expert. If the body is putrefied and the skin of the fingers are peeling off (degloving—see Fig. 5.24), then the skin of the pulps alone can be removed and put in separate bottles, in a flat position. Later, prints can be developed from the skin flaps.

## Face

Face will be livid and shows petechial haemorrhages in asphyxial deaths like hanging, strangulation, suffocation, etc. In corrosive poisoning with acids or alkalies, marks of corrosion may be seen around the mouth and other parts of the body. In all cases of poisoning, face, especially areas around the mouth should be examined carefully for the presence of violence which is indicative of forcible administration of poison. Bluish discolouration of the lips is a sign of asphyxia.

## Eyes

Examination of the eyes may provide valuable evidence as to the cause of death. Conjunctival congestion, proptosis, and petechial haemorrhages are signs of asphyxia. Conjunctivae will be pale in deaths due to haemorrhage. Suffusion of blood into the eyelids, commonly known as **black eye** is seen in injuries of head, fractures of base of skull, etc.

After death, eyes undergo various changes. The cornea becomes opaque due to drying. Two yellow triangles of discolouration of the sclera due to drying will appear on each side of the cornea. The colour will change to brown or black. This is known as **tache noire**. The eyeballs become sunken and collapsed. The pupils are slightly dilated and fixed immediately after death and may become constricted due to rigor mortis of muscles of iris later.

## Nostrils and Ears

The presence of froth at nostrils is an indication of fluid in the lungs (pulmonary edema). The froth may be blood-stained in severe pulmonary edema. Fine white lathery froth is an indication of waterlogged lungs in drowning. In insecticidal poisoning, the froth may have kerosene like smell. Discharge of cerebrospinal fluid (CSF) and/or blood is an indication of fracture of base of skull.

## Urethra, Vagina and Anus

In violent asphyxial deaths, relaxation of sphincters occurs with the discharge of semen, urine and faeces. If there is discharge of pus from the urethra, it could be a sign of venereal disease. Invariably in all female dead bodies, request the autopsy surgeon to conduct a vaginal examination to note the state of hymen and laxity of hymenal orifice/vagina.

Few vaginal swabs and smears for microscopical and chemical examination should also be collected. Injuries to genitalia and bleeding from vagina could be indicative of sexual assault. But in asphyxial deaths like hanging there could be bleeding from the urethra, anus and vagina due to increased pressure in the small blood vessels of those regions.

Examination of anal opening may provide evidence in cases of unnatural sexual offences. Injuries of the anal sphincter with dilatation of the anus may be seen in a passive agent of sodomy. Loss of tone of anal muscles, a patulous anal opening, presence of old fissures and scars are evidence of habitual anal intercourse. In suspected cases of sodomy, request the doctor to collect anal smears and swabs for microscopical and chemical examinations.

## Injuries

Injuries if any found on the body are to be recorded in detail. The shape, length and location of the injury should be noted. The distance from the nearest anatomical landmark should be measured.

Close up photographs of the major or significant injuries are to be taken after keeping a scale (Tailor's tape scale) by its side (Fig. 5.34). Life size images of the injury can be developed using the scale as a reference object. If a weapon is found thrust in the wound, it should not be removed without taking photographs and before developing latent fingerprints. It is better to keep the weapon in situ and despatch the body for autopsy, so that the doctor may be able to correlate the weapon with the injury. Injuries, blood stains and other salient features on the body can be marked in diagrams (Figs 5.35 and 5.36).

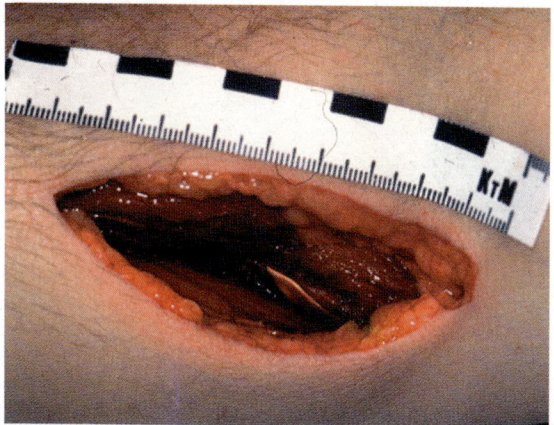

**Fig. 5.34:** Photographing a wound with a scale placed close by

In the case of death due to gun shot, the entry and exit wounds should not be wiped or cleaned as the gun powder residues will be removed (Fig. 5.37). The hands of the victim may also contain gun powder residues. After photographing the injuries, services of forensic pathologist and forensic scientist should be sought for collecting the trace evidence from the dead body and scene.

When a gun is fired, there will be leakage of explosive gases from the firing chamber of the gun. These gases containing the residues of the gun powder/explosive charge will stain the fingers of the person who fires the weapon. Detection of these residues in the fingers of the dead body will prove that the victim had fired

the gun. This finding will support the theory of suicide. The hands of the victim are covered with cotton gauze dipped in molten paraffin to form a glove-like covering. Later this is removed and tested with reagents to detect residues of the explosive charge. This test is known as **dermal nitrate test**. The details are given in Chapter 'Firearm and Explosive Injuries'.

## Evidentiary Materials

### Clothing and Personal Articles

Clothing and personal articles should be removed from the body and their detailed description noted. Clothing should be removed by cutting along the side seams. Before removing the clothing, a thorough search should be made to locate all foreign particles such as stains, fibres, hair, etc. sticking to the clothes and the body. The clothing should be dried in the shade before packing. The foreign materials should be collected and packed separately in polythene bags, labelled and sealed. Articles like ligatures, weapons, etc. which require an examination by the doctor should not be removed and kept in situ. In homicides and suspicious deaths, samples of hair from scalp, body and pubic areas should be taken wherever necessary. The scalp may be combed and loose hairs with roots may be taken. In putrefied bodies, hair can be pulled out as a tuft. The hairs are dried before packing them in separate polythene bags or bottles. Each container should bear descriptive labels.

### Finger Nails

Debris found underneath the finger nails may contain trace evidence including foreign DNA material. Finger nail scrapings can be collected in a clean paper or paper packet using a small wooden spatula or a swab. If it is not possible, finger nails can be clipped using a nail cutter, avoiding injury to fingers and contamination. The clippings are collected in small, clean glass bottles or polythene bags after drying.

### Blood

If there is extravasated blood in the scene, dip one or two pieces of clean white cloth in the pool of blood and dry it in the shade before packing them

Name.....................................................Crime No.....................Police Station...........................

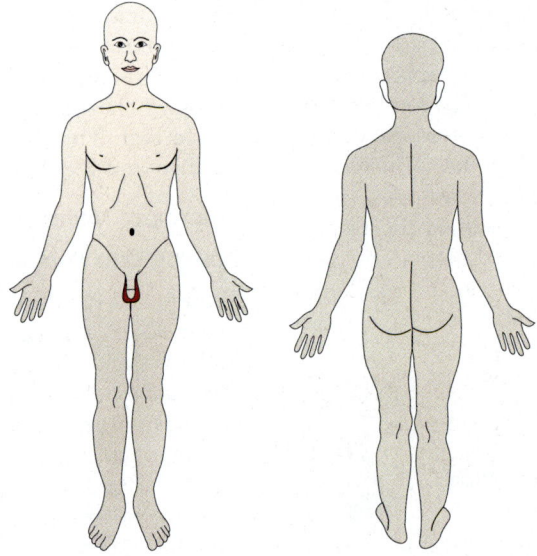

**Fig. 5.35:** Diagram to mark injuries, stains and salient features — front and back of the body

Name.....................................................Crime No.....................Police Station...........................

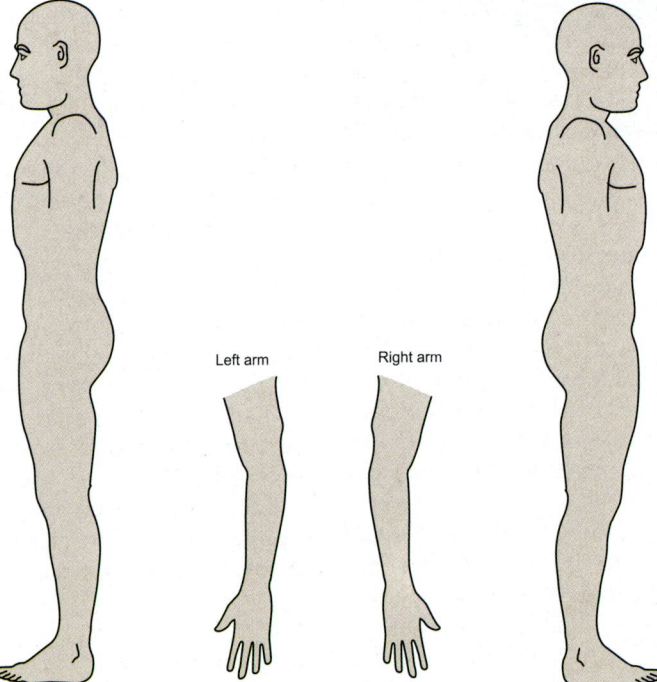

Left arm

Right arm

**Fig. 5.36:** Diagram to mark injuries, stains and salient features — left and right sides of the body

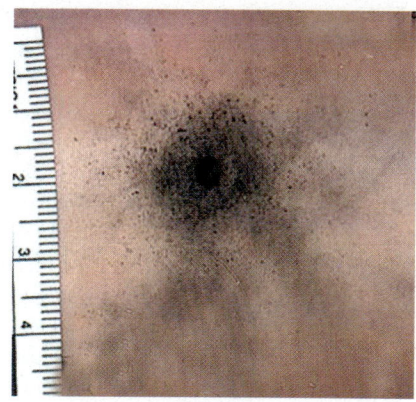

**Fig. 5.37:** Blackening and peppering around a gun shot injury

in clean glass containers or polythene bags. An unstained piece of cloth should also be packed as a control sample. Liquid blood is not suitable for grouping as it will decompose by the time it reaches the laboratory.

If there is no blood in the scene, it should be collected from the dead body (with the help of the doctor) for grouping. If blood stains are present in small articles, the articles are to be preserved as such. Dry stains from immovable articles should be scraped and preserved in a clean bottle for grouping. Methods of collecting and preserving blood stains and body fluids for DNA typing are discussed in Chapter on DNA Fingerprinting.

### Vomitus/Excreta

If there is any vomitus or excreta in the scene, the same may be collected in glass bottles after drying them thoroughly. Empty bottles and vessels containing remnants of food, drink or poisonous substances should be preserved in cases of suspected poisoning. This will be very helpful to find out the cause of death in cases of poisoning. In cases of food poisoning, remnants of food consumed by the victims, vessels used for cooking, remnants of uncooked food articles, etc. should be preserved for microbiological examination.

### PREPARATION OF INQUEST REPORT

Inquest is a preliminary investigation into the circumstances of death. The investigating officer has to examine the dead body and the scene of occurrence. As per **Section 175 (1) of Cr. P.C,** a police officer proceeding under **Section 174 Cr.P.C** may, by order in writing, summon two or more persons as aforesaid for the purpose of the said investigation, and any other person who appears to be acquainted with the facts of the case and every person so summoned shall be bound to attend and answer truly all questions other than questions, the answers to which would have a tendency to expose him to a criminal charge or a penalty or forfeiture.

The inhibition contained in **Section 162 of Cr.PC** also applies to statements recorded under **Section 174.** According to Section 162 Cr.PC, "No statement made by any person to a police officer in the course of an investigation under this chapter (XII), shall, if reduced to writing, be signed by the person making it; nor shall any such statement or any record thereof, whether in a police diary or otherwise, or any part of such statement or record, be used for any purpose, save as hereinafter provided, at any inquiry or trial in respect of any offence under investigation at the time when such statement was made:

Provided that when any witness is called for the prosecution in such inquiry or trial whose statement has been reduced into writing as aforesaid, any part of his statement, if duly proved, may be used by the accused, and with the permission of the Court, by the prosecution, to contradict such witness in the manner provided by **Section 145 of the Indian Evidence Act;** and when any part of such statement is so used, any part thereof may also be used in the re-examination of such witness, but for the purpose only of explaining any matter referred to in his cross-examination.

After the investigation, the investigating officer has to prepare a report. Inquest report is an important document. In the report, the appearance of the dead body and the scene are to be included in detail (**columns 7 and 8**). Detailed description of injuries, if any found on the body, are to be included. It is also necessary to state in what manner or by what weapon such wounds appear to have been inflicted (**column 12**). Apparent cause of death is noted under **column 11.** Opinion of the

Panchayatdars as to the cause and manner of death also finds a place in the report (**column 16**).

The inquest report also contains the statements of the persons present during inquest and questioned by the investigating officer. The facts thus ascertained by the investigating officer from those persons would not be admitted as evidence either for the prosecution or for the defence. But during the trial of a case, the defence counsel can cross-examine the prosecution witnesses based on the inquest report. The disclosure of the name of the accused is not mandatory in the inquest report. While conducting inquest, the investigating officer need not investigate and find out the person responsible for the death of the victim.

There should not be any delay in preparing the inquest report. It has to be prepared promptly and signed by the Panchayatdars and the investigating officer. The scope of the inquest report is to ascertain whether the person has died under suspicious circumstances. If the death is due to unnatural causes and if foul play is suspected, the dead body has to be sent for autopsy. If there is no foul play, the police has a discretion not to send the body for autopsy. But the discretion has to be exercised prudently and honestly.

The inquest report has to be forwarded to the executive magistrate concerned. A copy of the report has to be sent to the medical officer who conducts the autopsy. If the investigating officer is sending clothes, weapons, ornaments and other personal belongings of the deceased along with the corpse, the details of the same my be entered in the inquest report as well as in the requisition for postmortem examination. Proforma of the inquest report is given in (Proforma 5.1).

## FORWARDING THE DEAD BODY FOR AUTOPSY

After the inquest, if the police officer finds that the person has died under suspicious circumstances or that the death is an unnatural one, he forwards the dead body for autopsy. In sensational cases which require examination by an expert, services of a specialist in forensic medicine is sought for. Experienced doctors with postgraduate degree in forensic medicine are available in all the medical colleges. They are designated as police surgeons. Their duties and responsibilities are defined in the government orders-GO MS 123/66/Home dated 26-3-1966 and GO MS 364/68/Home dated 14-10-1968. The subordinate officers in the departments of forensic medicine are appointed as deputy and assistant police surgeons (GO MS/85/75/Home dated 1-7-1975 and GO MS/ 9/84/Home dated 3-2-1984). Jurisdiction of the units of the police surgeons has been defined (GO MS/87/84/Home dated 3-7-1984). They are paid honorarium and remuneration for conducting autopsies.

## Duties and Responsibilities of the Police Surgeon

- Police surgeon may conduct all medicolegal autopsies in the hospital to which he is attached and he will personally attend to cases of homicide, traffic accidents, suspicious deaths and other important cases.
- His assistants may conduct autopsies for all other simple deaths when the cause of death is reasonably certain.
- Autopsies at site will be conducted by the police surgeon or an assistant deputed by him as stipulated above.
- In cases of injury, poisoning, criminal miscarriage and other medicolegal cases, which may be dealt within the hospital to which he is attached, he will give consultant advice to the medical officer in charge of the case.
- He will provide consultant service to police officers in all medicolegal aspects of criminal cases.
- He will examine, in consultation with other specialists as may be required, articles of medicolegal nature furnished by investigating officers. Articles for medicolegal examination by other experts will be forwarded in consultation with him and through him.
- Cases where age is to be determined will also be forwarded to the police surgeon.
- He will appear as expert witness when called upon to offer second opinion in complicated criminal cases.
- He may delegate his duties to a competent officer working under him in straightforward medicolegal

**Proforma 5.1:** Proforma of Inquest Report

## KERALA POLICE

District:                    Circle:                    Station:

Report of investigation on the dead body of.................... .............Held at........... a.m/p.m. on the ...............................day of
............. .........(month) .....................(year)

Dated...................... Despatched ......................Received ...........................

## KERALA POLICE

District.......................................... Circle ......................... Station.....................................

## INQUEST REPORT

Report of investigation under section 174 Cr.P.C on the body of a person found dead at.....am/p.m ...................
on the.................. day of................(Month).....................(Year)

N.B      1.   In framing this report the questions below should be carefully answered.
         2.   Questions 20 to 26 apply to the Railway Police
         3.   The word "nil" should be written against the no. of any question which requires no answer.
         4.   Case diary forms should be used as inner sheets for answering these question.

1.   Name, calling and residence of persons composing the            :
     Panchayat, if any
2.   Name of the deceased, sex, age, calling, father's name          :
     and residence
3.   By whom first found dead, when and where?                       :
4.   By whom last seen alive, where and when and in whose            :
     company and whether he carried any valuable property
     with him
5.   Height, colour and descriptive marks                            :
6.   Married or single (if a male, was he living a pure              :
     or licentious life, if a female was she living with
     her husband or single, by reason of her being a widow or
     otherwise, if living singly, was she a good or bad
     character among the neighbours)
7.   State of corpse, its posture and exact state of limbs,
     eyes, mouth, etc.  If any wounds, particulars thereof, and
     list of all property found on the corpse.                       :
8.   Minute description of exact spot
     a.  Where corpse was found & if in water depth thereof           :
     b.  When body is found in a well, information on the
         following points should be given                            :
         i.  Is the well a public or private property,               :
             if the latter, to whom does it belong?
         ii. Is it near a public road or pathway?                    :
         iii. Does it have a parapet wall and float?                 :
9.   By which relative, body is recognised and their                 :
     statement given in short (blood relatives, such as parents,
     brothers, sisters always to be examined, if there are any)

*Contd...*

*Contd...*

| | | |
|---|---|---|
| 10. | Abstract of evidence of other persons examined. | : |
| 11. | Apparent cause of death | : |
| 12. | If by violence, apparently, by what weapon | : |
| | a. If any person is suspected, who and why? | : |
| | b. Was deceased insured in any company? | : |
| 13. | If corpse is not sent for medical examination, why? | : |
| 14. | If corpse is sent, for what purpose and by whose order, and no. of constable who went with it. (the date and hour when the body is sent should also be given here.) | : |
| 15. | By whose orders corpse was buried or burnt | : |
| 16. | Opinion of the Panchayatdars as to cause and manner of death | : |
| 17. | Signature of such of the Panchayatdars who concur with the above opinion | : |
| 18. | Station house officer's signature | : |
| 19. | a. If name and residence of deceased be unknown, state what steps have been taken to ascertain the same and secure identification. To what statements have proclamations been sent. | : |
| | b. Have fingerprints of the deceased been taken and sent to the finger print bureau concerned? | : |
| 20. | Was the body warm or cold when first found ? | : |
| 21. | If appearance shows that body has been dragged, was it by an up or down train? | : |
| 22. | Were suspected engines and carriages examined? if so by whom and with what result? | : |
| 23. | Circumstances under which the deceased met with the accident? | : |
| 24. | Reasons for supposing that body was run over by any particular train | : |
| 25. | Statements of driver and firemen of suspected train | : |
| 26. | Any reason to suspect foul play | : |
| 27. | Duration of investigation | : |

Investigation commenced at ..................Investigation closed at .........................................

Signature of witnesses...........................Signature of the Investigating Officer........................

cases or in other cases when he is unable to attend to them personally.

## Competent Authority to Requisition the Service of Police Surgeons (GO Ms 89/74/Home dated 6th June 1994)

- By the circle inspector of police in the district where the police surgeon's unit is located.
- By the superintendent of police in any district within the jurisdiction of the police surgeon. If the police surgeon concerned is not available, the SP can request the nearest available police surgeon after informing the range deputy inspector general of police and inspector general of police.
- The superintendent of police, crime branch CID in any district within the jurisdiction of the police surgeon. If the services of any other police surgeon is required, this may be secured through the deputy inspector general of police, crime investigation after informing the inspector general of police.
- By the Inspector General of Police (now the Director General of Police) any police surgeon anywhere.

Assistant surgeons of the general health services, possessing postgraduate degree in forensic medicine have been appointed as district police surgeons in some district hospitals. They conduct complicated, controversial and sensational medicolegal autopsies in the district hospitals of the respective districts.

At present, government has accorded sanction to the faculty of the departments of forensic medicine in the self-financing medical colleges to conduct medicolegal autopsies. The jurisdiction is limited to the local police stations.

To advise the government on medicolegal matters, the seniormost professor of forensic medicine of the state is appointed as the state medicolegal expert and consultant. Government of Kerala had also created a post of full time medicolegal adviser to the Kerala police.

## Requisition for the Conduct of Autopsy

A requisition in form no. KPF 102 (Proforma 5.2) is prepared and forwarded to the doctor along with the dead body. This form contains a gist of the findings of inquest. The requisition shall also contain directions for collecting viscera, blood, urine, hair, nail clippings or other materials from the dead body. Directions for forwarding the

original and copies of the postmortem certificates should also be mentioned in the requisition. It is better to forward a copy of the inquest report. The dead body will be entrusted to a police constable, who will accompany the dead body and hand it over to the doctor. He will identify the body as that of the deceased in the case.

## Autopsy at Site

If the body is putrefied or if it is difficult to transport it from the scene, autopsy can be conducted at site. The requisition for performing the autopsy at site has to be given by an officer not below the rank of a circle inspector of police. Necessary

**Table 5.1:** Jurisdiction of the police surgeons

| Government medical college | Jurisdiction (revenue district) |
|---|---|
| Thiruvananthapuram | Thiruvananthapuram, Kollam |
| Alappuzha | Alappuzha, Ernakulam |
| Kottayam | Kottayam, Idukki, Pathanamthitta |
| Thrissur | Thrissur, Palakkad, Malappuram |
| Kozhikode | Kozhikode, Wynadu |
| Pariyaram (self-financing) | Kannur, Kasaragod |

**Proforma 5.2:** KPF 102—Report to be Forwarded with the Body Sent for Autopsy

1.  Preliminary particulars

    Name ............................................................................... Male /Female

    Aged about ..........years

    Approximate height ............. cm

    Colour of eyes ..................colour of hair ...........length......cm

    Caste marks.............................................................................................................

    Other marks of identification .

    1..............................................................2..........................................................................

    Village ......................................... caste ...........................

    Found/Died at (hour) ..............a.m./p.m. on..................... at place ....................................

    sent by ........................................................................................... in charge of

    Head/Police Constable....................No......................on.........................at a.m/p.m..........

2.  State of body when found, its posture and other descriptions...............................................

3.  The spot where the body was found..................................................................................

4.  Injuries on the body, if any, their number and site .....................................................

*Contd...*

*Contd...*

5. The manner in which and the weapons or instrument (if any with which  the wounds and injuries mentioned in item 4 appear to have been inflicted)...................................................................

6. The circumstances of death ..................................................................................

7. If foul play is suspected, nature of foul play .................................................................

8. Apparent cause of death as per police inquest ..................................................................

9. The following articles are sent with the corpse:

   Clothes................................ Ornaments - jewelry.................

   Excreta ................................... Vomitus ...............................

   Weapons ......................................................................................

   Station.........................Dated...........................  Signature  of the Investigating Police Officer

---

To

Medical Officer,........................................................ Hospital

A postmortem examination may please be made on the body of the above person for the purpose of  investigation and the original of the postmortem certificate may be sent to ............................. (Magistrates having jurisdiction to enquire into the matter) and a copy sent to me.

Date......................        Signature............................................

                               Designation........................................

makeshift arrangements for the conduct of autopsy may be made in the scene. A temporary thatched shed may be built to protect the dead body (and the doctor too!!!) from sun and rain. Plenty of water may be provided for cleaning the body.

Autopsy on a disinterred dead body may be preferably conducted at site. Method of disinterring a body and conduct of autopsy are given in Chapter 'Forensic Taphonomy'.

## DIRECTIONS TO THE INVESTIGATING OFFICER

Investigation of unnatural deaths form a major share in police work. Many such cases get sensational coverage from the media and unwarranted allegations from the public. The investigation of unnatural deaths should be on a par with grave crimes. Valuable evidence may be obtained from the scene and the dead body during inquest. The scene of occurrence can be preserved for any number of days for further examination. But a dead body will be either cremated or buried after the inquest and autopsy. Therefore, the investigator should devote more time and attention for the examination of the dead body and collection of evidence. The investigating officer has to use his discretion in the collection of evidence depending on the nature of the crime suspected in each case.

Inquests are held during day time in broad daylight. Many pieces of valuable evidences will not be retrieved if sufficient light is not available. Similarly minute injuries and discolourations present on the dead body will be missed. This is the reason why autopsies are also conducted during day time. The time of starting and closing the inquest should be recorded accurately. The inquest report should be prepared at the scene itself. Signatures of the witnesses should be affixed at the end of the report.

## Crime Scene Survey

The investigator walks through the scene of occurrence and conducts a preliminary survey and mentally evaluates the findings. Preconceived notions should not affect his observations and inferences. He can mentally form different theories of reconstruction of the crime. He should also assess the requirements needed for investigation in terms of equipment, assistants and experts.

## Photographing the Crime Scene and Dead Body

Follow the procedure described in this chapter. Digital photography is the ideal for crime scene investigations. The images can be stored and retrieved easily with the help of computers. Problems are likely to be encountered in the admissibility of digital imaging evidence in the courts as the images can be easily manipulated. The dead body should be photographed from different angles and in relation to the articles in the crime scene. Close up pictures of the injuries should be taken.

## Videotaping the Crime Scene

In foreign countries, videotaping the crime scene has become a routine procedure. The videography should be on the same orientation as that of the scene survey. Panoramic view of the surroundings of the crime scene, roads leading to the scene, should be videographed first. Orientation of each article in the crime scene can be copied. Wide angle and closeup views should be taken. The audio of the description of the scene can be recorded along with the video. The tape should not be edited.

## Crime Scene Sketches/Floor Plan

The method of preparing sketches and floor plan of the crime scene is described in this chapter.

## Examination of the Dead Body

The rectal temperature, postmortem staining, rigor mortis, changes due to putrefaction, etc. are to be noted first. Clothes, foreign particles, samples of hair, swabs from stains, fingernail scrapings, etc. are to be collected. Documentation of the injuries should be done meticulously. Detailed description of the scene and dead body should be included in columns 7 and 8 of the inquest report.

# 6

# Trace Evidence

Detailed examination of the scene of occurrence will help the investigating officer to get valuable clues to solve the crime. First of all, he should take steps to isolate the area of the crime. Nothing in the crime scene should be touched, changed or altered. Bystanders are prevented from entering the scene. He should reach the scene without delay. If the officer is unable to reach the scene immediately, he should give proper instructions to his subordinates for guarding the scene to prevent access to unauthorised persons. It is necessary to install scene barriers to cordon the area.

Site of original criminal activity is the primary crime scene and subsequent crime scenes are called secondary crime scenes. For example, a person is murdered in a hotel room. Subsequently his body is transported in a car and dumped in a lake. The hotel room is the primary crime scene and the car and the lake area are the secondary crime scenes. Evidence is collected from all these areas. The main objective of crime investigation is to recognise, collect, preserve, analyse, interpret and reconstruct all the physical evidences collected from the scenes (Fig. 6.1).

## PRELIMINARY SURVEY

Before the survey of the crime scene, the investigator should obtain as much information as possible from the complainant and witnesses. During the preliminary survey, photography, videography, preparation of a rough sketch and documentation of the scene can be done (see Fig. 5.1). Evidences

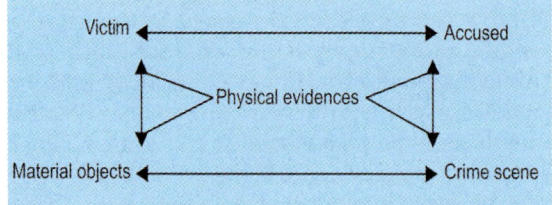

**Fig. 6.1:** Physical evidence links the victim and suspect to the objects and crime scene

which require immediate protection or processing should be identified and taken care of. From the preliminary survey, a plan of search for clues is decided. Then the leader of the team should give specific tasks for the other members.

## Search for Clues

Investigator must be careful and systematic in his search for clues. Proceed in any of the following fashion (Fig. 6.2). In a large outdoor scene, the whole area can be divided into strips, grids or zones and each area is assigned to a group. In a small circular area, the searchers can group at the centre and proceed to the periphery in a radial fashion.

In a crime scene without physical barriers, like open water, search can be conducted in a spiral fashion. In a limited area, choose an appropriate fashion; e.g. in a house, proceed from the entrance to the exit; in a room, proceed in a clockwise or anticlockwise fashion. In a field, wheel method is ideal. But all the methods are suitable in some way or other.

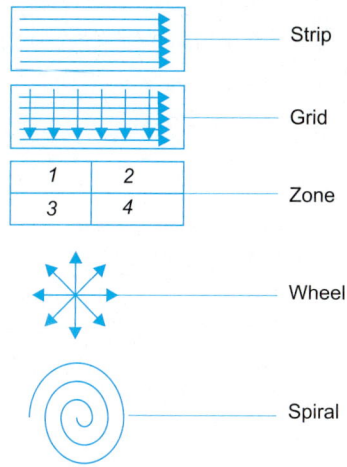

**Fig. 6.2:** Search methods

## Collection of Trace Evidence

Trace evidence is microscopic physical evidence. This comprises a large number of substances like body fluids, biological stains, paints, glass, fibres, soil, vegetations, etc. In every crime scene, there may be a large number of trace materials of evidentiary value. All physical evidences obtained from a crime scene may be significant.

The investigator must take extra care in preserving the trace evidence without contamination. Every person entering a crime scene is likely to contaminate the evidence. Therefore these evidences should be collected and preserved as early as possible. Several methods are employed in collecting the evidence. The investigator should use his discretion depending upon the nature of the material. Delicate and minute materials should be collected first. They can be picked by hands, or by vacuum suction or by using cellotapes. Different methods of collection and packing are needed for different types of materials. The general principle is that the evidentiary material should be placed in a primary container which is then placed in a secondary container. Outer container should be labelled with details such as crime number, nature of material, date and time of collection, name of collector, etc.

The majority of items will be solid and can be collected and packed without any difficulty. Liquid or volatile items should be placed in air tight, leak proof, unbreakable containers. Wet and moist articles should be dried in the shade and packed later. If there is no facility for drying in the scene, it can be collected, packed loosely, dried in a suitable place and repacked. Each item should be packed separately and sealed to avoid contamination and intermingling. Whenever needed controls should also be collected.

For despatching the articles to the forensic science laboratory, the labels on the packets should be numbered serially and should bear the signature of the forwarding officer with the number and date of his forwarding note. All the small packets should be sealed with the same metal seal and sealing wax. A letter of advice should be forwarded separately to the director of forensic science laboratory. A copy of the forwarding letter containing a sample seal should be enclosed in the parcel. The forwarding note is given in Proforma 6.1.

In the crime scene, an investigator must do the following:

- Investigator should observe the position and condition of doors, windows, furniture and other articles.
- He should search for fibres, hair, blood, semen, saliva, sweat, urine, vomitus, chemicals, paints, glass, empty vials, drinking glasses, utensils, remnants of food, footprints, fingerprints, tool marks, tyre marks, skid marks, weapons, implements and any article not likely to be seen at the scene.
- Take photographs of the scene from a number of angles to establish the exact position of things and their condition.
- When photographs are taken, a scale should be placed near the evidentiary material to indicate the size.
- Prepare a sketch of the scene, marking the position of various articles in relation to one another and note down the measurements. The articles can be numbered and a description may be appended.
- Do not touch the articles. Prepare short notes regarding their position and condition before removing them. Remove them carefully by holding the articles by such parts which are unlikely to have been touched by the criminal.

## Certificate

Certified that the Director, Forensic Science Laboratory ............................................................ has the authority to examine the exhibits sent to him in connection with the case of State versus ........................ u/s .............. of .................... Police Station and if necessary to make them to pieces or remove portions for the purpose of the said examination.

Place...............................

Date ..............................

Seal...............................

Signature and designation of
the forwarding authority

---

### I. Nature of Crime

---

### II. List of Articles Sent for Examination

| Sl. No. | Description of exhibits | How, when and by whom found | Source of exhibits | Remarks |
|---------|------------------------|------------------------------|--------------------|---------|
|         |                        |                              |                    |         |

---

### III. Nature of Examination Required

---

**Forwarded To**

Director,
State Forensic Science Laboratory

Specimen seal impression

Signature of the forwarding officer

Designation of forwarding officer

- Pick out trace evidence like fibres, hair, etc. by forceps. Use a hand lens for the search. Always wear rubber gloves when collecting trace materials to prevent contamination.

## Physical Clues

Fibres and fibrous material : Textile fibres, human hair, animal hair, feathers, wood splinters, fragments of paper

Stains : Blood, semen, urine, sputum, chemicals, paint, oil, grease

Documents : Handwritten and typed documents

Dust : Any form of dust, vegetable materials like grass, seeds sticking to clothes, metal filings, glass fragments

Marks : Fingerprints, footprints, tool marks, tyre marks, teeth marks, cut or broken articles.

Firearms : Firearms, cartridges, cartridge cases, bullets, pellets, wads, fire effects on clothes, powder marks on hands and fingers

Poison : Vomitus, faeces, remnants of food and drinks, drinking glasses, chemicals, seeds

*Always remember the dictum—"Never leave any stone unturned"* The scene of occurrence should be thoroughly examined for collecting physical evidence. Assistance of forensic scientists and fingerprint experts may be sought for this. Footprints, latent fingerprints, paint, grease, fibres, hairs, glass pieces, tyre marks, weapons, spent bullets, cartridge cases, drinking glasses, remnants of poison, food materials, etc. are to be collected depending upon the nature of the case. The dictum is "**all unnatural deaths should be treated as homicides unless otherwise proved.**"

## Directions for Collecting and Preserving Different Types of Exhibits

### Weapons/Tools

Weapons/tools stained with blood will rust easily. Therefore they should be sent as early as possible. The weapons/tools are secured to a board with strings. This board is placed in a box with a lid, closed and sealed. Labels should be affixed on the container and not on the weapon or tool.

### Hair and Fibres

If hair and fibres are found sticking to an object, the whole object should be sent. Loose hair/fibres are picked up with a forceps, wrapped with a filter paper, put in a container and labelled. A polythene packet is better than a filter paper. From a living person, hair can be collected by combing or clipping with scissors close to the root. Hair should not be pulled out.

### Dust/Soil

The samples are collected in a filter paper, folded and placed in a suitable container. Vacuum cleaners can be used for collection of dust, filings, etc. Soil is collected with a scalpel or spoon. These have to be collected in clean glass containers and labelled.

### Blood/Blood Stains

Blood and blood stains have to be dried at room temperature before packing. Liquid blood should not be collected as such. A piece of gauze is dipped in the blood, dried and put in a polythene packet. A sample of the gauze material is to be sent as control. A clean white cloth can be used instead of gauze. The stained fabric is dried in the shade. Sandwich the fabric between clean white papers, pack and enclose in a polythene packet. In the case of blood-stained clothes, the whole clothe has to be sent. Stained areas should not be cut out or marked.

Dried stains found on solid objects have to be scraped out and collected in a test tube or glass bottle. If it is difficult, moist a filter paper with 0.9% saline and apply it to the stain for sometime to transfer it. Then it is dried and packed in a polythene packet. If blood stains are found in the earth, the stained soil is collected, spread on a paper to dry and then packed with clean white paper or put in glass bottles.

Blood-stains from the body of a person are removed by applying a moist filter paper till the stain is transferred. The paper is then dried and packed. If stains are suspected to be present in the nails, the nails have to be clipped and collected in glass containers. Care should be taken not to injure the fingers while the nails are clipped.

## Seminal Stains

Stained clothes and articles are allowed to dry at room temperature before packing. When the clothes stained with semen are packed, care should be taken not to fold the stained areas. Clean white paper should be placed between the folds and it can also be used for packing. Pubic hair matted with semen have to be clipped, dried and packed in glazed paper. Dried seminal stains from the body are transferred to moist filter paper, dried and packed.

## Saliva

Clothes stained with saliva are dried and packed. Control samples of saliva from the victim and accused are to be collected in clean test tubes and placed in an ice box. From the dead bodies, swabs from the mouth are taken, dried and put in test tubes and closed with a plug of cotton wool.

## Tissues

Tissues for grouping, species specific test or DNA typing are not to be preserved in formalin or spirit. They have to be dried at room temperature and collected in glass bottles.

## Arson Cases/Burns

Remnants of clothes and debris containing inflammable material are to be put in glass bottles and closed with airtight stoppers.

## Tool Marks

The whole tool is to be sent if possible. Several impressions of the tool on similar materials are made using the marking area of the tool. The tool mark should be protected by covering with soft paper and with strong wrapping paper. The whole thing should be put in a box and packed.

## Firearms

Labels containing the description of type, make, serial number and calibre have to be affixed on the box used for packing the firearm. Cartridge cases, spent bullets, etc. are to be recovered from the scene and forwarded. They should never be tampered with. The muzzle end of the barrel should be capped with clean cloth or a cork. The firearm should be separately wrapped with clean paper, tied with thread and kept in a wooden box with packing material such as cotton waste. The ammunitions like cartridge cases, spent bullets, etc. are to be covered with cotton, wrapped with paper and put in envelopes.

Tissues surrounding the firearm wounds should be removed, preserved in rectified spirit and sent in lead free containers. Clothing have to be packed in polythene packets without disturbing the tears, holes and fire effects like burning, blackening and peppering. Clean paper may be placed above the area.

## BLOOD STAINS

### Shape of the Stain

Collection of a large pool of blood near the dead body may indicate that the victim had sustained the injuries and died at that spot. However, if a large blood vessel is cut, blood may ooze from a dead body following the law of gravity. Spurting, splashing and spraying of blood will be due to injury involving an artery (Fig. 6.3). Flow of blood from a vein will be steady oozing. Blood falling

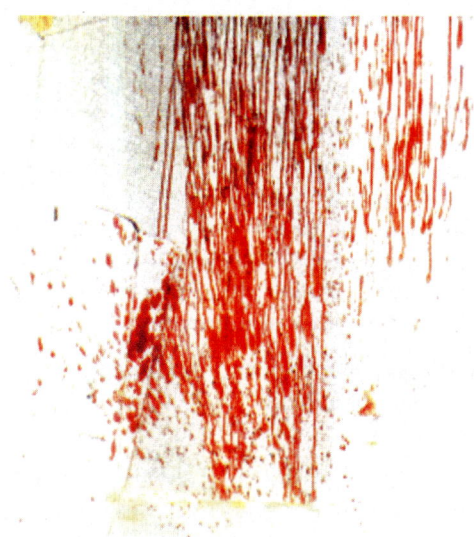

**Fig. 6.3:** Spurting of blood when an artery is injured

on a flat surface will form circular stains (Fig. 6.4) and as the height of fall increases, the margins of the stain will become prickly or stellate (Fig. 6.5). Blood falling on a surface in a slanting manner will produce an oval-shaped stain with a tail (Fig 6.6).

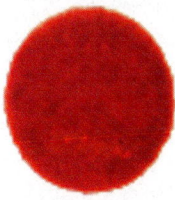

**Fig. 6.4:** Shape of a drop of blood falling vertically on a smooth surface (margin is circular and smooth)

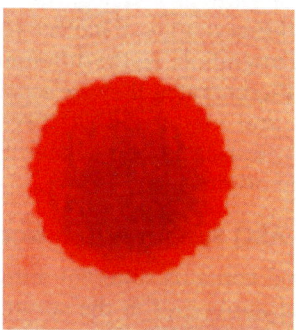

**Fig. 6.5:** Shape of a drop of blood falling vertically on a rough surrface (margin is crenated)

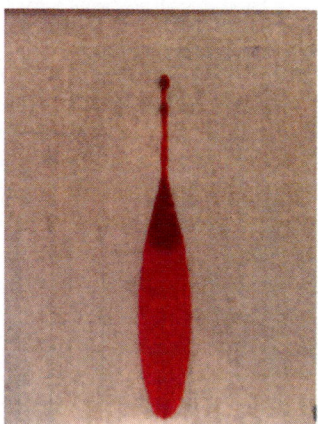

**Fig. 6.6:** Shape of a drop of blood falling on a surface in a slanting manner

## Age of the Stain

Fresh stains of blood will be bright red in colour. The colour will change to reddish brown in 24 hours. Old stains will be brown or black. In coloured garments, stains are not easily visible. Examination under an ultraviolet lamp will reveal the presence of stains. Rust, dyes, vegetables and mineral stain will resemble blood stains.

## Screening Tests for Blood

### Benzidine Test

This test will indicate that a particular stain could be blood. Place a small piece of stained material on a porcelain tile. Add a drop of saturated solution of benzidine in glacial acetic acid. Then one drop of hydrogen peroxide is added to it. If blood is present, an intense blue colour develops. **A negative reaction is more valuable as there can be false positive reactions with pus, saliva, milk, rust, etc.** Benzidine is now recognised as a carcinogen and is seldom used in the laboratories.

### Tetramethylbenzidine (TMB)

This test nowadays is used instead of benzidine. Now test strips containing TMB reagent are available. A moist swab is applied to the blood stain and then applied to the reagent strip. Presence of blood is indicated by a green or bluish green colour change.

### Chemiluminescence Tests

Tests using chemicals producing luminescence and fluorescence with blood stains are widely used. They are now considered as the best presumptive tests. **Luminol,** a chemical will luminesce when it is oxidised by the blood stain in an acidic or alkaline medium. The method is to spray a chemical mixture of luminol on a suspected blood-stained area in situ and the luminescence is observed in darkness or reduced light. Similarly, fluorescein is oxidised by the blood into fluorescein which fluoresces in the presence of ultraviolet light or with an alternate light source. This test should not be done if the blood stain is visible. Materials like house bleach can give a deceptive positive reaction with luminol.

## Microscopical Examination

Microscopical examination of fresh stains will show intact red cells. If the red cells are nucleated ones, the blood may be amphibian, reptilian or avian. Mammalian RBCs are non-nucleated. Crystal tests like 'haemin' (**Teichman test**) or 'hemochromogen' (**Takayama test**) will prove the presence of haemoglobin in blood. These are confirmatory tests for blood.

## Spectroscopy

The principle of the spectroscope is that when light passes through a transparent material like a thin solution of blood and then through a prism, rays of certain wavelengths get absorbed in the substance, whereas rays of other wavelengths pass through unabsorbed. The areas of the spectrum with rays absorbed by blood appear as dark bands. For example, hemoglobin and its different forms appear as dark bands in different zones of the spectra. Spectroscopic examination of blood will detect the presence of oxyhemoglobin, reduced hemoglobin, carboxyhemoglobin, methemoglobin, etc.

Spectroscopy is a confirmatory test for the presence of blood in a stain. The test is also helpful to confirm whether death was due to antemortem burns. The victim may inhale carbon monoxide during conflagration. Carbon monoxide will combine with hemoglobin and carboxyhemoglobin will be produced. A sample of blood is taken from the dead body and subjected to spectroscopy for the presence of carboxyhemoglobin. Cyanhemoglobin bands can be prepared and identified in cases of cyanide poisoning.

## Species Specific Tests for Blood

The following tests will prove that a blood stain is of human origin.

## Ring Precipitin Test

This test is an immuno-precipitation test. Antiserum is prepared from rabbits inoculated with human serum. Antiserum contains antibodies (gamma globulins) against human proteins. When antiserum and human proteins are made to contact with each other, a precipitin reaction occurs. In this test, simple diffusion occurs between anti-serum and extract of the sample blood stain inside a test tube. Antiserum is placed in a test tube and the stain extract is layered over the dense antiserum. A fine ring of precipitate is formed if the stain is of human origin.

## Immuno-electrophoresis

Human serum contains five different types of proteins: albumin, alpha 1 globulins, alpha 2 globulins, beta globulins and gamma globulins. Electrophoresis is employed in identifying the protein fractions. Proteins are caused to migrate in an electric field in a suitable support medium (starch gels, cellulose acetate membrane, etc.) under controlled conditions of temperature, pH, voltage and time. Positively charged molecules will migrate to cathode and negatively charged to anode. Individual charges of molecules play a role in the rate of migration. As the different molecules migrate at different rates, they are separated. They are stained and visualised. At present, rapid immunoassay test strips are available to determine the species of origin.

## Grouping—ABO System—Fresh Blood

Human blood contains different antigens in the red cells and antibodies in the serum. Based on this, blood is divided into four groups: A, B, AB and O. Apart from this, many blood group substances like M, N, S, Rh, etc. are identified. But due to the unavailability of specific antisera, it may not be possible to identify these rare groups in all the laboratories. For practical purposes, identification of ABO and Rh system would suffice. The important aspect of blood grouping is that the blood group of an individual remains unchanged throughout his life. But certain diseases like leukemia can bring about alterations in the blood group. But this is a very rare occurrence. Detection of the group from blood stains will be very helpful in establishing the involvement of the criminal with the crime. But a negative finding is more valuable than a positive one.

## Rh Factor Blood Grouping System

An antigen named Rh factor is present on the surface of red cells of 85% of people and they are called Rh+ve. Those who do not have this factor are called Rh-ve. A person with Rh-ve blood can develop Rh antibodies in the plasma if that person receives a transfusion of Rh+ ve blood. An Rh+ve person can receive Rh-ve blood without any problem; but an Rh-ve person will develop reaction if he receives Rh+ve blood. So people are classified according to both systems. For example, 'AB Rh+ve' (AB+), or 'O Rh-ve'(O-), etc. Rh factor is an important factor during pregnancy. If the mother is Rh-ve and the father is Rh +ve, and if the baby inherits Rh+ve factor, the mother can develop antibodies against the baby's blood and its blood can lyse resulting in hemolytic jaundice of the newborn.

## Grouping of Dry Blood Stains

If dried blood stains are present in immovable objects, the stain may be scraped off using a knife and collected in a clean glass bottle. If the stained object is small, the same may be packed and transmitted to the forensic science laboratory. The stained area should not be marked or indicated with ink or other substances. This will interfere with the tests. To determine group of dried blood stains is a laborious process. One of the modern methods is **lattes crust method.** In this method, several portions of blood stained crusts are allowed to react with known red cell suspensions. Aggluti-nation (clumping)observed microscopically will indicate the presence of isoagglutinins in the sample. Other methods are absorption-elution, absorption inhibition, mixed agglutination, etc. Determination of blood group from dried blood stains can yield wrong results due to decom-position of the stain and prolonged storage of the sample at high temperature. Chromatographic separation of the stain is advised before grouping. Atypical results are possible with absorption elution method. Therefore, the results are to be interpreted with caution.

## Secretors

Blood group can be determined from the exami-nation of secretions like saliva, sweat, semen, stools, tears, nasal secretions, etc. Group specific substances are present in the body secretions of 75 to 80% of individuals. They are called secretors. Their blood and body fluid will be of the same group. But there are aberrant secretors with different groups.

## Disputed Paternity

Blood grouping is applied in cases of disputed paternity also. Here also a negative finding is more valid. Blood groups of parents and possible groups of children based on the ABO system are given in Box 6.1. In the case of disputed paternity, blood groups of the parents and the child are determined. It is not proper to establish the paternity based on a positive finding, but an individual can be conclusively excluded as being the father of a child based on a negative finding.

**Box 6.1:** Blood groups of parents and possible blood group of children

| Blood group of parents | Possible blood group of children |
|---|---|
| A × B | A, B, AB, O |
| B × B | B, O |
| O × AB | A, B |
| A × AB | A, B, AB |
| B × AB | A, B, AB |
| AB × AB | A, B, AB |
| O × O | O |
| O × A | A, O |
| O × B | B, O |
| A × A | A, O |

## DNA Typing/Fingerprinting

DNA typing is the epoch making discovery which revolutionised crime investigation and paternity testing. Typing can be done from blood, semen, bone marrow, hair roots, tooth pulp and tissues. Several techniques are available now for the analysis of DNA. Typing of DNA is the conclusive method available at present to determine the identity of the accused in a crime and the paternity of a child. DNA typing is done from the blood of the child, mother and the putative father. The technique is done in most of the forensic science laboratories of the country. Centre for Cellular and Molecular Biology (CCMB) Hyderabad is the pioneer institution under the leadership of Dr. Lalji Singh, a veteran molecular biologist who developed the technique in India.

## Source and Pattern of Blood Stains

Blood extravasated from an artery will be bright red in colour. Blood from a vein is dark. Menstrual blood has got a disagreeable smell; and on microscopical examination vaginal and endometrial cells can be seen. Vomited blood will be coffee brown in colour and acidic in reaction because of the interaction with the acid in the stomach. Frothy blood is usually from the lungs in case of hemoptysis. Blood is six times more viscous than water. The specific gravity is also higher than that of water. But surface tension is less. These physical properties are responsible for the pattern of flow of extravasated blood and shape of the drops.

One drop of blood is approximately 0.05 ml. When it falls from a height of six inches, it produces a circular stain of 13 mm. When the height is 7 feet, the diameter will be 21.5 mm. When the blood drop falls on a hard, smooth nonporous surface such as glass or smooth tile, there will not be any splatter in contrast to a rough surface like concrete or wood. Rough surfaces rupture the surface tension and produce irregularly shaped stains. If the angle of impact is 90°, the resulting stain will be circular. If the angle is less than 90°, it will produce elliptical stains. From the pattern of the splattered blood stains, position of the victim, mechanism of splatter, location of origin of blood, etc. can be found out. Impact splatters of blood in case of gun shot, stab injuries, beating, etc. can produce different patterns.

Bleeding from an artery produces peculiar spurting/spraying patterns. These vary according to the severity of the injury to the artery, clothing covering the injured area, etc. When an object like knife wet with blood comes into contact with a surface, a transfer pattern occurs. From this pattern the nature of the object can be inferred. Blood stains found on the cloth of the accused can provide information based on flow pattern, splatter pattern, etc. (Figs 6.3 to 6.6).

## Determining the Sex of the Individual From Blood

Each of the cells in our body contains 46 chromosomes; 22 pairs of autosomes and 2 sex chromosomes. In the male, the sex chromosomes are XY and in the female they are XX. The XX pattern can be made visible as sex chromatin, if the cells are stained with Leishman or hematoxylin-eosin. When neutrophils in the females are examined, they appear as spherical masses extending from a lobe of the nucleus by a slender-stick-like structure giving the appearance of a drumstick. They are called 'Davidson's bodies' (Fig. 6.7). In buccal epithelial cells, sex chromatin is identified as plano-convex masses inside the nucleus just beneath the nuclear wall. These bodies are called 'Barr bodies' (Fig. 6.7).

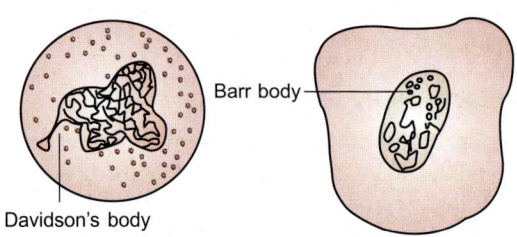

**Fig. 6.7:** Sex chromatin in the white blood corpuscle

## Chemical Examination of Blood

Chemical analysis of blood will reveal the presence of poisons. Quantitative estimation of the poison is also possible. Spectroscopic examination of blood will detect the cause of death in carbon monoxide and cyanide poisoning. Deaths due to irrespirable gases can be confirmed by blood examination. Chronic lead poisoning will cause changes in the blood such as basophilic stippling of red cells, anisocytosis, poikilocytosis. Chemical analysis of blood will reveal the presence of poisons. Quantitative estimation of the poison is also possible.

## SEMINAL STAINS

Semen is the fluid ejaculated by males during orgasm. About 2 to 5 ml is voided normally each time. Semen consists of sperms and seminal fluid rich in sugars, proteins and enzymes. In vasectomised and sterile persons, semen will not contain sperms. Detection of seminal stains is an important aspect in the investigation of cases like rape, sodomy, etc.

## Appearance

Freshly voided semen will be viscous, dirty white in colour and has a musty odour. In white clothes, it produces a light yellow stain with starchy feel on drying. In coloured clothes, stains may be visible only in ultraviolet light. The stains give a blue fluorescence under UV light. Pus, egg albumin, starch, leucorrhoeal discharge, etc. resemble seminal stains. Florence test, Barberios test, acid phosphatase test, etc. are based on the reaction of certain reagents with various constituents of semen. If they are positive, species-specific test can be done to confirm human origin.

## Chemical Tests

### Florence Test

This is a screening test for semen. A small piece of stained material is placed on a slide, a drop of acidulated distilled water is added and allowed to stand for 1–2 minutes. A drop of Florence reagent is added to the edge of the dissolved specimen and covered with a coverslip. Brown rhombic crystals of choline periodide will be formed if semen is present.

### Barberios Test

A small portion of stained material is placed in a test tube and soaked in 2% trichloracetic acid for one hour. The tube is then centrifuged and a drop of the clear supernatant fluid is added to a drop of saturated aqueous solution of picric acid. Yellow rhombic crystals of spermine picrate are formed if the stain contains semen. Choline and spermine are the constituents of seminal fluid.

### Acid Phosphatase

Human semen contains high levels of enzyme acid phosphatase, produced by the prostate gland. This enzyme is readily soluble in aqueous media. A filter paper or cotton swab moistened with sterile water is applied to the suspected stain. Brentamin, fast blue reagent is added to the paper or swab. An intense purple colour develops if semen is present. A strong reaction within 30 seconds is diagnostic for the presence of semen. Vaginal secretions, perspiration, faeces, urine, etc. may show a positive reaction. Therefore, prostate, specific antigen is used as a standard.

## Confirmatory Tests

### Microscopical Examination

Microscopic identification of spermatozoa is the absolute proof that the suspected stain contains semen. Semen contains 60–150 million sperms per millilitre. Human spermatozoa will survive for about 6–8 hours at room temperature. In the vagina, sperms may survive up to 24 hours. Dead sperms have been found up to 96 hours in some cases. If they are not seen, further tests are to be done. The smear of stain can be stained with hematoxylin-eosin, picro-indigo-carmine (PIC) and nuclear fast red dyes (Fig. 6.8). Before staining the sample, enough quantity should be preserved for DNA typing. If the stain is dry, a piece of the stained material is placed in a watchglass and soaked in sterile water for 10 minutes. It is picked up with a forceps and smears are prepared on microscopic slides. Slides are dried and stained.

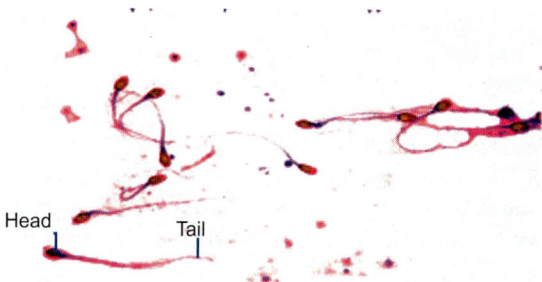

**Fig. 6.8:** Human spermatozoa stained with nuclear fast red dye

### Prostate-specific Antigen (PSA)

The antigen secreted by the prostate gland is an ideal marker for the presence of semen. This antigen can be detected by electrophoresis, which is time consuming and not very sensitive. There is a screening test based on antigen–antibody reaction, developed by Hochmeister in 1999. Test kits are available now. A small portion of the stained material is immersed in sterile water for 10 minutes, centrifuged and placed in the well of the test kit. Development of a band is confirmatory for semen.

## Serological Tests

Serological tests confirm the origin of semen as human. In **precipitin test**, specific antiserum is made to react with the seminal fluid. The antiserum is prepared by injecting rabbits with human seminal fluid or testicular extract. Antiserum is prepared from the serum of the animal. Antiserum (0.1ml) is added to the same quantity of stain extract. A positive test will confirm human origin. Gel precipitin test, chromatography and electrophoresis are the other tests to detect species specificity.

## Grouping

Semen can be grouped using the anti A and anti B sera used for blood grouping. The stain should be fresh and uncontaminated.

## DNA Typing

Even from one intact spermatozoa, DNA typing can be done. But in a sperm, only half of the genetic information will be available. At least 80 sperms are needed to generate a full male DNA profile. Therefore, it is important to preserve enough samples for DNA analysis before utilising the sample for other tests.

## SALIVARY STAINS

Saliva is the secretion from the salivary glands situated near the oral cavity. The secretion flows through ducts from the glands opening into the mouth. Detection of salivary satins is important in cases of strangulation, hanging, smothering, sexual offences, theft, etc. Saliva consists of water, salts and various enzymes. Amylase is the important enzyme present in saliva. Detection of the enzyme amylase is the basis of tests for salivary stains.

## Starch–iodine Test

Amylase converts starch into dextrose and glucose. Starch-iodine test is based on this principle. In the presence of iodine, starch appears blue. When material containing saliva is added to starch stained with iodine, the blue colour disappears as the amylase in the saliva breaks down starch. Presence of proteins like albumin and gamma globulin present in other body fluids like blood

and semen can cause false positive reaction. Faeces also contain, amylase.

## Phadebas Reagent

This is a commercial product in which starch is linked to a dye molecule to form an insoluble complex. Starch is cleaved from the dye by amylase present in the salivary stain. The dye molecule becomes soluble producing a coloured product which can be measured with a spectro-photometer. The degree of colouration is proportional to the amount of amylase present. A limitation of this test is that it is not very sensitive.

## Microscopy

Stains can also be examined microscopically for the presence of buccal mucosal cells. For this, the stain is extracted and centrifuged. A smear is made from the bottom layer and stained with hematoxylin-eosin.

## DNA Typing

Tests for identifying a salivary stain will be detrimental to DNA analysis. Swabs from bite marks, envelope flaps, stamps, cigarette buds, etc. can be subjected to DNA and the identity of the owner of saliva can be found out. Species specific tests and grouping can also be done with salivary stains.

## URINARY STAINS

Urinary stains can be detected by chemical tests. Detection of urine relies on identifying urea and creatinine. These are present in sweat, saliva, semen and blood. But urea is present in very high concentration in urine (1400 – 1500 mg in 100 ml). Quantity of creatinine present in 100 ml urine will be 100 – 200 mg. Urease enzyme breaks down urea and releases ammonia and carbon dioxide. Ammonia is detected by an indicator chemical, Nesslers reagent (mercuric iodide in potassium iodide). Creatinine is identified by applying a saturated solution of picric acid in toluene or benzene to a stain extract. A coloured product, creatinine picrate is formed. Urinary stains contain very little cells and hence not suitable for DNA typing. Species specific tests cannot be done with urine. Grouping is also difficult because urine seldom contains group specific substances.

## FAECES

Faeces are the end products of digestion of food after the absorption of nutrients. Faeces consist of undigested food residues, mucosal cells, bacteria, breakdown products of bile pigments, breakdown products of amino acids like indole, skatole, etc. Faecal stains can be identified by microscopical examination for the presence of undigested matter like plant material, starch grains, meat fibres, etc. Faeces contain stercobilin and urobilinogen, which can be detected by chemical tests. Species specific tests cannot be done with faeces.

Grouping can be done using absorption elution method. Because of the inhibitory effect of bile pigments, nuclear DNA testing is unsuccessful. Bacteria and digestive enzymes also degrade the DNA. But mitochondrial DNA testing can be done.

## VOMITUS

Vomitus contains food material, stomach acid and digestive enzymes. The vomitus will be acidic due to the presence of stomach hydrochloric acid. Acidity can be determined by estimating the pH. Microscopy of the contents will reveal the presence of food materials.

## VAGINAL SECRETIONS

Vaginal secretions have to be examined in cases of sexual assault like rape, introduction of foreign articles into the vagina, etc. When a suspect in a case of rape is apprehended, his penile swabs or washings can be examined for the presence of vaginal secretions. Vaginal swabs and smears taken from the victim of a case of rape will contain semen as well as vaginal fluid. The vaginal secretions are identified by the presence of vaginal epithelial cells. The cells contain glycogen. *Periodic acid-Schiff* (**PAS**) reagent stains the glycogen in the cells giving a bright magenta colour. It can also be stained by Lugol's iodine. Vaginal smear on a microscopic slide is placed upside down over a petri dish containing Lugol's iodine for 5–10 minutes. The vaginal cells take up a chocolate brown colour from the iodine vapour.

The amount of glycogen varies during the menstrual cycle. During ovulation period, glycogen content will be more. Glycogen will be absent in prepubertal and post-menopausal females. Glycogenated epithelial cells may be present in small numbers in the urethral tract and mouth of males also. If the vaginal secretions are to be subjected to DNA typing, PAS staining or Lugol's iodine should not be resorted to especially if the sample is minimal.

## MENSTRUAL BLOOD

Menstrual blood will be acidic in reaction and will contain endometrial cells, epithelial cells and bacteria. The stain is extracted and a smear is prepared. It is stained with hematoxylin-eosin and examined under the microscope. If endometrial cells are identified, the blood can be confirmed as of uterine origin. Menstrual blood contains fibrinolysin and fibrinolytic activity can demonstrated by converting insoluble fibrin to soluble fibrin by electrophoresis.

## HAIR

Examination of human hair can provide valuable information for the crime investigator. It will supply evidence regarding the accused in case of murder, sexual offences, theft, etc. The following information can be obtained from the examination of hair.

### Human or Animal?

Microscopic examination of the hair will confirm human origin. Human hair has got a thin interrupted medulla containing pigments and a thick cortex having an outer scaly layer (Fig.6.9). Animal hairs have a thick medulla and thin cortex (Fig. 6.10). The diameter of the shaft of human hair is usually 100–150 microns. The diameter of the medulla is only one-third of that of the shaft. This ratio is called medullary index and can be found out by taking the cross-section of hair and subsequent microscopical examination. The pattern of distribution of pigment and cuticle are also studied and this helps in comparison (Fig. 6.11). Microscopical examination of hair can yield information as to body location as well as the race of the individual.

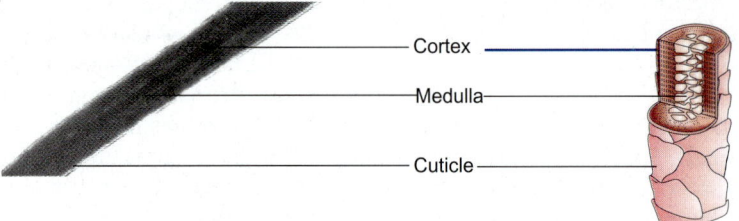

**Fig. 6.9:** Structure of human hair

**Fig. 6.10:** Structure of animal hair

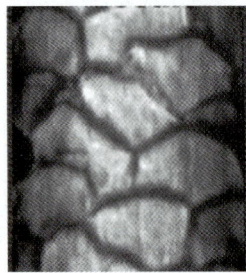

**Fig. 6.11:** Cuticular pattern of human hair

### Source of Hair

If the hair is found to be human, the part of the body to which it belonged has to be found out. This is based on the physical appearance and microscopical examination. Hair from the eyebrows, eyelashes, moustache, beard, chest and pubis have characteristic features which will help in identification.

### Age and Sex of the Individual

Determination of the age of the person from hair is difficult. Greying of hair cannot be taken as an index of age. Sex can be determined if a whole strand of hair with the root and bulb is available.

Sex chromatin can be identified in the cells surrounding the bulb in females' hair. But the length and refractive index together will be indicative of sex.

### Identity

Identity is established mainly by comparison. Hair obtained from the crime scene is compared with the sample hair of the suspect. Cuticular pattern, medullary index, pattern of distribution of the pigment, refractive index, etc. are helpful criteria in comparison.

The modern technique **neutron activation analysis (NAA)** is very helpful in establishing the identity. The inorganic elements present in the hair are detected by bombarding them with neutrons and the emission spectrum is analysed with the help of scintillation counters. Hairs of an individual will have similar elemental pattern. The constituents of the hair vary from person to person. Toxicological analysis can also be done using this technique. Identity of hair can be established unequivocally by DNA typing. Cells of the hair root sheath are a source of mitochondrial DNA from which typing can be done.

### Other Information

Microscopic examination will show whether a hair has been cut, crushed, pulled out or burnt. Stains, dyes, blood, etc. if present on the hair can also be detected by modern analytical methods. Time of death can be found out from the growth of hair, if the time of the most recent shaving of facial hair is known. Hair grows at the rate of 0.3 to 0.4 mm/day. By absorption–elution method, grouping of the hair is also possible to establish the identity of the individual.

## FIBRES

Detection of fibres in the crime scene will be helpful in cases of murder, rape, theft, etc. Fibres of animal origin, vegetable origin and synthetic nature can be identified by microscopy, solubility tests, refractive index, spectroscopy, etc. Fibres obtained from the scene of crime can be compared with fibres of the fabric or those obtained from the body of the suspect. In a case of suicidal hanging, fibres of the ligature material may be detected in the hands of the deceased. Cellophane tapes, affixed on the palms of the deceased are subjected to microscopy for detection of fibres and comparison with those of the ligature material and those found on the suspension point. The investigating officer has to send the ligature and the cellophane tapes to the forensic science laboratory for analysis.

Trace evidence is analysed qualitatively and quantitatively using modern sophisticated analytical methods and devices. Microscopical examination is limited to the morphology of the article. Constitution of the material is detected by elemental analysis and study of the molecular spectra. In forensic analysis, different types of microscopes, chromatography, electrophoresis, spectrography, etc. are employed.

*Microscopes:* Compound binocular microscope, polarised light microscope, stereo-binocular microscope, comparison microscope, electron microscope.

*Chromatography:* Column chromatography, paper chromatography, thin layer chromatography, gas chromatography, liquid chromatography.

*Electrophoresis:* Capillary electrophoresis, gel electrophoresis, paper electrophoresis.

*Spectrometry:* Ultraviolet and infrared spectroscopy, mass spectrometry, atomic absorption spectrophotometry, plasma-mass spectrometry, neutron activation analysis, X-ray diffraction analysis, energy dispersive X-ray spectroscopy.

## REQUESTING THE DOCTOR TO VISIT THE SCENE OF OCCURRENCE

The doctor who conducts a medicolegal autopsy can furnish the cause of death without much difficulty. It is the duty of the police officer to find out the manner of death by conducting a detailed investigation. The doctor will be able to help him to arrive at a conclusion by providing useful clues gathered during autopsy and by examining the scene of occurrence. The investigating officer should request the doctor to visit the scene of occurrence either before conducting the inquest or after the autopsy or at a later stage.

The doctor will be able to fix the time of death by noting the temperature of the cadaver, extent of rigor mortis and fixation of postmortem lividity. If injuries are present, he can conduct a preliminary examination to ascertain the nature of the weapon as well as the mode of infliction of the injury. Examination of a scene of occurrence will always be helpful for a doctor to arrive at conclusions regarding the cause and manner of death. The doctor will be able help the investigating officer in the reconstruction of the crime.

A crime can be reconstructed by correlating the findings of autopsy with versions of the witnesses and findings in the scene of occurrence. For example, in a case of murder, the factors such as relative positions of the victim and the assailant, evidence of a scuffle, attempts of warding of the inflictions, the place where a particular injury was inflicted, volitional activities, etc. may be found out. In cases of death due to hanging, accessibility to the point of suspension, nature of the stepping device if any, presence of stains, etc. can be found out. In traffic accidents, examination of vehicle and scene of occurrence may help to reconstruct the crime by correlating the injuries caused by the impact of the vehicle and the damage sustained to the vehicle. The doctor can also guide the investigating officer regarding the collection of material objects which will be helpful in the detection of the crime.

## DIRECTIONS TO THE INVESTIGATING OFFICER

The main objective of examination of the crime scene is to identify, collect, preserve and interpret physical evidence from the scene of occurrence. These evidences are examined by the scientists in various laboratories. The results will provide the investigator information to reconstruct the crime and help to solve it. The "Locard's law" states that whenever two objects come into contact, mutual exchange of matter will take place between them. Trace evidences collected from the scene, victim and suspect will be helpful to connect the suspect with the vicitm and the crime. Evidence in the crime scene may be contaminated or altered due to the entry of unauthorised persons. Therefore, it is highly essential to cordon the crime scene and access should be restricted. Crime scene examination is a team work. The investigator should seek the help of the forensic pathologist, forensic scientist, fingerprint expert, photographer, dog squad and other appropriate experts.

## Crime Scene Search

Several methods of search have been described in this chapter. Each method has advantages and disadvantages. Practically a combination of methods may be used in a crime scene. All the members of the search team should be instructed not to touch, handle or move articles which may reveal latent fingerprints. The items detected should be photographed and documented. The dictum of crime scene search is **"never leave any stone unturned"**.

## Collection and Preservation of Trace Evidence

Procedure of collection and preservation of trace evidences has been dealt with in this chapter. There is no hard and fast rule regarding the collection of evidence. Those evidences which are likely to perish easily should be collected first, e.g. biological stains,vomitus, tissues, etc. Wet artcles should be thoroughly dried in the shade before packing to prevent decomposition or fungal growth. The material objects are to be collected in separate packets or containers and labelled. All the individual containers can be enclosed in a large box, labelled and sealed.

## Reconstruction of the Crime

Crime scene reconstruction is a scientific experiment useful for the successful detction of the crime. This procedure can either confirm a theory or rule it out. In order to conduct a crime reconstruction, data obtained from the autopsy surgeon, forensic specialists, laboratory analysis and statements of witnesses is necessary.

*"Always remember that forensic medicine, forensic science and allied specialities connected with crime investigation are abstract sciences. False positive results are possible in the laboratory analysis. There may be several alternatives and variations for a particular finding or result. Therfore scientific evidence should not be always accepted as fool proof and absolutely reliable. Scientific facts which correlate or corroborate with the facts revealed during field investigation, can only be accepted."*

# Medicolegal Autopsy

The word autopsy is derived from ancient Greek which literally means to "view for oneself." In common usage, it means postmortem examination of a body. It includes external examination and dissection of internal organs to find out the pathological changes. "Dead men tell tales", this axiom will be found true if a postmortem examination is carefully carried out. Apart from finding out the cause of death, many valuable clues pointing to the manner and circumstances of death will also be obtained in an autopsy. The doctor performs the autopsy assisted by one or two attenders. The main objectives of a medicolegal autopsy are to:

- Identify an unknown body
- Find out the cause of death
- Find out the time since death
- Find out the clues which will help to determine the manner of death, viz. accidental/suicidal/homicidal
- Find out the intrauterine age of a foetus and determine whether it was live born/stilborn/dead born (foetal autopsy).

## TIME OF PERFORMING THE AUTOPSY

There is no statute regarding the time limits for the conduct of a medicolegal autopsy. The general convention is that, an autopsy should be conducted in broad daylight and not in artificial light. The principle is that many colour changes on the dead body such as jaundice, cyanosis, postmortem staining, bruises and minor injuries are liable to go unnoticed and undetected in artificial light. Hence it is always better to conduct the autopsy between 7 am and 5 pm. In suspicious deaths, autopsies will never be conducted at night as important findings will be sometimes missed. Police inquests are never conducted at night except in situations where law and order problems arise.

Government of Kerala, vide circular no.18023/H2/86/Home dated 4th September 1986, have given instructions to all district collectors, superintendents of police, revenue divisional officers and district police surgeons that postmortem examination should be conducted in daylight and not in artificial light as far as possible and that it should be as thorough and complete as circumstances permit. This will ensure credence to the postmortem certificates by courts as well. The government vide letter no. 4494/Spl.2/86/H and FWD have given further instructions that dead bodies should be received only up to 4 pm, as it will take one to one and a half hours to complete an autopsy. Therefore, the dead body should be sent to the doctor for autopsy sufficiently early to avoid inconvenience to the relatives of the deceased.

Most of the Government hospitals have mortuaries. Medical college hospitals have modern mortuaries with cold chambers, where dead bodies can be preserved for days without decomposition. If such a facility is not available, it is better to conduct the autopsy at the earliest as putrefactive changes will vitiate the findings. If autopsy is performed at site, the body should not be exposed to sun.

57

A temporary shed or covered area may be made available at site to guard the dead body (and the doctor too!!) from the sun and the rain.

The doctor receives the dead body from the police constable who is in charge of the copse. Doctor gives him a receipt. The constable has to identify the dead body as that of the deceased in the particular case and sign in the postmortem detailed note. After the autopsy, the constable receives the dead body from the doctor after giving him a receipt. The police constable then hands over the body to the relatives for funeral after obtaining a receipt from them. This entire procedure is to maintain the legal chain.

If there are no relatives to claim the dead body immediately after the autopsy, it has to be kept for 72 hours in the cold chamber. If there are no claimants, the local administration authorities have to be intimated for the disposal of the copse. The appropriate authority can give the body to the nearest medical college as per the Anatomy Act.

Before proceeding to dissect the body, the doctor reads the requisition from the police carefully. It will provide him an account of the circumstances and apparent cause of death. If the deceased was under treatment, the hospital case sheet is perused and salient points are noted for future reference. Investigating officer may also obtain a copy of the hospital case record for future reference, especially in cases where there is an allegation of medical negligence. If the doctor requires any further information about the deceased, it should be provided by the investigating police officer.

Only authorised persons should be present at the time of autopsy. The investigating police officer can be present, if he so desires. The doctor performs a complete autopsy. All the cavities are opened, all the organs are dissected and examined even if the cause of death is obvious. The postmortem findings are recorded in detail. An assistant takes down notes during autopsy. Otherwise the doctor will use a voice activated tape recorder to record the data. After the autopsy, the data is copied in the detailed notes. Permanent detailed notes are kept in every case. From the detailed notes, a postmortem certificate is drafted incorporating the salient findings. Doctor will forward the original of the

certificate to the court concerned. The copy will be sent to the investigating officer.

If the doctor has collected viscera/other material objects during autopsy for chemical and laboratory examination, the investigating officer has to depute a constable for transmitting the materials to the laboratories concerned. If the results of the laboratory examination are required urgently for the investigation of the case, the investigating officer may send a written request to the laboratory concerned for expediting the analysis. This may be necessary in murder cases and suspicious deaths as the results of laboratory examinations are usually delayed. The reason is that the material objects are analysed chronologically in the order of receipt. This can sometimes cause problems in the smooth investigation of the case. For example, in a case of suspected homicidal poisoning with cyanide, if there is delay in the analysis of viscera and body fluids, cyanide will disappear due to decomposition. Ethyl alcohol will vapourise from the material objects, if analysis is delayed. Therefore, it is the duty of the investigating officer to identify the cases where a speedy analysis is required and request the scientist to give priority for analysis.

## EXTERNAL EXAMINATION OF THE DEAD BODY

The body is placed on the autopsy table, with wooden blocks placed under the shoulders and buttocks, so that the neck is extended and the back of head touches the table. The clothing if present, are removed. Shirts, blouse, etc. are removed by cutting the sleeves along the seams. If the dead body is that of an unknown, unidentified person, a detailed description of the apparel and other personal belongings are recorded. In the case of homicides, positions of blood stains, tears or rents caused by weapons, bullets, pellets, etc. are recorded. Photographs of the injuries are taken. If gun powder residues are present in the clothes, detailed description of the pattern of the residue is recorded and the clothes are handed over to the investigating officer. Normally in such cases, the investigating officer may record the details and preserve the clothes during inquest.

Clothing, ornaments, personal belongings, etc. found on the body are removed and handed over to the police constable in charge of the corpse. A receipt has to be given to the doctor. Length and weight of the body are recorded. For taking the length, a 7 feet long wooden scale or a flexible metal tape is used. This is important especially in murder cases, traffic accidents and hanging where the height of the deceased will be a material point in the reconstruction of the crime.

Various types of stains will be found on the body, such as blood, semen, etc. Foreign particles such as mud, sand, weeds and maggots will be present in some cases. Location and nature of these stains and particles are recorded. Relevant materials are collected in suitable containers and labelled. Afterwards, the body is thoroughly cleaned using a sponge and plenty of water. Skin of a dead body will be pale due to cessation of circulation. Skin will be lax due to loss of elasticity. The postmortem changes such as cooling, postmortem staining, rigor mortis, decomposition, etc. are noted.

Injuries, if any are present, are measured and a detailed description is recorded. Injuries are marked in appropriate diagrams. Patterned injuries are photographed with a scale. Doctors have to collect foreign particles or trace materials present in the wounds or in their vicinity.

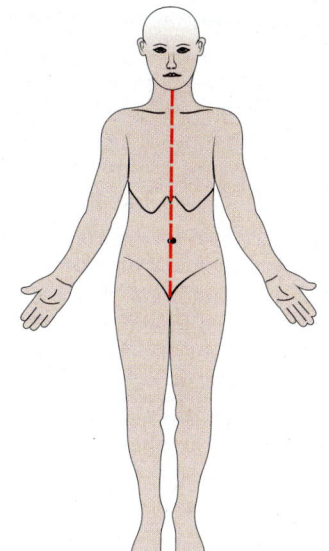

**Fig. 7.1:** Primary incision

## Dissection—Primary Incision

There are different types of incisions to cut open the dead body. The common incision is one starting from the chin to the symphysis pubis (Fig. 7.1). But if a bloodless field is required for the dissection of neck, as in the case of hanging, strangulation, etc. the incision begins from the root of neck to symphysis pubis. In this method, after removing the thoracic and abdominal organs, the skull is opened and brain is removed. By this time, blood might have been drained from the vessels and the neck can be dissected. The incision is extended from the root of neck to chin to examine the neck structures.

The primary incision is deepened up to the breast bone in the thoracic region and up to the sheath of the rectus muscle in the abdominal region (Fig. 7.2). Using scissors, the rectus sheath and the lining membrane of abdominal cavity (peritoneum) are

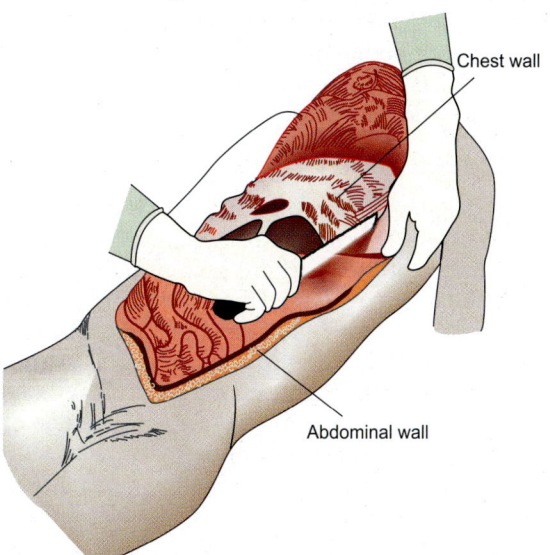

**Fig. 7.2:** Opening the abdominal cavity

cut guided by the fingers, so that injury to intestine is avoided. Then the peritoneum is opened up to the pubis. The attachments of the rectus muscles are cut and skin of the chest wall is reflected on both sides by cutting the chest muscles.

Abdominal cavity is examined first. If there is any blood or fluid, the quantity is measured, and the nature noted. Measuring is done by dipping a sponge in the fluid and squeezing it into a measuring jar. For opening the thoracic cavity, the skin of the chest wall is reflected sideways up to axillae. At this stage, testing for air in the chest cavity (**pneumothorax**) is conducted. Pockets are created by the reflected skin flaps below the axillae. Water is filled in the pockets and chest wall is punctured with a scalpel through one of the intercostal spaces under water. If pneumothorax is present, air will escape as bubbles. An alternate method is to fill a syringe with water and little water is injected into the pleural cavity. When the plunger is slowly withdrawn, bubbles will appear in the water in the syringe if air is present in the pleural cavity.

### Thoracic Cavity

The thoracic cavity is opened up by cutting through the cartilaginous portions of the ribs with a rib/cartilage knife (Fig.7.3). The sternum is lifted up and chest cavities are to be examined at this stage, before removing the sternum. If any fluid or blood is present in the pleural cavity, the quantity and nature are noted.

### Pericardial Cavity

The covering of heart (**pericardium**) is opened up with scissors. The contents of the pericardial sac and the surface of the heart are examined. Normally 20–50 ml of straw coloured fluid will be present and pericardial surface will be smooth and glistening. Frank blood may be due to the rupture of heart from trauma or natural disease. Rapid collection of 300–400 ml of blood or fluid can cause compression of heart (**cardiac tamponade**) and death. In stab injuries involving the heart, death is often due to cardiac tamponade.

### Air Embolism

Air embolism is a condition which causes death in cut throat injuries, criminal abortion, etc. When a considerable volume of air enters the venous channels and reaches the right side of the heart, the air mixes with blood to form a froth which obstructs the pulmonary flow like an air lock. To cause death, 100–150 ml of air is sufficient. Air embolism is tested by filling the pericardial cavity

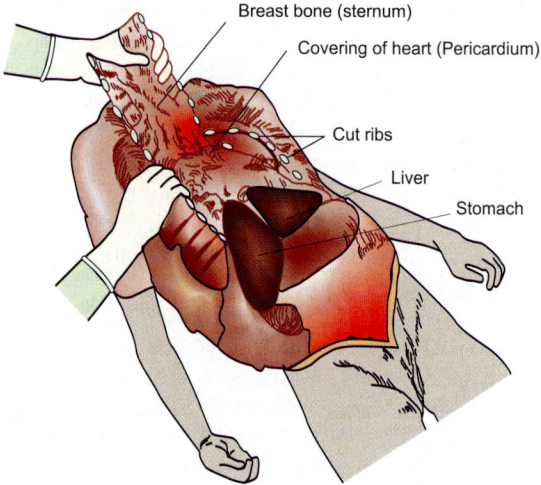

Breast bone (sternum)

Covering of heart (Pericardium)

Cut ribs

Liver

Stomach

**Fig. 7.3:** Opening the chest cavity

and puncturing the right lower chamber (right ventricle) of heart with a scalpel under water. Escape of air is an evidence of air embolism provided the body is not putrefied, as gases of putrefaction will give a false positive result.

### Pulmonary Embolism

Fatal pulmonary embolism is a complication of incapacitating injuries. Tissue damage will increase the clotting tendency of blood. Forced bedridden state will have pressure effect on the calf muscles which in turn will reduce the flow of blood in the veins. These factors will lead to formation of blood clots (thrombus) in the deep veins. **Deep vein thrombosis (DVT)** is also seen in passengers of long distance air travel or old people who sit for a long time on hard chairs. Injury to the tissues of legs and pelvis can also lead to local venous thrombosis. Contused muscles, fractures of leg bones and pelvis are some of the causative injuries. Pelvic vein thrombosis is also associated with pregnancy, abortion and delivery. The blood clot in the calf veins spread proximally to the major veins. Many blood clots detach and are carried to the right side of the heart. They reach the major artery (pulmonary artery) to the lungs, cause obstruction to the blood flow and cause death.

The medicolegal significance is that even trivial injury can lead to fatal pulmonary embolism. The victim develops pulmonary embolism during the recovery period, several days after the trauma. Death is sudden and clinical diagnosis and treatment may not be possible. If pulmonary embolism is suspected during autopsy, the pulmonary artery should be palpated for the presence of blood clots. If a clot is felt, the right ventricle of heart and pulmonary artery are opened in situ and the size and extent of pulmonary embolism are noted. In case of pulmonary embolism, origin of the thrombus is found out by exploring the calf veins, pelvic veins and the inferior vena cava.

## REMOVAL OF ORGANS

### Intestines

The first part of the small intestine is identified (it is the fixed loop) and a double ligature is placed around it and severed. The intestines are completely removed and taken out by placing a double ligature around the rectum and severing it (Fig.7.4). The surface of the intestines is examined for the presence of injuries or other changes. The small intestine and large intestine are opened up and the cavity is examined for changes due to diseases. The intestines can be injured either by penetrating injuries or by blunt force. Blunt violence like fisting or stamping need not cause contusions externally. The skin of the abdomen may be normal; but the force will be transmitted in all directions internally and intestines may be

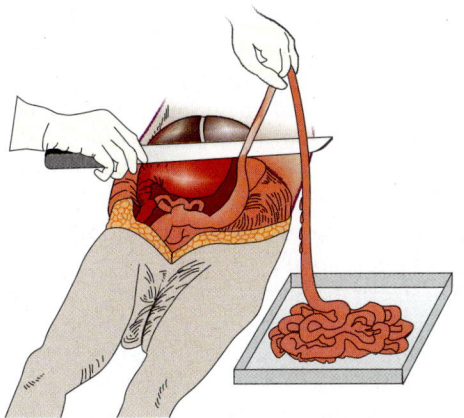

**Fig. 7.4:** Removal of intestines

contused or ruptured. Contusion of intestine will be bluish black in colour and should not be confused with postmortem staining. The area can be incised and the infiltration of blood in the wall of the intestine can be seen. Contusions are small and localised; but postmortem staining involves many dependent loops.

Microscopical examination can be done to confirm. If the contusion is associated with crushing of the wall of intestine, later the wall will be damaged and perforation can occur. Penetrating injuries of abdomen like stabbing can involve the blood vessels or intestines. If blood vessels are injured, death can be imminent due to bleeding, unless prompt treatment is given. If the intestinal wall is penetrated, infection (peritonitis) will ensue. Pus (purulent peritonitis) can develop in 36 hours after the injury. In blunt injuries to the abdomen, death will be delayed if peritonitis has occurred due to the rupture of intestines. Very often, there will not be any history or external signs. Hence, if a perforation is detected, it has to be ascertained whether it is due to injury or natural disease. Microscopical examination will confirm the nature of the lesion.

### Stomach

After removal of the intestines, the stomach is removed by clamping the cardiac and duodenal ends (Fig.7.5). It is placed in a tray and opened; so that the contents are not lost. The stomach is opened and the contents measured. The details of the food particles present are recorded. Time of death can be found out if the time of last meal is known. Emptying of stomach starts within half an hour and is completed by 4–6 hours after a meal. Emptying will be delayed in unconscious persons. If there is any unusual colour or smell of the contents, the details are noted. Many of the poisons have characteristic smell. Organophosphorus insecticides have kerosene-like smell. Cyanides will emit a smell similar to crushed tapioca leaves.

### REMOVAL OF OTHER INTERNAL ORGANS

The internal organs are removed en bloc or one by one. The organs are washed and placed in a tray for dissection. The inner aspect of chest and abdominal cavities are mopped clean. Ribs are

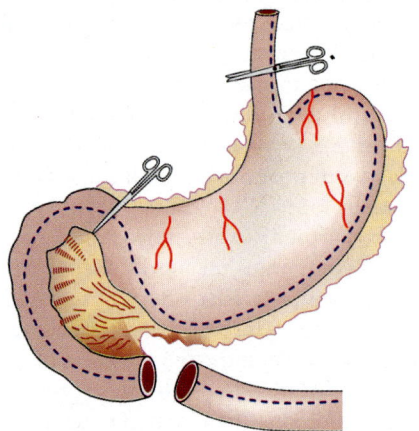

**Fig. 7.5:** Removal of stomach

## DISSECTION OF ORGANS

Adrenal glands are removed and dissected first. Right adrenal gland is triangular in shape and is situated just above the kidney, very close to the lower surface of liver. Left adrenal is semilunar in shape and is situated above and medial to the left kidney. These organs are sectioned and the cut sections are examined. They are enlarged in burns. Adrenal haemorrhage is seen in septicaemia, hypertension, eclampsia, etc.

Then both kidneys are examined. With a large knife, each kidney is bisected. If the capsule strips easily, it can be inferred that kidney is free from inflammatory lesions. If the kidneys appear abnormal, they are preserved for microscopical examination.

Prostate and seminal vesicle are removed along with the bladder at this stage. Testes are examined by incising the abdominal wall in the region of the inguinal canal. The spermatic cord is located and the incision is enlarged enough to introduce two fingers into the scrotal sac. The testis is located and pulled into the abdominal cavity along with the epididymis. When it has come out of the inguinal canal, it is either removed or examined in situ. Disease or injuries like contusions can be noted by sectioning the testis. In this method, scrotal skin will remain intact.

In female bodies, uterus, ovaries and fallopian tubes are removed and examined. The size of the uterus is measured. The vaginal wall is examined for injuries and diseases. The mouth of uterus **(cervix)** is examined. A mucus plug in the cervical opening (os) indicates that there has been no mechanical interference for inducing abortion for the past 24 hours. In women who have not delivered (nulliparous women), the os will be circular and in women who had delivered it will be either slit-like or irregular in shape. Injuries will be present in the vagina, cervix and uterine wall in cases of criminal abortion.

The size of the uterus is measured. The uterus is opened and the uterine cavity and lining of uterus (endometrium) are examined for the presence of injuries, infection, products of conception, etc. In asphyxial deaths, endometrium will be congested and haemorrhagic. This can be misinterpreted as

examined for fractures. Usually the site of fracture can be identified easily by the presence of surrounding infiltration of blood. But if crack fractures are suspected, the muscles in between the ribs (intercostal muscles) are cut lengthwise, ribs are freed and then examined. Dislocation and fractures of vertebrae can also be detected.

Organ en bloc is placed on a dissection table and firstly the major blood vessels are examined. The aorta is slit open along its posterior wall up to the arch and examined for changes due to diseases. The renal arteries are probed for excluding stenosis. Then they are also opened up to the kidneys. Constriction of renal arteries is some times seen in hypertension. The iliac veins and inferior vena cava are opened to search for blood clots (thrombi). Ureters are palpated for stones.

The oesophagus **(food passage)** is slit open and examined for injuries, foreign bodies, corrosion of mucosa, dilated oesophageal varices (swollen veins— a sign of disease of the liver like cirrhosis), etc. Presence of food particles in the oesophagus has no significance as it may be an agonal finding. In corrosive poisoning, mucosa will be corroded. Foreign bodies like fish bones and ENT procedures can cause perforation of oesophagus. If oesophageal varices are suspected, the stomach is not removed prior to the dissection of oesophagus, as the varices will collapse. After the examination, the oesophagus is separated from the surrounding structures using scissors.

menstruation. In suspected cases of abortion, bits should be taken from the uterus for microscopy. Uterus and appendages can be sent for chemical analysis, if use of abortifacient is suspected. Section of ovaries are made with a sharp knife. Presence of a large corpus luteum of pregnancy may be seen, even if the products of conception are evacuated in a case of abortion. Twisted ovarian cyst and ruptured ectopic pregnancy are conditions which can cause sudden death.

## Midline Structures of Neck

The tongue is examined for injuries. In suspected violence of the neck, the neck-structures are examined in a bloodless field. If a contusion is suspected, serial cross-sections are taken to find out the extent of the bruise. The soft tissues surrounding the midline structures are examined for bruising. The hyoid bone is examined for fractures. The thyroid, cricoid and tracheal rings are also examined for the presence of fractures. The larynx and wind pipe **(trachea)** are examined. Glottic edema will be seen in death due to anaphylactoid reactions.

The bronchi (air passages) are opened as far into the lungs as possible. Foreign bodies such as mud, sand, weeds, etc. may be found in drowning. Presence of soot in the bronchioles is an indication of death due to antemortem burns. Frothy fluid is an indication of pulmonary edema. Presence of food particles in the trachea could be due to agonal regurgitation or due to the pressure of gases of putrefaction. But an isolated bolus or a chunk of meat or other foreign bodies stuck in the larynx or trachea with signs of asphyxia will be suggestive of choking.

## Dissection of Lungs

The lungs are removed by cutting the bronchi and pulmonary vessels at the hilum. The lungs are dried by a sponge and the surface is examined. Then the lung is bisected with a brain knife. Usually the lower lobes and posterior aspects are dark due to postmortem staining. This can be misinterpreted as contusion. Bruising of the lungs are seen as isolated dark patches and on incising them, infiltration of blood can be detected.

Petechial haemorrhages are seen in asphyxia, poisoning, etc. Pneumonic consolidation should be suspected, if there is a liver-like feel. A bit of lung taken from that area will sink in water. Lungs are sectioned along its lateral margins. The cut sections are wipe dried and examined. Exudation of frothy fluid on pressure is indicative of pulmonary edema. Dark colour is due to venous congestion.

Collapsed lung will be small in size and will have no air. Collapse of the lungs may be due to hemopneumothorax (blood and air in the chest cavity). If injuries are seen in the lungs, the position and nature are noted. Measurements of injuries on the lungs are not significant as they will vary due to the collapse of the lung. Finding the direction of a stab injury of the lung by connecting the external wound and wound in the lung will also be fallacious to some extent. In such cases, an inference as to the general direction of the wound track can only be made. When a lesion is suspected, bits are preserved for microscopical examination.

In drowning, bits of lungs are preserved for demonstration of foreign particles in the air passages microscopically. Along with bone marrow, bits of lungs are also preserved for 'diatom test' for the demonstration of diatoms, which are unicellular algae present in water. **Diatom** detected in bone marrow is a definite proof of drowning. Diatom tests are done in the state forensic science laboratories (biology division). There is a view that diatoms found in the lungs have no significance as diatoms can percolate to the air passages even after death. Lungs of quarry workers may contain diatoms.

In deaths due to poisonous or irrespirable gases and anaesthetic deaths, lungs are preserved in bottles with a layer of molten paraffin poured over it to prevent the escape of gases. In anaesthetic deaths and deaths due to gaseous poisons, bits of lung tissue are collected in nylon bags, preserved in a frozen state and sent for chemical analysis. Even a lung can be removed after tying the main bronchus and blood vessels at the hilum and preserved in the aforesaid manner. Volatile gases will be lost if the organ or tissues are collected in the routine fashion.

## Dissection of Heart

The epicardial surface of heart is examined for evidence of pericarditis, infarcted areas, etc. A recent infarct is softer than the surrounding tissues and will be red or grey. There will be a small amount of fibrin on the pericardial surface. Old infarcts are clay/white coloured and the myocardium will be thinned. The chambers are opened in the direction of the blood flow. Atrial appendage is examined for mural thrombi. Bits are taken from the appendage to detect Aschoff nodules in rheumatic carditis. Right atrium is examined for thrombi. The endocardium, papillary muscles, chordae tendinae and valve cusps are inspected. The valve cusps may show thickening in stenosis or vegetations in endocarditis. Endocardium is examined for infarctions, fibroelastosis, thrombi, etc. The semilunar pulmonary valves are examined.

The mitral valve is examined and a finger is passed through the orifice to exclude stenosis. The thickness of the left ventricular wall is noted. When the aorta is opened, the coronary ostia can be seen above the aortic valves. In atherosclerosis and syphilitic aortitis, ostia will be narrowed. The heart is held at the apex by the left thumb and left index finger and placed on the dorsum of left hand. The course of left and right coronary arteries can be seen on the epicardial surface. Left artery gives the anterior descending and circumflex branches. Right coronary artery has got a main posterior descending branch. With a brain knife, coronaries are sectioned serially at every 3–5 mm (Fig. 7.6). The patency of the lumen is examined. The segment with the myocardium is taken as one piece for histology. Finally, the heart is placed on the dissecting board with the walls spread out and epicardial surface upward. Serial sections are made to note whether there is any intramural infarct, fibrosis or calcification.

## Removal and Dissection of Brain

An incision is made from one ear to the other across the scalp. The scalp is reflected in both directions from the line of incision, i.e. towards the orbital region and towards the occipital region (Fig. 7.7). In a hairy head, injuries like contusions may not be visible but corresponding hematomas can be detected in the scalp.

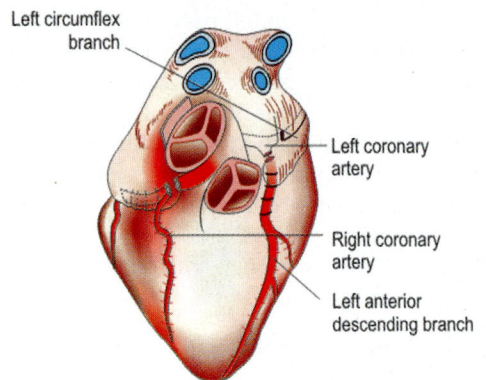

**Fig. 7.6:** Dissection of coronary arteries of heart (The arteries are cut serially to examine their lumen)

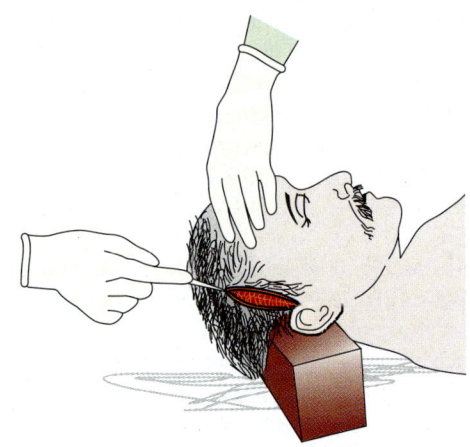

**Fig. 7 .7:** Incising the scalp to expose the skull cap

Skull cap is removed by sawing through the bones in a line more or less horizontal to the sides. A hand saw or electric saw is used. If any blood clot is present above the coverings of brain (extradural haemorrhage), its site, size and colour are noted. The dural covering is removed to find out whether there is a blood clot beneath it (subdural hematoma). Sometimes subdural hematomas of various stages of organisation or a chronic subdural hematoma may be seen.

It is possible to assess the age of the subdural hematoma by observing the changes that develop in it in the course of time. This is necessary to corroborate with the history of a previous trauma to head. The pia mater and arachnoid coverings of brain are inspected next. Subarachnoid bleeding or any other exudate can be visible under the pia-arachnoid. Flakes of pus and purulent exudate are found in the arachnoid space in leptomeningitis. In cerebral edema, the brain will appear to be dry with flattening of the sulci and narrowing of gyri. Grey nodules are present in the base in tuberculous meningitis. The brain is removed (Fig. 7.8) and dissected.

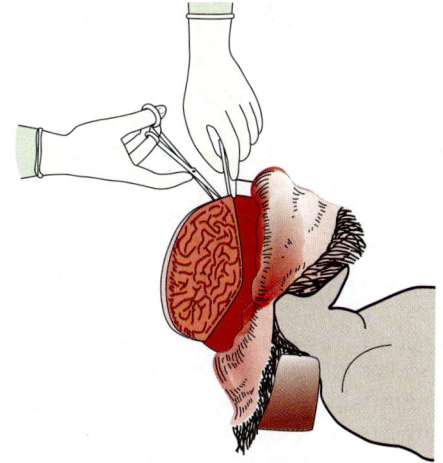

**Fig. 7.8:** Cutting the dura and removing the brain

The dura is stripped completely and the base of the skull is made visible. Removal of the dura from the base will reveal extradural clots, if any, present at the base. Fracture of the base of skull will also be visible when the dura is removed. The brain is examined for the presence of diseases, injuries, bleeding in its substance. As the brain is soft, it is better to fix it in formalin before dissection. The cerebrum, cerebellum, midbrain, pons and medulla are sectioned serially and examined. The important structures like ventricular system, thalamus, caudate nucleus, basal ganglia, internal and external capsules are examined.

## Dissection of Liver, Duodenum, Pancreas and Spleen

The duodenum is opened; mucosa wiped and examined. When the gallbladder is pressed, bile can be seen coming through the sphincter of Oddi in the duodenum if the bile duct is patent. The pancreas is removed, palpated for fibrosis/stones and then serially sectioned.

The spleen is removed, sectioned and the cut surface examined. The pulp is usually soft and cannot be scraped away easily if it is normal. Spleen will be found enlarged in portal hypertension, leukaemia, kala-azar, malaria, etc. A blunt impact on the abdomen can easily rupture such a spleen. Spontaneous rupture of an enlarged spleen is also possible.

Serial sections of liver along its long axis are made and findings like venous congestion, abscesses, tumours, etc. are noted. The cut surface will be yellow and greasy in fatty liver and nodular in cirrhosis. If any pathological change is suspected in any of the organs, bits from those organs are preserved for microscopical examination. The bits are preserved in 10% formalin; ten times the volume of the bit.

## Dissection of Spinal Cord

Exposure and dissection of spinal cord is required to examine fractures of vertebral column and injuries of the spinal cord. In all cases of sudden and suspicious deaths, the cervical spines are definitely examined. Fractures and dislocations above the level of third cervical vertebrae can cause respiratory paralysis and sudden deaths due to involvement of phrenic nerve (originates from the fourth cervical segment). Sudden flexion or extension of neck can cause sudden deaths due to cord injury.

After evisceration, the anterior surface of the spine will be clearly visible. Fracture sites can be distinguished by the presence of infiltration of blood around the fracture site. Dislocations can be identified by abnormal mobility of the spine. To find out the extent of the injury, the entire spine has to be exposed and spinal cord examined.

The body is placed in a prone position, with a wooden block under the chest. If the entire spinal cord has to be examined, an incision from the occipital protuberance up to the sacrum is made. If it is possible to locate the injured area or site of lesion from the anterior aspect after the removal of thoracic and abdominal organs, incision on the back is made for that particular area alone.

The subcutaneous tissues and muscles are cut through along the sides of spinous processes. Once the soft tissues are separated, the laminae are cut on both sides by an electric saw or a chisel and hammer. The spines and laminae are lifted up and extradural parts of spinal nerves are severed. The cord is removed gently from the cauda equina up to the cervical cord. The dura of the cord is gently slit open with scissors and cord is examined. In fracture/dislocations of vertebral column, laceration/haemorrhage in the cord can be noted. If necessary, cross-sections are made (Fig. 7.9).

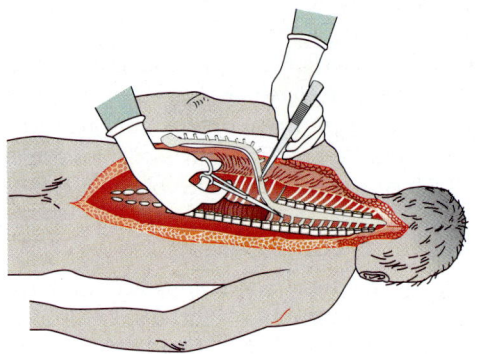

**Fig. 7.9:** Exposure of spinal cord

## CLEANING AND STITCHING

Once the autopsy is completed, the body cavities are mopped clean. The dissected organs (including brain) are squeezed dry and placed in the thoracic and abdominal cavities. If the body is to be kept for disposal for a long time, the dissected organs are put back after treating them with formalin or embalming fluid. The cavities are packed with cotton soaked in embalming fluid. The skull cavity is packed with cotton and the skull cap is placed in position. The reflected scalp is sutured using a large needle and black thread. Continuous sutures are put with the needle threaded from the inner layer of scalp outwards, so that the sutures are not visible outside. The breast bone is put back in position and the reflected skin flaps of abdominal and chest cavities are sutured in a similar fashion. After suturing, the body is washed, dried and dressed up before handing over to the relatives. A dead body should not be mutilated and should be given back to the relatives in a good

condition so that they can perform the last rites. The body is given to the police constable and a receipt is obtained. Clothes, ornaments and other material objects, etc. are returned and receipt obtained. The police constable will hand over the body to the relatives after obtaining a receipt from them.

All unidentified and unclaimed bodies should be kept for 72 hours. If there are no claimants, body can be given to municipal/corporation authorities for disposal.

## COLLECTION OF BODY FLUIDS

### Blood

For chemical analysis and other laboratory investigations, blood and other body fluids have to be collected from the dead body. Ideally, blood sample should be taken from the femoral artery or vein by percutaneous puncture. Blood is collected in fresh glass or Bakelite screw capped containers. Ten milligrams sodium fluoride or potassium flouride per milliliter of blood is the ideal quantity for best preservation. Blood should not be collected from the paracolic gutter, as it will be contaminated with gut contents, urine, etc. Sample from heart is also not suitable for toxicological examination as there is a possibility of seepage of poison from the stomach and lungs.

### Urine

Urine is obtained from direct puncture of the exposed bladder with a syringe and needle, or by catheterisation before autopsy. If urine is collected after incising the bladder, there is a possibility of contamination with blood. If there is delay for more than 2 hours for analysis, it is better to add a preservative to prevent bacterial overgrowth and decomposition. Several chemicals like boric acid, acetic acid, toluene, etc. are used as preservatives. These can interfere with toxicological and microbiological analysis. Therefore, it is better to use sodium fluoride (10 mg/ml).

### Cerebrospinal Fluid

For special investigations, it is necessary to obtain cerebrospinal fluid. It is difficult to obtain CSF from a dead body by the conventional lumbar puncture. CSF can be taken easily by a cisternal puncture. The neck is flexed and atlanto-occipital membrane is palpated in the midline. Using a syringe fitted with a lumbar puncture needle, CSF is collected by inserting the needle directed towards the bridge of the nose. Sodium fluoride is used as preservative.

### Vitreous Humour

Vitreous humour is the fluid in the anterior chamber of the eyeball. For special investigations, this fluid is collected. A syringe fitted with 17 or 15 gauge needle is used to collect vitreous humour. The eyelids are retracted and the sclera is punctured at a latitude of 60°, considering the pupil as the north pole. The needle is directed towards the centre of the eyeball. Aspiration is done gently. Fluoride is used as the preservative.

### COLLECTION OF VISCERA FOR CHEMICAL ANALYSIS

Viscera and body fluids are collected from the following medicolegal cases subjected to autopsy.
- All cases of suspected poisoning.
- All cases of sudden death.
- Dead bodies recovered from water when conclusive evidence of drowning is absent.
- Traffic accidents and homicides when the stomach contents have smell of alcohol.
- All cases of death where no definite cause of death is detected.
- All cases of death where an unusual smell, colour or an unidentifiable material is detected in the stomach contents.
- Deaths due to hypersensitivity reaction to drugs/food.
- Anaesthetic deaths.
- When the investigating police officer requests to forward the viscera irrespective of the cause of death or opinion of the medical officer.

### Materials Collected

- Stomach with contents (entire stomach).
- Small intestine (first part of jejunum) 30 cm in length with contents.
- 500 gm of liver and one kidney or one half of each kidney (whole liver, if less than 500 gm),

- Blood — 30 ml.
- Urine — 30 ml (if the bladder contains less than that, take as much as possible).

### Method of Collection

During autopsy, stomach is removed after tying or clamping the cardiac and pyloric ends. It is transferred to a clean tray and slit open along the greater curvature. After recording the nature of the contents and also the changes in the mucosa, the stomach is transferred to a clean wide-mouthed glass bottle of one litre capacity. The contents of the stomach are then added. If the contents are too much, they are collected in a separate bottle. If any peculiar unidentifiable substance, undissolved tablets, etc. are detected in the stomach, they are collected in separate bottles.

Similarly 30 cm of the first part of jejunum is also tied or clamped and removed. This loop of the intestine is slit open and put into the bottle (Fig. 7.10A) containing stomach. After the dissection of the liver, 500 gm of sliced liver is transferred to another bottle of one litre capacity. In the case of an infant's liver the whole of the liver is sent if it weighs less than 500 gm. But the liver is sliced before transferring it into the bottle. Both kidneys are dissected and one-half of each kidney or one kidney alone is put into the bottle containing the pieces of liver (Fig. 7.10B).

In all types of poisoning, blood (Fig. 7.10 C) and urine (Fig. 7.10D) are collected invariably. Extraction and detection of poisons from the viscera is a laborious process and sometimes will yield negative results. This is true especially in a

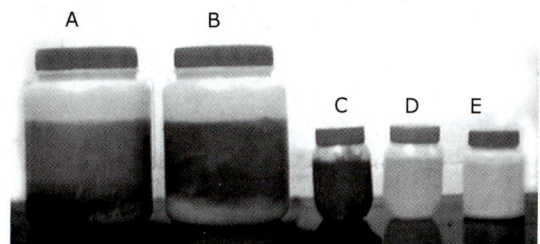

**Figs 7.10 A to E:** Collection of viscera and body fluids (A. Stomach and part of intestine, B. Part of liver and one kidney, C. Blood, D. Urine, E. Sample preservative)

hospital-treated case of poisoning in which the poison present in the stomach might have been eliminated by stomach wash.

Even in treated cases, traces of poison will be present in the blood and urine. By employing the modern analytical methods like chromatography and spectrophotometry, detection of poison is possible. But in putrefied bodies it will be difficult to collect blood sometimes, as it will be lysed. In such cases, unlysed blood clots or blood-stained fluid if present is collected.

## Preservation

In order to prevent decomposition of the viscera, preservative, is added. Rectified spirit (90% ethyl alcohol) is the ideal one. But it is not used as a preservative if the presence of alcohol is suspected. In cases of suspected poisoning with phenol, paraldehyde, phosphorus and acetic acid, rectified spirit is contraindicated as it will react with the poison. Methylated spirit should never be used. Saturated solution of sodium chloride is used. Purified common salt powder will be sufficient for this purpose. Whatever be the preservative used, a sample of the preservative (Fig. 7.10E) should accompany the materials collected (Fig. 7.10).

## Labelling

All the bottles are labelled properly (Fig.7.11). The label will contain the reference number of the case, name of the deceased, nature of the material, nature of the preservative and the signature of the Medical officer with the date of collection. A copy of the label is sent to the chemical examiner for verification purpose.

## Packing and Sealing

After affixing the labels and tightly closing with the screw caps, the bottles are wrapped with packing paper. Using country twine, each bottle is tied vertically with the final knot coming on the top of the bottle. Sealing wax is melted and applied to the knot and all the junctions of vertical ties. A metal engraved official seal is used for sealing. If the sealing is improper, the chemical examiner will not accept the viscera under the presumption that there could be tampering. The wrapping, tying and sealing are done in such a manner that the bottle cannot be opened without breaking the seals (Figs 7.12 to 7.14).

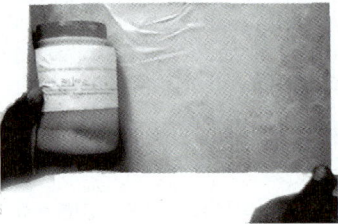

**Fig. 7.12:** Packing with paper

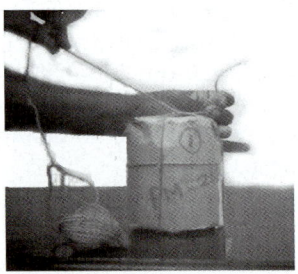

**Fig. 7.13:** Tying with country twine

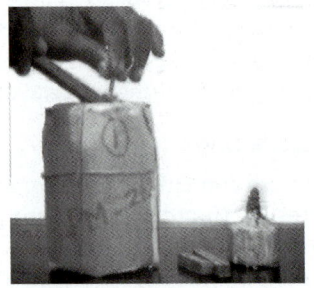

**Fig. 7.14:** Affixing the seal with wax

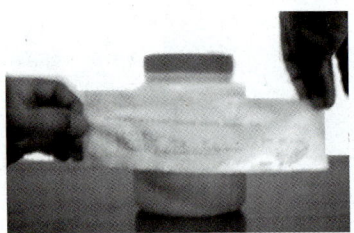

**Fig. 7.11:** Affixing label

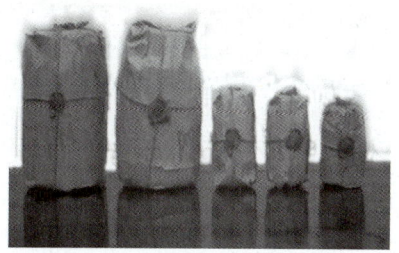

**Fig. 7.15:** Labelled, packed and sealed material objects

## Forwarding the Material Objects

The labelled, packed and sealed material objects (Fig.7.15) are enclosed in a card board box and transmitted to the chemical examiner's laboratory. To identify each bottle the postmortem number and bottle number are written on each packed bottle. The best method of forwarding the material is through a police constable. The material objects are handed over to the constable when he reports before the medical officer with an authorisation by his superior police officer. The packed and sealed material objects are handed over to the constable along with a letter to the chemical examiner. This letter contains all the relevant details of the case. The name and number of the constable are also entered in the letter. This letter is placed in an envelope, sealed and handed over to the constable. A register is kept by the medical officer regarding the despatch of these articles. Details such as the reference number of the case, number of bottles, date of collection, date of despatch of the articles, name, number and signature of the police constable who receives the articles for transmission, etc. are entered in the register.

In many states the chemical analysis of viscera and body fluids are conducted in the chemistry division of the state forensic science laboratory. In some states like Kerala, chemical examiner's laboratory is an independent establishment under the home department. In Kerala state, the chief chemical examiner's laboratory is situated in the capital. There are regional laboratories at Ernakulam and Kozhikode district headquarters.

The material objects will be accepted by the chemical examiner's laboratory, only if the articles are well preserved, packed, labelled and sealed.

If the seals are absent or found broken, the articles will be returned. Therefore, proper care is taken in packing, labelling and sealing of the material objects. In order to obtain the result of the analysis in murder cases and other sensational cases, the investigating officer has to request the chemical examiner to give priority for the examination.

## RECORDING THE AUTOPSY FINDINGS

Autopsy findings are recorded in a dossier. When the doctor is performing the autopsy, he dictates the findings and an assistant notes them in the printed dossier. If there is no assistant, the doctor can use a voice operated tape recorder for recording the data. After the autopsy, the data is copied in the dossier. The injuries are marked in appropriate diagrams with legends.

## AUTOPSY CERTIFICATE

After the autopsy, a certificate is drafted from the findings noted in the detailed notes. All positive findings are included in the certificate; but salient negative findings are also added sometimes. Autopsy certificate is a very important document. Basically, a medicolegal autopsy report differs from a hospital pathology report in its objectives and significance. Medicolegal autopsy report is perused by persons who are unfamiliar with medical jargon. Therefore, as far as possible, medical terms are substituted by common terms.

The certificate will contain a preamble consisting of preliminary details regarding the case, the name of the deceased, time and place of conduct of autopsy, etc. The general findings are narrated next. Identifying features are included next in the case of unidentified bodies. After this, postmortem changes are described. Injuries are described in a descending order beginning from the head to the feet in an orderly manner. Lengthy, ambiguous descriptions should be avoided. Then the salient internal findings are included.

The report is concluded with the well-formed opinion as to the cause of death. It is always expressed in morbid anatomical terms. Four copies of the certificate are prepared. Copies are either written or typed. A specimen copy of an autopsy certificate is given in Proforma 7.1. The autopsy certificate is sent to the authorities concerned at the earliest, within 24 hours.

## Legal Aspects

Autopsy certificate is a very important piece of evidence. The certificate is a substantive evidence and it has to be proved by the person who prepared and signed it. It is not admissible in evidence, if it remains unproved.

It is not a public document within the meaning of **Section 74 of the Indian Evidence Act.** Therefore, the accused is not entitled to inspect it or get a copy of it during investigation of the case. Opinion of the autopsy surgeon in the certificate is to aid the investigating officer in the investigation of the case. The report cannot be considered as a record of his official act for the use of the public.

The findings observed by the doctor during autopsy are recorded in the autopsy certificate. When he narrates the findings while tendering evidence, he acts as a witness of fact. His observations may help to corroborate the testimony of the eye witnesses. When he expresses opinion on the findings observed, he acts as an expert witness. It can be said to be an independent testimony, as it may help to establish facts of the case apart from other oral evidence.

For example, the eye witness testifies that A stabbed B with a knife on the left side of the chest and B died imminently. Autopsy surgeon testifies that there was an incised penetrating wound on the left side of the chest injuring the heart which could have been caused by the weapon recovered by the investigating officer as per **Section 27 of the Indian Evidence Act**. The doctor also opines that the injury of the heart is imminently fatal. The testimony of the doctor corroborates the oral evidence of the eye witness and scientifically proves that the injury was imminently fatal as defined under **Section 300 of Indian Penal Code**. Therefore, it can be considered as direct evidence of the facts discovered on the dead body of the victim.

The copy of the autopsy certificate is sometimes needed by the heirs of the victim for several civil purposes. To obtain a copy of the certificate,

the legal heir shall apply to the doctor/hospital. This application is forwarded to the Investigating police officer for verification and approval. After obtaining a 'no objection' certificate from the Police officer, a xerox copy is issued to the relative after realising a prescribed fee.

When the report of chemical analysis is received by the doctor, he forwards the original to the Court concerned and a copy to the Investigating officer along with a certificate of final opinion as to the cause of death (Proforma 7.2).

## DIRECTIONS TO THE INVESTIGATING OFFICER

## Questioning the Doctor U/S 161 of Criminal Procedure Code

As per this Section, any police officer making an investigation under this Chapter (XII), or any police officer not below such rank as the state government may, by general or special order, prescribe in this behalf, acting on the requisition of such officer, may examine orally any person supposed to be acquainted with the facts and circumstances of the case. Such person shall be bound to answer truly all questions relating to such case put to him by such officer, other than questions the answers to which would have a tendency to expose him to criminal charge or to a penalty or forfeiture.

The police officer may reduce into writing any statement made to him in the course of an examination under this Section; and if he does so, he shall make a separate and true record of the statement of each such person whose statement he records.

No statement made by any person to a police officer in the course of an investigation under this chapter, shall, if reduced to writing, be signed by the person making it; nor shall any such statement or any record thereof, whether in a police diary or otherwise, or any part of such statement or record, be used for any purpose, save as hereinafter provided, at any inquiry or trial in respect of any offence under investigation at the time when such statement was made.

It is better to examine the doctor immediately after the autopsy. The objective of questioning is to

**Proforma 7.1:** Specimen Copy of an Autopsy Certificate

### Autopsy Certificate

Autopsy No. 20/08

Hospital....................................
Date..........................................

(Body was that of an unknown male with early putrefactive changes)

I, Dr. Thomas Abraham, MBBS, Asst. Surgeon, P.H.Centre, Pulincunnu, certify as hereunder:-

On 12-4-2008, at 13.00 hours, I received the dead body of an unknown male aged about 40 years, deceased in Crime 38/06 of Pulincunnu Police Station from police constable no 2434 with a requisition no. Cr. 38/08 dated 12-4-2008 of the sub inspector of police, Pulincunnu for autopsy and report.

The dead body was identified by P.C. No. 2434 as that of the deceased in Crime 38/08 of Pulincunnu Police Station. Autopsy commenced at 13.10 hours in the mortuary attached to the hospital and concluded at 14.30 hours on the same day.

### Autopsy Findings

Dead body was that of a well-nourished, circumcised male of dark complexion. Height was 1.7 mtr. and weight 70 kg. Body was in an early stage of putrefaction. Different shades of putrefactive discolouration were seen on the body. Skin showed blebs and was peeling off in places. Marbling was present here and there. Face and external genitalia were bloated. Abdomen was distended. Eyeballs, tongue and rectum were protruded. Pinkish froth was coming through the mouth and nostrils. Nails were blue. Other body orifices were normal. No antemortem injuries were seen on the body.

### Identifying Features

1. A. Black mole, 2 mm diameter on the right side of face, 4 cm in front of the tragus of right ear.
   B. Scar 3 x 0.5 cm on the left side of forehead, 5 cm above the middle of left eyebrow.
   C. Tattoo mark of a crescent and star in the middle of the left forearm.
2. A. Scalp hair-black in colour — 10–12 cm long, clipped
   B. Moustache-black, 1–2 cm long — beard – recently shaven
   C. Axillary and pubic hair — black and rich.
3. Teeth — Total 32 in number — all permanent — caries of lower 1st molar teeth
   Teeth stained due to chewing.
4. Ossification — cranial sutures fused inside — started fusion outside.
   Manubrium and xiphoid not fused with the body of sternum.

Air passages contained pinkish froth. Lungs were soft and dark. Stomach contained 200 ml of brown fluid with kerosene-like smell. The stomach mucosa was congested and haemorrhagic. The intestinal contents also had kerosene-like smell. All the other organs were in varying stages of putrefaction; otherwise normal.

The following materials were collected for chemical analysis:
1. Stomach and part of intestine with contents
2. Part of liver and one kidney
3. Blood
4. Urine

### Cause of Death

Postmortem appearances are consistent with death due to poisoning. However, final opinion is reserved pending the report of chemical analysis.

The age of the person could be 35–45 years:

PH Centre                                                                Signature of Medical Officer
Pulincunnu                                                              Dr. Thomas Abraham
13-4-2008                                                               Assistant Surgeon
Forwarded to: (Original is forwarded to the court concerned)
Copy to: (Investigating Police Officer)

**Proforma 7.2:** Autopsy certificate — Final Opinion as to the Cause of Death

**Autopsy Certificate — Final Opinion as to the Cause of Death**

Autopsy. No. 20/08                                P.H. Centre, Pulincunnu

Dated: 20.5.08

As per requisition from S I of police, Pulincunnu Police Station dated 12.4.08, an autopsy was conducted on the body of an unknown male aged about 40 years involved in crime 38/08 of Punlincunnu Police Station and the opinion as to the cause of death was reserved in the autopsy certificate no.20/08 dated 13.4.08 issued by the undersigned.

The certificate of chemical analysis no. 206/08 dated 17.5.08 received on 19-5-08 from the chemical examiner to government is enclosed herewith:

Other Laboratory Findings: Nil

**Opinion**

Based on the autopsy findings and the result of chemical analysis, I furnish my final opinion as follows:

"Death was due to poisoning with parathion, an organophosphorus insecticide."

Signature:

Dr. Thomas Abraham

Assistant Surgeon

Forwarded to: (Original certificate to the court concerned)

Copy to: (the Investigating Officer)

obtain information regarding the cause of death, time of death and probable manner of death. This will help him to start the investigation without delay in the proper direction. In the light of the medical evidence, questioning other witnesses will be an easy task. After receiving the autopsy certificate, the IO should question the doctor again. This time the objective of recording a statement is to obtain clarification of the facts noted in the autopsy certificate. Most often the certificate will contain medical/technical jargon which may not be properly conceived by the investigating officer.

An autopsy certificate has mainly two parts; a record of the morbid anatomical changes seen in the dead body and the opinion as to the cause of death expressed by the doctor. For example, in the case of a dead body recovered from water, the doctor observes certain changes in the dead body and he records them in the autopsy certificate. Based on those findings, he arrives at a conclusion that death was due to drowning. This opinion also finds a place in the certificate.

The investigating officer should ask the doctor about the salient findings and how he had arrived at the cause of death. He should also elicit the opinion of the doctor regarding the manner of death. It may not be possible for the doctor to provide definite opinion as to the manner of death in most of the cases. But he may be able to discuss the various possibilities and help the investigating officer to find out the truth, which is the main objective of crime investigation.

One should not rely heavily on the opinion of experts like the autopsy surgeon. More importance should be given to evidence collected through the tedious and exhaustive process of interrogation, verification, etc. The medical and scientific opinion has to be appreciated and evaluated in conjunction with the evidence collected during field investigation. There are many instances when investigating officers had gone astray following medical evidence alone.

In homicides, when the weapon used for inflicting injuries is recovered, the investigating officer should invariably show it to the doctor and obtain a statement regarding the possibility of inflicting the injuries with the weapon recovered. It is better to draw an outline of the weapon on a sheet of paper and record the measurements like length, breadth, etc. A copy of the statement recorded and the drawing of the weapon may be given to the doctor. The doctor can acknowledge receipt of the same by signing in the original. There is no provision in the Cr.PC to provide a copy of the statement to the witness examined. But this will be helpful for the doctor to refresh his memory when he is summoned to give evidence before the trial court at a later date. No witness can deny that he has not been examined orally by the investigating officer.

It is better to prepare a set of questions before examining a doctor. No relevant point will be missed if this method is followed. Experienced doctors are conversant with the method of recording the statement. They will be able to furnish a statement containing all the relevant information. If the investigating officer needs further clarification, he can pose questions to the doctor on those points. There is a tendency among some officers to fabricate a statement after recording in the case diary that the doctor was examined orally. Needless to say that this practice is illegal, irregular and dangerous. It is also not desirable to depute a subordinate officer to record the statement of the doctor.

# Forensic Taphonomy

The term 'Taphonomy' is derived from the Greek word 'Taphos' which means burial or grave. Taphonomy deals with the history of changes of a body after death. Forensic taphonomy derives inputs from many disciplines such as archaeology, anthropology, entomology, geology, botany, etc. Many processes alter the condition of human remains.

## CHANGES IN THE BURIED DEAD BODY

The buried body undergoes decomposition, skeletonisation and disarticulation. The internal organs, teeth, nails, hair and clothing also undergo various changes. Changes in the dead body are dependent on individual factors like age, physique, etc. apart from environmental factors like temperature, moisture, pH and properties of the soil. Temperature is the most important as the chemical and biological changes of decomposition are regulated by this factor. Decomposition will be hastened in bodies exposed to the sun than those buried or remaining in water. Usually bodies exposed to the sun can skeletonise in 1 month. It may take 2 months to 1 year for the buried bodies to undergo skeletonisation.

Animals, rodents, insects, maggots and bacteria destroy human remains. Jackals, dogs, cats and rats attack dead bodies. In forest areas, many wild animals also take part in scavenging dead bodies. Soft parts are eaten and bones are gnawed. The bones will be carried away and will be found scattered over a wide area. Dead bodies in rivers, lakes and sea are destroyed by fish. Flies and beetles lay eggs on the decomposing dead bodies. These eggs hatch out into larvae. The larvae are called maggots.

Maggots feed on the dead tissues and undergo moulting three times before developing into pupae. From the pupae, adult flies emerge. Estimation of the rate of development of maggots and pupae provides information regarding time since death. Samples of eggs, maggots and pupae are preserved in 75% ethyl alcohol for entomological examination. Live samples can also be collected. These should be put in a vial containing a small quantity of beef liver and air.

Plants including algae and fungi play a role in the decomposition process. Bodies lying in the open will be covered with plant debris. Roots can invade buried bodies. Roots also provide an environment for microbial activity. Botanical evidence will help in determining the season and time of occurrence of death. Samples can be collected in plastic containers and sent to a botanist for examination and report.

## LOCATING A GRAVE

Sometimes, crime investigators experience difficulty in locating the grave where the dead body of a crime victim is buried. Several methods are available in locating the burial place. Initial phase of search is based on the information gathered from investigation. Statements of the witnesses, geological maps of the possible locations, aerial survey and photo-

74

graphy will be helpful to identify an area as the burial place. The next step is to locate the exact spot of burial. The surface will be disturbed when compared to the surroundings. The disturbance will have a number of effects on the vegetation. Initially there will be destruction of the vegetation. The soil becomes loose and more aerobic due to digging. Later decay of the human remains provides nutrients to the vegetation which will show a luxurious growth. If the dead body is encased in a coffin or covered in materials like plastic or if the grave is filled with stones, this will not occur (Fig. 8.1).

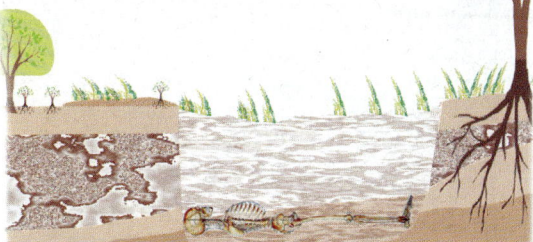

**Fig. 8.2:** Disturbed layers of earth in the place of burial. (The area is depressed due to compaction of the filling of the grave. The vegetation above the grave is disturbed and new growth of plants is also seen.)

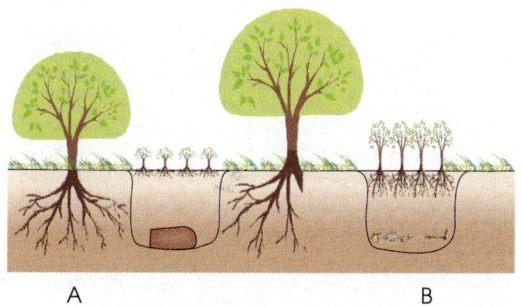

**Fig. 8.1:** Growth of vegetation above the place of burial (A. Sparse growth of vegetation in the case of a covered dead body, B. Luxurious growth of vegetation above the place of burial of an uncovered body).

When a grave is dug, the soil is dumped in the surrounding ground surface. As the sub-surface layers of the earth varies in texture, colour and other physical properties, the dug out earth will also show these properties. Examination of the soil will reveal remnants of deeper constituents like clay or rock.

After the burial of the dead body, the grave is filled with the soil dug out earlier. There may be excess soil, producing a mound over the grave. This mound will gradually sink due to consolidation of the grave infills and decay of the body. A depression or concavity may appear in the burial area due to the compaction of soil. The size of the compaction will be almost similar to the outline of the grave (Fig. 8.2).

Another method to confirm whether human remains are actually buried in a particular site, is to employ **cadaver scent dogs**. These dogs, specially trained to identify the smell of decomposed bodies will be able to locate the place of burial.

The methods employed in geophysical survey can be made use of in identifying a burial place. **Magnetometry** will detect disturbances in the soil causing changes in the local magnetic field. **Ground penetrating radars** are used to detect changes in the density of the sub-surface earth. Metal detectors will detect metallic objects buried along with the corpse. Probing the area using a rigid pipe for identifying soil disturbance, emission of methane gas from the putrefied body is also useful. As the decaying body generates heat, new technique of thermal imaging is also employed in detecting the site of burial.

## Exhumation

Exhumation means the digging out the dead body from the grave (Figs. 8.3A to D). This is usually done:
- To detect secret homicides,
- When foul play is suspected after burial, and
- For the purpose of establishing identity of the corpse in disputed cases.

## DIRECTIONS TO THE INVESTIGATING OFFICER

Under section 176(3) of Criminal Procedure Code, order for exhumation can be given by the district collector, additional district magistrate, sub-collector, RDO, tahasildar, or deputy tahsildar. They are the executive magistrates. Investigating police officer has to request the executive magistrate concerned to conduct exhumation. The doctor has to be informed about the exhumation sufficiently early so that he can be available during

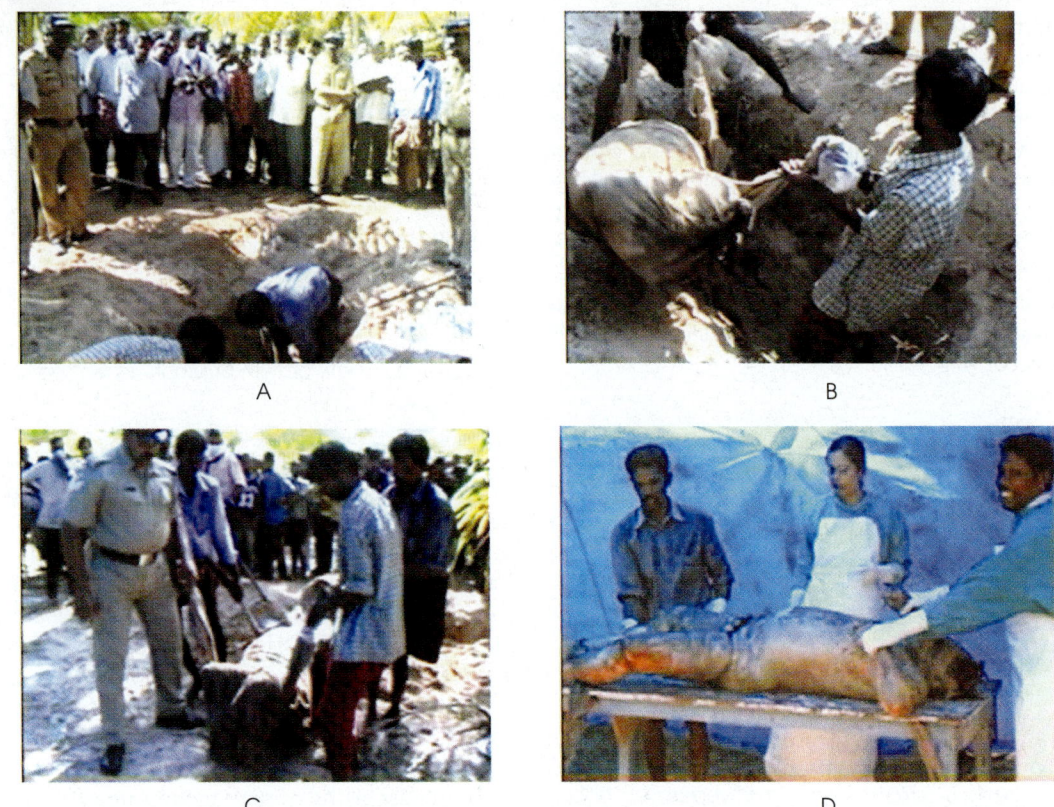

**Figs 8.3 A to D:** Exhumation and autopsy at site. A. Digging the grave  B. Removing the sack containing the dead body of the murdered victim,  C. Removing the dead body for inquest and autopsy  D. Autopsy at site (*Courtesy:* Dr. K. Sreekumari, Dr. N. Rajaram)

the procedure and examine the exhumed body at site.

The executive magistrate holds the inquest in the presence of respectable inhabitants/relatives, etc. Evidence from the persons who were present at the time of burial is also taken at the time of inquest. They help in identifying the grave and the corpse. In case of secret homicide, site of burial is identified as per the admission/confession recorded by the accused under the provisions of Section 27 of Indian Evidence Act.

## Technique

Once the site of burial is identified, the next step is to recover the dead body. Recovery of the buried body should be done carefully. Three types of activities are involved in burying a dead body. Firstly, soil is removed during digging a grave. Then the body is deposited in the grave and the grave is filled. During disinterment, these processes are done in the reverse order. After identifying the boundaries of the grave, additional space all around the boundaries should be marked for easy excavation. A lateral access is considered better. For preserving the integrity of the grave, shoring the sides with planks can be done. It is better to remove half of the filling in the long axis of the grave initially. The filling should be removed in layers using trowels.

The removed soil should be examined for the presence of evidentiary materials like body parts, personal articles, remnants of clothing, wrappings, weapons, etc. Each article should be preserved for examination, noting the location from which it was recovered.

Articles should be photographed in situ. All evidences should be packed and labelled at the scene itself. The excavation should be done slowly till the entire dead body is exposed. Usually, the burial may not be very deep in secret homicides. The body remains should be photographed in situ. A sketch should be prepared showing the relative positions of the remains, if they are found scattered.

The next stage is the lifting of the dead body out of the grave. If the body is entire, removal will not be difficult. The body can be lifted up by placing a strong canvas sheet or tarpaulin underneath the body. If the body is skeletonised, the bones will be loose and found scattered. As many bones as possible may be retrieved from the pit. In that case, it is better to make an extension trench by the side of the grave pit as a work area. Sitting in that area, the doctor can collect and examine all the bones. Search for bullets, weapons or metallic objects can be done with the help of a sensitive heavy duty metal detector.

In some cases, the dead body or skeletal remains may be found on the surface. Scavenging animals can cause scattering of bones over a wide area. If the skeletal remains are found scattered, the entire area should be searched systematically. Each piece should be photographed in situ. Each photograph should show a scale and the indication of the magnetic north for knowing the location of the remains. The bone pieces should be examined, documented, labelled and packed. The area can also be tested with a metal detector.

Facilities for conducting autopsy at site may be arranged by the IO. A temporary shed, table and sufficient quantity of water may be provided for the examination of the corpse or skeletal remains.

# Human Skeletal Remains

Very often police officers have to encounter skeletal remains or highly decomposed dead bodies during the investigation of unnatural deaths. In such instances, establishing identity is an important factor, apart from finding out the cause of death. The examination of the skeleton is warranted in the following instances:

- Exhumations, when suspicion of foul play arises after burying a body,
- Murder and secret disposal of dead bodies,
- To support a presumption of death, a set of bones may be produced which are alleged to have belonged to a particular individual,
- In case of accidents like air-crash, fire, natural calamities, etc. and
- Examination of foetal bones in the case of concealment of birth/infanticide.

In all the above mentioned situations, services of the forensic surgeon and forensic scientist should be obtained. Particular care should be taken in retrieving and examining as many bones as possible. But sometimes if the body is buried without a coffin, it may not be possible to retrieve small bones such as carpal, tarsal, phalanges, etc. For establishing identity, the skull with mandible, pelvis, long bones such as femur and tibia are essential. From the examination of these bones, sex, age, stature, time since death, etc. can be found out with 95% accuracy.

## ARE THE BONES HUMAN OR NOT?

If the bones are intact and complete, it is not difficult for a doctor to find out that they are human bones, based on the anatomical configuration. But in the case of smaller bones, or fragmentary bones, it may be very difficult to distinguish between human and non-human. The same difficulty will be experienced with charred or mutilated bones. Microscopic bone structure is basically the same in all the mammalian bones. However, it may help to identify a small fragment of unknown origin as a bone.

To confirm human origin, the bones should be subjected to a **precipitin test**. Species specific proteins are extracted from the bones and tested against specific antisera prepared by immunising a rabbit against proteins derived from blood. The drawback of the test is that the test cannot be applied to bones that have been burnt or dead for more than 5 to 10 years. Precipitin test is being done in Chemical Examiner's laboratory or state forensic science laboratory. Using different antisera, many species can be identified.

If the bones are fresh, DNA analysis can be done from the marrow cells for species identification.

## TIME OF DEATH

Assessing the time of death is purely presumptive, because skeletonisation of a dead body depends upon the circumstances under which it has been found. In the ordinary course, if a dead body is lying in the open, it may take 1 to 2 months for skeletonisation. A completely skeletonised body will be devoid of soft tissues, ligaments and cartilages. They will be without much odour. Body buried in earth without a coffin will be skeletonised in 2 to 6 months. Encasing in a coffin or a tomb will retard the process of putrefaction. Bones buried long since may be chalky-white in colour and the time of burial can be determined by radioactive carbon (C-14) estimation.

## Radioactive Carbon Estimation

On account of cosmic radiation, atmospheric nitrogen is broken down to an unstable isotope of carbon (C-14). This becomes attached to the organic molecules of plants through photosynthesis. Animals eating these plants absorb C-14. This process of ingesting C-14 continues as long as the animal is alive. C-14 in an animal is continually decaying to stable carbon isotopes. Since the organism is absorbing more C-14 during its life, the ratio of C-14 to C-12 remains the same as the ratio in the atmosphere. When the organism dies, the ratio of C-14 in its body decreases gradually. The rate of decrease is half of the quantity at death every 5730 years. This is the half-life of C-14. The quantity of C-14 at the time of death is calculated from the ratio of C-14 to C-12. The sample is analysed with suitable instruments and C-14 content is assessed. From this, the time since death can be found out. In recent years, scientists have developed a new approach to radiocarbon dating using a device called an accelerator mass spectrometer (AMS). This device directly counts C-14 atoms, rather than counting rate of disintegration. Accelerator mass spectrometry can date even a small sample. This method can date items that are up to 90,000 years old. These tests are done in the atomic research station at Trombay. Bones should be despatched through one of the central forensic science laboratories.

## Racial Difference

Determination of the race becomes a material point in the identification of human skeletal remains in the event of a mass disaster like the crash of an international airliner carrying people of many races. As there is an admixture of races of the world at present, the populace is not homogeneous as in the past. Racial differences are observed in the skeleton, most pronounced in the skull and facial bones. In forensic anthropology, there are three traditional classifications, viz. caucasoid (white),

mongoloid (East Asian, Amerindian) and negroid (black). Though there is some admixture, most humans belong to one of these categories.

## DETERMINATION OF SEX

The sex can be determined fairly well from the bones, especially the skull and pelvis. In the skeleton, sex differences appear only after puberty and will reach the maximum between 15 and 20 years. Pelvis is the best bone to determine the sex with 95% accuracy. Unfortunately, morphologic features are not always consistent. Many factors like environmental influences, endocrine conditions, etc. influence the morphologic dimorphism. The main drawback of morphologic approach is that the differentiation of sex is based on visual assessment. Experience becomes an essential component.

Sexual differences in prepubertal skeleton are not marked and it is not possible to form an opinion based on morphologic or osteometric approaches. In immature skeleton, mandible shows more distinct sexual dimorphism than skull or pelvis. It is possible to identify sex from the skull with 93% accuracy. The adult male skull shows well-defined characteristics (Fig. 9.1). The anatomical landmarks like the supraorbital ridges, glabella, malar bones,

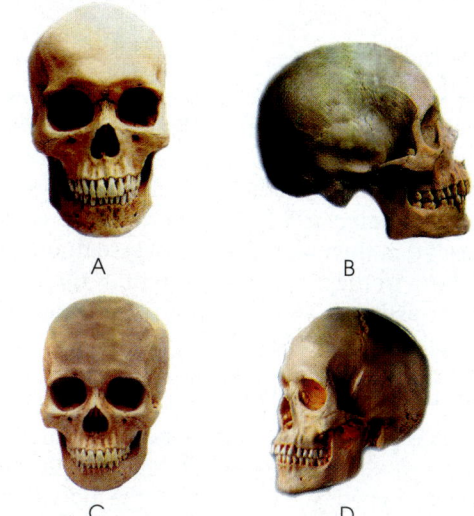

A                    B

C                    D

**Figs 9.1A to D:** Sex difference in the skull. There are more than twenty features to differentiate a male skull from that of a female. A. Male skull—frontal view, B. Lateral view C. Female skull—frontal view D. Lateral view

occipital protuberance, etc. in the male skull are more prominent than those of a female skull. Like the skull, male mandible also shows well-defined features (Figs 9.2A to D). The square-shaped chin and everted angle of the male mandible are unique features of a male.

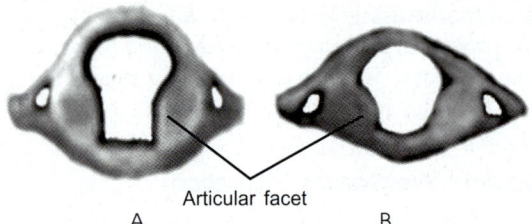

Figs 9.3 A and B: Sex difference in the atlas: A. Male, B. Female

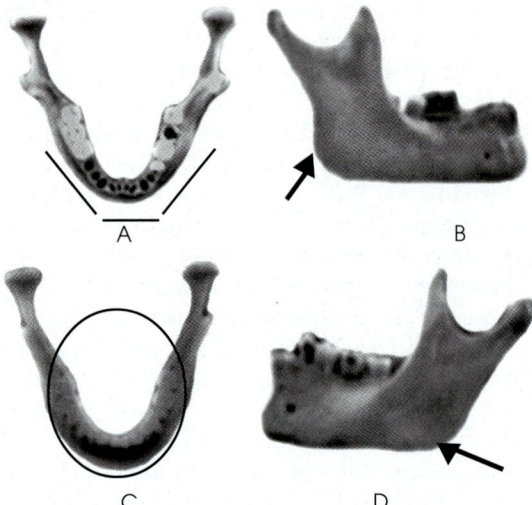

**Figs 9.2 A to D:** Sex difference in the jaw bone: A and B Male —The outline is square-shaped and the angle is evereted. C and D Female — Circular outline with smooth angle

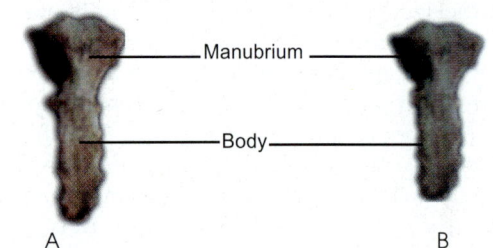

**Figs 9.4A and B:** Sex difference in the breast bone (sternum) A. Male, B. Female

be >149 mm in the male and <149 mm in the female (Figs 9.4A and B).

### Vertebral Column

The vertebral column in the male is massive when compared to that of the female. Mean length of spine is 70 cm in the male and 60 cm in the female. Lumbar lordosis is exaggerated in the female. Atlas, the first vertebra is more massive in the male. The transverse diameter is >76 mm in the male and <76 mm in the female. Upper articular facet is larger in the male than the female (Figs 9.3A and B).

### Sternum (Breast Bone)

Sternum is composed of three bones: manubrium, body and xiphoid process. Sternal measurements provide a good clue to the sex of the individual.

In the male, the body is more than twice the length of the manubrium. In females, the length of body is less than twice the length of manubrium. The total length of the manubrium and body will

### Femur (Thigh Bone) and Humerus (Upper Arm Bone)

Generally, the long bones of females are shorter, slender and smoother when compared to those of the males. Muscular attachments are rough and prominent in males. Heads of humerus and femur are larger in male (Figs 9.5 and 9.6).

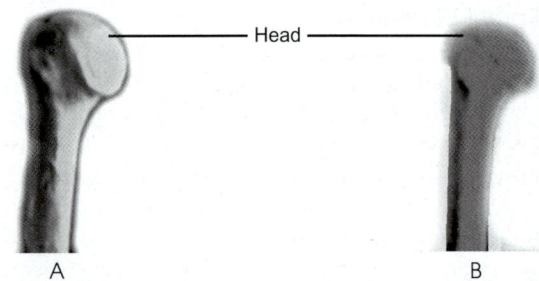

**Figs 9.5 A and B:** Sex difference in the humerus (A. Male, B. Female)

## Thigh Bone (Femur)

Head of femur will be large in males (diameter >4.5 cm) and smaller in females (diameter <4.5 cm). In males, the neck makes an obtuse angle with the shaft while the angle will be less obtuse in females. The angulation is less inclined in males and more inclined in females (Figs 9.6A and B).

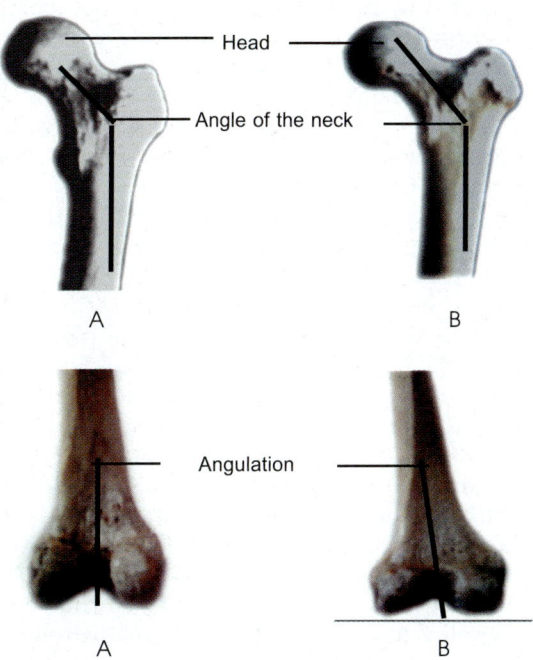

**Figs 9.6 A and B:** Sex difference in the femur— A. Male, B. Female

## Hip Bone (Pelvis and Sacrum)

Hip bone is formed by the union of three bones; ilium, ischium and pubis. Sex can be determined with 95% accuracy from the examination of the pelvis. Post-pubertal pelvic bone shows well-defined sexual characteristics, especially in the females (Figs 9.7A and B). Even though the identification of the sex is based on the subjective impression of the forensic expert, various measurements are taken for confirmation. Sacrum is a part of the pelvis and it also exhibits marked features in the female. There are more than 15 bony features which will help to identify sex in the hip bone.

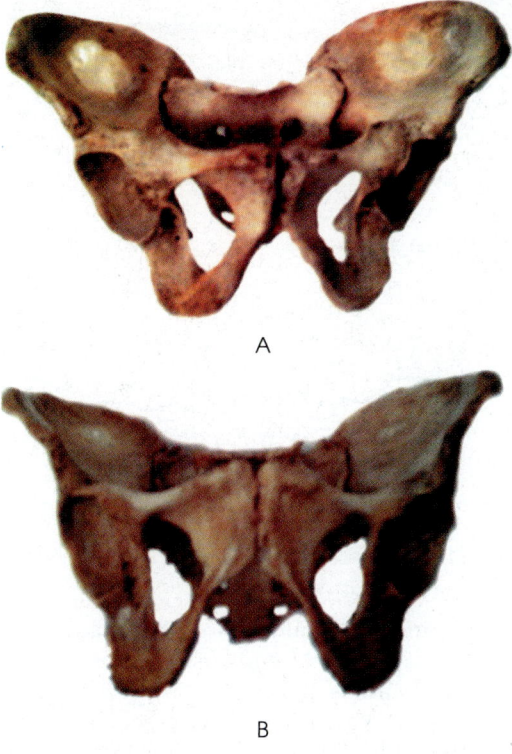

**Figs 9.7 A and B:** Sex difference in the pelvis— A. Male, B. Female

## Estimation of Age from Skeleton

From conception to adulthood, age can be determined by the growth and development of the skeleton. The appearance of ossification centres, tooth formation and eruption, union of epiphyses, closure of skull sutures, etc. are helpful in determining the age up to adulthood. Afterwards, bones like pubic symphysis undergo degenerative changes which will help to estimate the age to a certain extent.

First of all, the teeth sockets are counted and age is ascertained. From a single tooth, especially incisors, age can be determined by Gustafson's technique. Age is determined from the skull by observing the closure of sutures at various sites. Generally speaking, sutures in the inner aspect of the skull start closing between the ages of 25 and 35 years. In the outer aspect, suture closure starts between 35 and 45 years. As there are so many variations seen individually, this assessment is not accurate (Fig. 9.8).

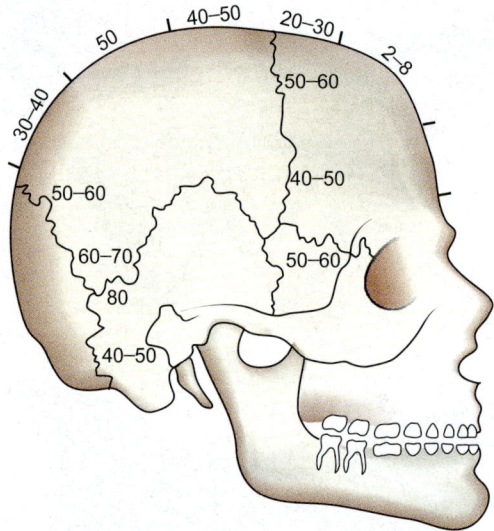

**Fig. 9.8:** Determination of age from closure of skull sutures

Age can be determined more or less accurately from the appearance and fusion of ossification centres of various bones. From the hip bone, age up to 19–21 years can be assessed. From the changes in the sacral vertebrae, age from puberty to 20–25 years can be found out. The four pieces of the body of the breast bone (sternum) fuse with one another from below upwards. The 3rd and 4th fuse at the age of 14, fusion between the 2nd and 3rd and the 1st and 2nd occurs between 14 and 25 years. The xiphoid process fuses at the age of 40. Manubrium fuses at the age of 60 or still later. To assess the fusion, the sternum is bisected and examined.

After the second decade, the symphysial face of pubis exhibits morphological changes related to the advancement of age. Age from 20 years up to 70th year, can be estimated by observing the changes in the symphysis pubis. But this is not an accurate estimation. The inner end of the collar bone **(clavicle)** fuses between 20 and 22 years. From the appearance and fusion of long bones, age can be assessed up to 17 years.

## Estimation of Stature from Skeleton

It is possible to estimate the height of an individual from the length of long bones. If the entire skeleton

is available, the bones are arranged with anatomical contiguity, total length is measured and 2.5–3.5 cm can be added to estimate the height. Rough estimates can be done if skull or one hand alone is available. Eight times the height of skull gives the approximate height. Height of the skull is the vertical distance between the top of head to the tip of chin. Stature can be calculated from the foot length (from footprints). Stature can be calculated by multiplying maximum foot length in centimeters by 100 and dividing it by foot length-stature ratio index which is about 15 (Abraham Philip-1989).

As a general rule, the height of a person is approximately the measurement between the tips of middle fingers of outstretched hands. If only one arm is available, the stature is calculated by multiplying its length by 2 and adding 34 cm for the length of clavicles and width of sternum. More or less accurate assessment of stature can be made using regression formulae like Karl Pearson's, Trotter and Glesser's, etc. For this, length of femur, tibia, humerus and radius are measured using an osteometric board or using two wooden blocks fixed on a graph paper. Karl Pearson's formula (French) is suitable for calculating the stature in south Indian population (Table 9.1). Formula to assess the height from foetal bones is given in Table 9.2.

It is better to avoid the measurements of humerus and radius to get a correct estimate of the stature. The accuracy of the estimate will be +/- 3 cm.

## Whether the Bones Belong to One or More Individuals

This is ascertained by aligning the individual bones in their respective anatomical position and reconstructing the skeleton if possible. There should not be any disparity in the age or sex. The bones forming joints should articulate very well. For example, the thigh bones should articulate with the sockets in the hip bone and the jaw bone should articulate with the skull.

## Determining the Cause of Death

If the body is completely decomposed, injuries to soft parts, disease of organs, etc. cannot be made out. The skeleton is to be thoroughly examined for

**Table 9.1:** Karl Pearson's formula to calculate the height from the length of long bones

| Bone (L=length) | Male | | Female | |
| --- | --- | --- | --- | --- |
| | Dry | Humid | Dry | Humid |
| Humerus | L × 2.894+ 70.164 | L × 2.894+ 70.714 | L × 2.754+ 71.475 | L × 2.754+ 72.046 |
| Radius | L × 3.271+ 89.925 | L × 3.271+ 86.464 | L × 3.343+ 81.224 | L × 3.343+ 82.189 |
| Femur | L × 1.880+ 81.30 | L × 1.880+ 81.231 | L × 1.945+ 72.844 | L × 1.945+ 73.163 |
| Tibia | L × 2.894+ 78.664 | L × 2.376+ 78.807 | L × 2.352+ 74.774 | L × 2.352+ 75.369 |

**Table 9.2:** Formula to assess the height from the length of foetal bones

Height = Length of diaphysis of femur × 6.71 cm.

Height = Length of diaphysis of tibia × 7.63 cm.

Height = Length of diaphysis of humerus × 7.6 cm.

Height = Length of diaphysis of radius × 9.2 cm.

the presence of antemortem fractures. An antemortem fracture will show staining of the edges as well as infiltration of blood into the layers (lamellae) of the bone. Fracture of skull, hyoid bone, ribs, etc. may give evidence of a fatal assault. The bones are subjected for chemical analysis to exclude poisoning. This is done as a routine in all cases. Thigh bone (femur) is the ideal bone to be sent for chemical analysis. It is packed, labelled and despatched to the chemical examiner's laboratory. Drowning can also be proved by doing a diatom test. The marrow from the sternum or a long bone is taken for this test and is done in the chemical examiners laboratory, forensic medicine departments and forensic science laboratories.

### Establishing the Identity of the Skeleton

It is a difficult task to pinpoint the identity of the individual. If dental or bony peculiarities are detected and identified by the relatives beyond doubt, part of the problem is solved. Irregularities of the teeth, extractions, filling and other dental work are some of the helpful features. Tobacco smoking and chewing will impart staining to the teeth. Recent fractures, prostheses, diseases and atrophy of the bone, etc. may sometimes help in establishing the identity.

### SUPERIMPOSITION TECHNIQUES

### Photographic Superimposition

Photographic superimposition can be attempted to establish the identity, provided a recent photograph of the missing person is available. This is based on the principle that the shape of the face is related to the bony contours of the facial part of skull. Life size enlargement of the photograph of the face is copied on a transparent dispositive (cine) film. This is superimposed on the life size enlargement of the photograph of the skull copied on another film. To find out the life size of the face, reference objects like spectacles, patterns in clothes, etc. seen in the original photograph should be still available. The negative of the original photograph is mounted on an enlarger and the photograph is enlarged to such an extent that the measurements of the original reference object tallied with those seen in the enlarged photograph of the missing person. For example, in the photograph of the missing person, the distance between two button holes is 1 cm. The same shirt is recovered and the distance between the two button holes is measured. If the distance is 10 cm the negative should be enlarged to such an extent that in the

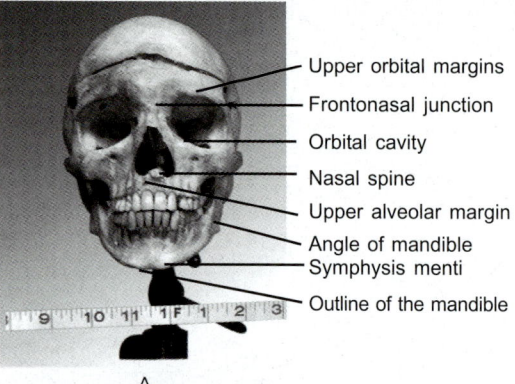

Upper orbital margins
Frontonasal junction
Orbital cavity
Nasal spine
Upper alveolar margin
Angle of mandible
Symphysis menti
Outline of the mandible

A

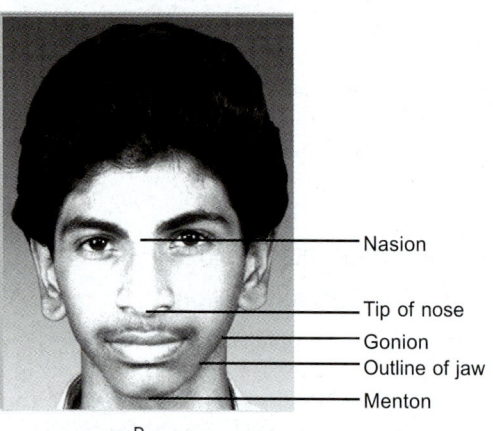

Nasion

Tip of nose
Gonion
Outline of jaw
Menton

B

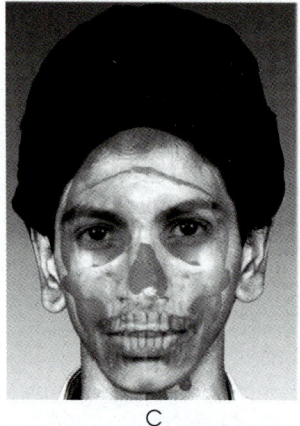

C

**Figs 9.9 A to C:** Photgraphic superimposition (A. Skull of the deceased, B. Photograph of the missing person, C. Superimposed photograph)

enlarged photographs, the distance between the two button holes is 10 cm (Figs 9.9A to C).

If no reference object is available, life size enlargement can also be made by taking the interpupillary distance as a reference measurement. Interpupillary distance is determined by measuring the distance between the midpoints of the orbital cavities of the skull. Midpoint can be found out by drawing outlines and diagonals in the image of the orbital cavities in a life size paper print of the photograph of skull. The photograph of the face is enlarged according to the interpupillary distance thus found out. Average interpupillary distance in human beings is 7 cm. The skull and mandible are mounted on a stand giving appropriate tilt similar to the tilt of the face in the photograph. The skull and mandible are photographed with a scale. That negative is enlarged to life size using the scale as the reference object. When these two photographs are superimposed, anatomical landmarks should correspond to anthropological landmarks (Box 9.1).

**Box 9.1:** Anatomical landmarks and corresponding anthropological points

- Eyeballs should be within the orbital cavities.
- 'Nasion' should correspond to the frontonasal junction.
- 'Menton' should correspond to symphysis menti.
- Nasal spine should be above the tip of nose
- Eyebrows should correspond to upper orbital margins.
- Upper alveolar margin should be just below the tip of the nose.
- 'Gonion' should correspond to angle of mandible.
- Outline of the mandible should be congruous with the outline of jaw, granting due allowance to the thickness of soft tissues.

When all these points agree, it can be assumed that the skull belongs to the person in the photograph. This is a good corroborative evidence accepted by the Hon. Supreme Court. However, a negative result is more conclusive. This technique is done in the forensic science laboratory. For this, the skull and mandible, a recent photograph of the missing person and reference objects, if any, should be despatched to these institutions.

## Video Superimposition

There is another method of conducting super-imposition with the help of a video system consisting of two video cameras, a monitor and a videomixer. One camera is directed at the skull and the other directed at the photograph of the face. The skull is fixed with the same orientation of the face in the photograph. This can be achieved by fixing it on a rotatable universal stand or on a cork ring placed on the floor. The photograph is also placed parallel to the skull. Both images are projected on a monitor placed near the skull. In this position, adjustments of the position of the skull can be made. By performing a series of 'blending, fading and sweeping' the photograph and the skull image are superimposed and analysed for conformity. Vertical, horizontal and diagonal sweeps are performed for analysing the superimposition. Point by point comparison of the anatomical and anthropological landmarks is possible by this method. Video superimposition is an exclusionary method rather than one of positive identification. However, in the presence of other evidences, this technique will provide good corroborative evidence.

## Computer-assisted Superimposition

At present, computer-assisted superimposition has become popular with the advancement of computer technology. The basic procedure is to digitise the skull and facial photograph using a computer with suitable software and then to compare the two images morphologically by image processing. Establishing a scale for the digitised skull image is performed by converting the actual measurement between the anthro-pological landmarks into the number of pixels in the monitor. For assessing the anatomical consis-tency between the digitised skull and face, the distance between the anatomical and anthro-pological landmarks and the tissue thickness are measured by means of pair dots by the computer mouse. The software allows for fade in and fade outs, wiping and sweeping the face and skull in a vertical or horizontal plane for comparing them. Experimental studies have proved that a positive opinion can be given if both frontal and lateral

photographs are compared with the skull. But it is not possible to get two such photographs in all cases. If the anterior teeth are present in the skull and images of the same are visible in the photo-graph, a positive comparison of these will provide definite consistency between the skull of the missing person and his photograph (Figs 9.10A and B).

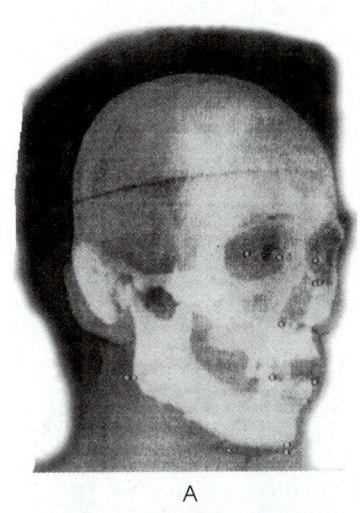

A

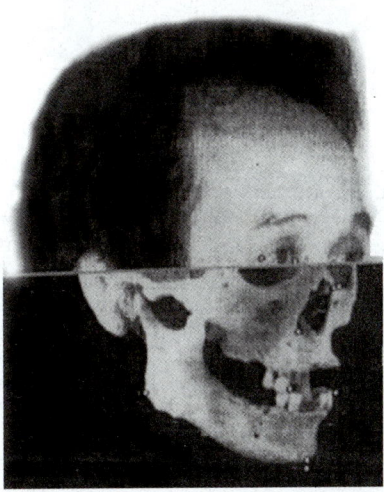

B

**Figs 9.10 A and B:** Computer-assisted superimposition—A. Total superimposition of digitised skull and photograph, B. Horizontal sweep of facial image over the skull. The dots represent the anatomical and anthropological landmarks (*Courtesy: Yoshino and Seto*)

## RECONSTRUCTION OF FACE FROM SKULL

### Sculptural Reconstruction

If a recent photograph of the deceased is not available, superimposition cannot be performed. In that case, the face can be reconstructed from the skull and mandible. This is also based on the principle that the shape of the face depends upon the shape of facial bones and mandible. Though, eyes, ears and nose are individualistic, shape of the face is the basis of personal identity. Depths of tissues at 15 important anatomical points on the face are determined from dead bodies of both sexes.

According to average thickness of tissues at various points on the face, clay or paper pulp is applied on the skull and mandible. The face thus reconstructed will have close resemblance to the actual face of the deceased (Figs 9.11A to G). The shape of the nose, ears and hair style are not based on scientific data. These factors are not relevant, as the shape of the face is the most important aspect to fix the identity. Even if those factors are not congruous with the actual shape and size, acquaintances of the deceased will be able to identify the reconstructed face as that of the deceased. However, there are norms to calculate the size and shape of these features.

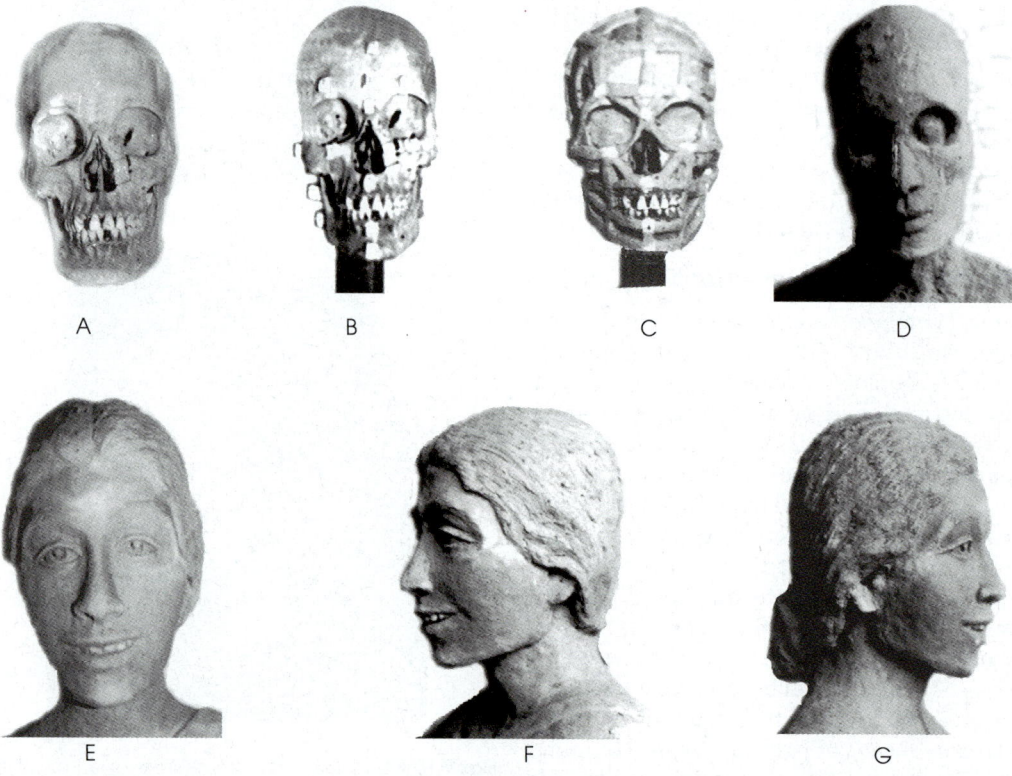

A   B   C   D

E   F   G

**Figs 9.11 A to G:** Sculptural reconstruction of face: A. Skull of the deceased—frontal view, B. Blocks having the same thickness of tissues fixed on facial landmarks, C. Blocks of paper pulp connected by bridging with the same material, D. The gaps filled with paper pulp and face is reconstructed, E. Face is reconstructed by including eyes, nose, ears and lips. Hair style is purely imagination of the artist. The picture reveals the prominent upper central incisor teeth, F. Left profiles, G. Right profile

## Two-dimensional Method

The first step is to take a life size picture of the skull in both frontal and lateral views using a digital camera. A scale is kept by the side of the skull. This will be a useful reference object for enlarging the image of the skull to life size. The picture is captured in a computer. Facial thickness can be marked on the picture of the skull at known landmarks. These marked dots are connected to each other to make a general outline of the face. The face is drawn from this image using suitable computer software like Coral draw, photoshop, etc. (Figs 9.12A to C). Suitable modifications are made according to age, sex, race, etc. Another method is to take a paper print of the life size image of skull and drawing the face manually according to tissue thickness.

## Computerised Facial Reconstruction Three-dimensional Method

There are several methods of computerised three dimensional (3D) facial reconstruction which are faster and more accurate than the traditional plastic methods using plasticine or modelling clay. The basic procedure is to capture a 3D image of the skull using a laser scanner and computer. Using a predefined set of tissue thicknesses and the facial reconstruction software, the face is reconstructed.

Before attempting the reconstruction, a general assessment of the skull for sex, age and race is made. The skull is placed on a rotating platform which is rotated through 360° under computer control (Fig 9.13). A low power, low intensity thin laser beam is used for scanning the skull. The skull

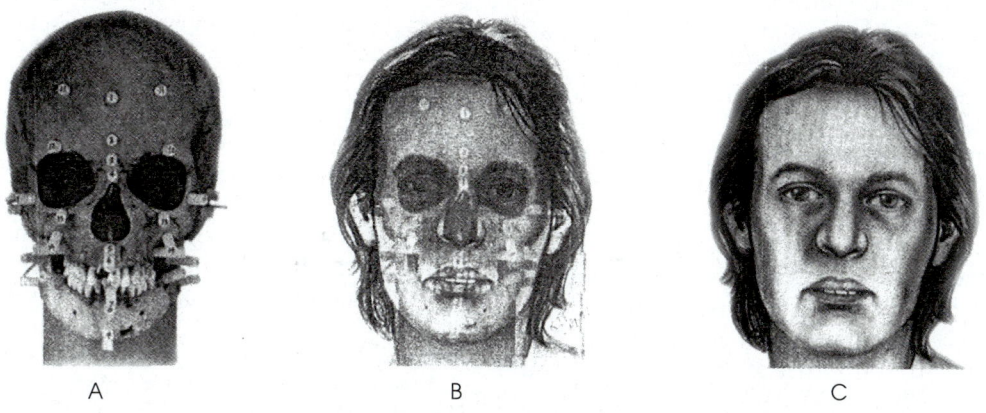

**Figs 9.12 A to C:** Two-dimensional facial reconstruction: A. Life size image of skull fixed with tissue depth markers, B. Drawing the facial features according to tissue thickness, C. Completed drawing of face (*Courtesy:* Karen T Taylor)

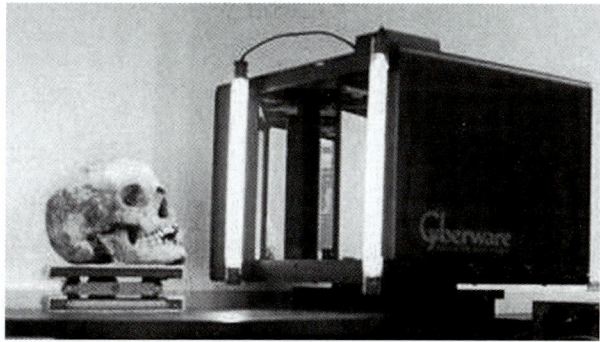

**Fig. 9.13:** Laser scanner and computer work station. The skull is placed on a rotating platform and scanned by a laser scanner

profiles are captured by a video camera. The data from the scanner is stored in the form of a 'Laser scan multiple' file. These measurements are converted to coordinates by the special software. The software is capable of viewing the skull and face, position the corresponding landmarks on them and perform a reconstruction. Associated with each landmark, is a set of tissue thicknesses taken from subjects. To make a database of tissue thickness, CT scan, MRI scan, ultrasound scan, etc. are used. The soft tissue thicknesses are represented as lines projecting from the landmarks. Forty anthropological and anatomical landmarks are used.

The next stage is the selection of facial template from the database of faces. A face with standard average features is chosen. Landmarks are placed on the face which correspond to those of the skull. The relative position and distance between these points will be the tissue thickness chosen. The next process is to move every point on the original face to a new position.

Using a 3D transformation termed a warp. The warp is then applied to every point on the original face, producing the reconstructed face. The skull can be superimposed to find out whether there is proper alignment. The major problem with the reconstruction process is to add eyes, ears, lips, nose and hair style. These features are imported from a police identikit system such as CD-fit or E-fit. The features are added according to the sex, age, race, etc. If any information regarding the appearance of the

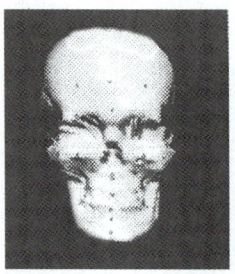 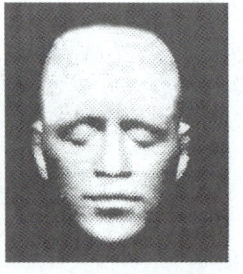

|  A  |  B  |

**Figs 9.14A and B:** 3D reconstruction of face: A. Digitised images of skull, B. Reconstructed face (*Courtesy:* Vanezis et al)

person is available, similar characteristics can be added (Figs 9.14A and B).

One of the advantages of computerised facial reconstruction is the speed with which it can be conducted. Sculptural plastic reconstruction of the face needs lot of time and attention. Picture of the reconstructed face can be published in papers with available data on physical features and relevant information about the case. Relatives, friends or acquaintances of the deceased will be able to identify the face and provide clues to the investigators.

## DIRECTIONS TO THE INVESTIGATING OFFICER

When an unknown dead body is highly decomposed and skeletonised, all efforts should be taken to establish the identity of the deceased. Clothing and personal belongings should be removed and preserved for further examination and identification. When it is difficult to remove and transport highly decomposed bodies, the doctor concerned may be requested to conduct autopsy at site. Necessary facilities may be arranged. But it is always better to transport the body to a well-equipped mortuary for autopsy. A large thick plastic sheet may be tucked underneath the body by rolling the body on to its side. Then it becomes easy to lift the body using the plastic sheet. The body may be foul smelling and covered with flies and maggots. Never spray any deodorant or insecticide on the body. It can interfere with the chemical analysis of body fluids and viscera.

If skeletal remains are discovered, services of a forensic pathologist is required. Only a forensic specialist will be able to examine the set of bones and furnish opinion regarding the sex, age and stature of the deceased. When a body buried long since is exhumed, it will be a difficult task to retrieve all the bones except with the help of an expert. From the skull, pelvis, mandible and few long bones sex, age and stature can be identified. But sometimes valuable clues which can throw light on identity and cause of death may be obtained if all the bones are available for examination. If the forensic pathologist is not available, a local government doctor may be requested to assist in the collection of skeletal remains and conduct a preliminary examination. The doctor can make an inventory of the bones collected and forward the materials to the forensic pathologist for detailed examination. The bones can be put in a plastic cadaver bag and transported to the specialist along with a copy of the inventory.

During investigation, if the investigating officer has come to the conclusion that the skeletal remains could be that of a missing person, he has to ascertain the following facts with the help of the Forensic specialist:

1. Whether the sex, age and stature of the missing person tally with that of the skeleton?
2. Whether the time since death ascertained from the skeletal remains tallies with the missing of the person?
3. Are their any dental peculiarities which could be recognised by relatives?
4. Are there any bony peculiarities, deformities, diseases or injuries which could help in identifying the missing person?

If there are positive findings, the next step is to conduct special investigations to establish that the skeletal remains could be that of the deceased. Photographic/video/computerised superimposition can be conducted, if a recent photograph of the missing person is available. The technique is done in the state forensic science laboratory. If no recent photograph is available, plastic reconstruction of face from the skull can be attempted. At present, 2 D and 3 D computerised facial reconstruction of face from skull is possible.

If there are no obvious signs of violence in the skeleton, a long bone like thigh bone (femur) may be sent for chemical analysis. Heavy metal poisons like lead, mercury, arsenic, etc. can be detected from the bones. Diatom test can be done from the bone marrow to prove death due to drowning.

To establish identity by DNA typing can be done and compared with the DNA profile of parents, children and siblings of the deceased. Marrow, tooth pulp, hair with roots, soft tissues, etc. can be utilised for isolating DNA.

**Proforma 9.1:** Sample Certificate of Examination of Skeletal Remains

Department of Forensic Medicine                                No 12/ML/07
Medical College, Thiruvananthapuram                            Dt 20-10-2007

### Medicolegal Report

Reference: Requisition no Cr 156/07 from Circle Inspector of Police, Kulathupuzha, dated 12/10/2007

Material objects brought by police constable no 2345

Date and time of examination: Commenced from 13-10-2007 and concluded on 18-10-2007

1. History of the case: Skeletal remains were recovered from the Sankili Forest, Kulathupuzha
2. Number of bones — inventory:
   a. Skull -1
   b. Pelvis -1
   c. Humerus — Left and Right
   d. Femur — Left and Right
3. Description of individual bones
   a. Skull — showed human male features, total teeth — 32, permanent, stained yellow, skull sutures fused inside, started fusion outside. There was a depressed fracture 8 × 2 cm obliquely placed on the left parietal bone — edges of the fractured bone showed infiltration of blood.
   b. Pelvis — showed human male features. All ossification centres were fused. The sacral vertebrae were fused. The heads of two thigh bones articulated well with the sockets (acetabulum) of the hipbone (pelvis).
   c. Humerus (Lt & Rt) — showed human male features
   d. Femur (Lt & Rt) — showed human male features. There was irregular thickening of the shaft of left femur, 10 cm above its lower end (evidence of a healed fracture)
4. Stature: Stature was calculated using Karl Pearson's formula and the result was 168 cm (+/- 3)
5. All the bones were devoid of soft tissues and emitting foul smell
6. No duplication of bones. No discrepancy of sex, age and articulation

Right femur was sent for chemical analysis to exclude poisoning. Diatoms test was conducted and the result was negative.

*Contd...*

*Contd...*

### Opinion

Based on the above findings, I am of opinion that all the bones could belong to:

1. A human male
2. Aged about 35–45 years
3. Height could be 168 +/-3 cm
4. Time of death could be minimum six months prior to this date
5. Cause of death could be a blunt injury of head which resulted in fracture of skull. It is highly probable that the brain could have sustained fatal injuries.
6. The following identifying peculiarities were noted
    a. The teeth were stained yellow, probably due to smoking
    b. The deceased could have sustained a fracture of the shaft of left thigh bone 1–2 months prior to his death.

Thiruvananthapuram  
Date 20-10-2007

Signature........................................  
Designation.....................................

Forwarded to The Subdivisional Magistrate, Kottarakkara

Copy to The Circle Inspector of Police, Kulathupuzha (The bones are kept under safe custody. Kindly depute a Police Constable for onward transmission to the Court)

# 10

# Mechanical Injuries

Injury related offences are covered by the following sections of the Indian Penal Code.

*Section 44 I.P.C:* Injury—The word 'injury' denotes any harm whatever illegally caused to any person, in body, mind, reputation or property.

*Section 349 I.P.C:* Criminal force—If any person by his bodily power or by disposing any substance or by inducing any animal uses force to cause fear, annoyance or injury to another person is said to commit criminal force.

*Section 351 I.P.C:* Assault—Whoever makes any gesture, or any preparation intending or knowing it to be likely that such gesture or preparation will cause any person present to apprehend that he who makes that gesture or preparation is about to use criminal force to that person is said to commit an assault.

*Section 319 I.P.C:* Hurt—Whoever causes bodily pain, disease or infirmity to any person is said to commit hurt.

*Section 320 I.P.C:* Grievous hurt—The following kinds of hurt are designated as grievous:

| | |
|---|---|
| **First** | Emasculation |
| **Secondly** | Permanent privation of the sight of either eye |
| **Thirdly** | Permanent privation of the hearing of either ear |
| **Fourthly** | Privation of any member (organ or limb) or joint |
| **Fifthly** | Destruction or permanent impairing of the powers of any member or joint |
| **Sixthly** | Permanent disfigurement of the head or face |
| **Seventhly** | Fracture or dislocation of a bone or tooth |
| **Eighthly** | Any hurt which endangers life or which causes the sufferer to be during the space of 20 days in severe bodily pain, or unable to follow his ordinary pursuits. |

*Section 324 I.P.C:* Voluntarily causing hurt by dangerous weapons or other means.

*Section 326 I.P.C:* Voluntarily causing grievous hurt by dangerous weapons or other means.

*Section 336 I.P.C:* Rash and negligent act endangering life or personal safety of others.

*Section 337 I.P.C:* Rash or negligent act causing hurt endangering life or personal safety of others.

*Section 338 I.P.C:* Rash or negligent act causing grievous hurt endangering life or personal safety of others.

## MECHANISM OF WOUNDING

Medicolegally, wound means injury inflicted by mechanical force upon living tissues. Physical laws are involved in the causation of mechanical injuries.

"Every object remains in its state of rest or uniform motion until that state is disrupted by an external force"—Newton's first law.

Similarly wounds are produced when a moving object changes the state of rest of tissues or when the motion of tissues is changed by meeting a force of resistance. When force is applied to any part of the human body, the cellular components of the tissues are set in motion and are replaced from their original position resulting in a discontinuity or wound. Nature and severity of the wound depend upon the properties of the injuring force such as its velocity, mass, shape, etc. as well as the peculiarities of the area affected such as its elasticity, toughness, etc.

The formula, **Force = Mass × 1/2 Velocity²**, plays a crucial role in the mechanism of wounding. If a stone weighing one kilogram is pressed against the head, no injuries will be produced. But the same stone thrown against the head at a velocity of 10 km/hour may fracture the skull. In the place of the stone, if a tomato is thrown even at 50 km/hour nothing will happen to the head. When a car moving at a low velocity hits a person, it produces more severe injuries than a paper weight moving at the same velocity. But a pointed object having low velocity can penetrate the tissues. A rough and hard object can produce more harm than a smooth object. Whatever be the nature of the agent, adequate mechanical force applied to tissues, can produce a wound (Fig. 10.1).

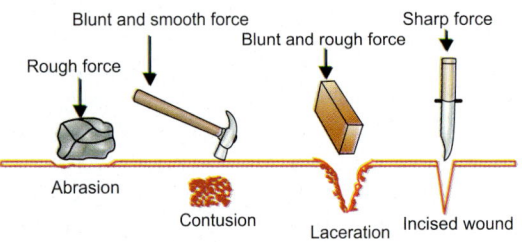

**Fig.10.1:** Causative forces of injuries

Nature of injury depends upon the area over which the force acts. This is why a narrow striking surface of a blunt weapon will produce severe injuries than one with a broad surface. The force derived from the mass and velocity concentrated on a smaller area will cause more damage to tissues. The same principle applies to the causation of incised and punctured wounds. The kinetic energy is concentrated on the sharp edge and tip of the weapon, causing incised or punctured wounds.

## CLASSIFICATION OF INJURIES

*Blunt force injuries:*   Abrasion, contusion, laceration, fracture

*Sharp force injuries:*   Incised wound, punctured wound

*Firearm injuries:*   Caused by the projectiles and fire effects of various firearms

*Explosion injuries:*   Caused by the sharpnels, explosive charge and blast effects of various explosive devices such as bombs, grenades

## BLUNT FORCE INJURIES
### Abrasion

It is an injury involving the superficial layers of skin (epidermis and/or a part of dermis) produced by a sharp or a rough object coming into forcible contact with the skin or vice versa. The mechanism of production of abrasion is shown in Fig. 10.2. Depending upon the mode of causation, abrasions can be classified as follows.

#### Scratches

These are linear abrasions caused by a sharp or pointed object passing across the skin removing the epithelial layer in its track (Fig.10.2). Fingernails, thorns or the tip of a knife can cause scratches. Direction of the infliction can be sometimes detected by the presence of heaped up epithelium in the terminal part of the scratch. Fingernail marks are seen as crescentic abrasions, if the pressure is steady as in throttling.

Rodents, ants and insects invade a dead body and produce injuries similar to an abrasion. Excoriations caused by ants are called **ant erosions**. They are seen in and around eyeballs, nostrils, ears, corners of mouth, armpits, groins, genital regions, etc.

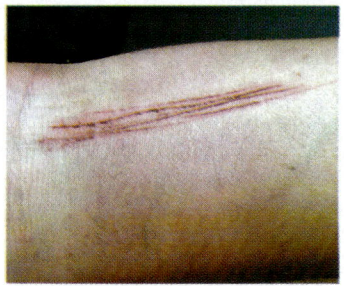

**Fig. 10.2:** Scratch abrasion

Because of the invasion of small blood vessels, blood will be seeping from these injuries, simulating antemortem injuries. But there will not be any scab formation and the exposed dermis will be pale.

### Graze Abrasion

These are abrasions produced when a hard and rough object comes into contact with the skin in a sliding or scraping fashion. These are commonly seen in the case of fall on a rough surface or when the body is dragged over a rough surface. Abraded area will show multiple linear furrows (Fig.10.3).

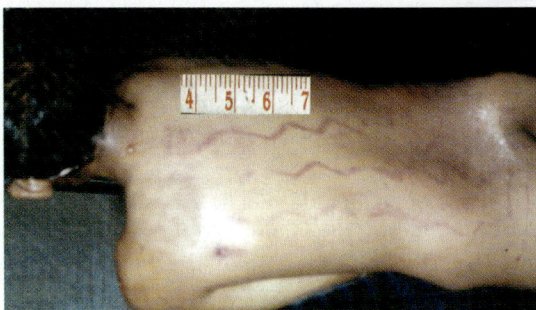

**Fig. 10.4:** Patterened pressure abrasion-tyre marks (When a patterned injury is photographed, a scale should be placed nearby)

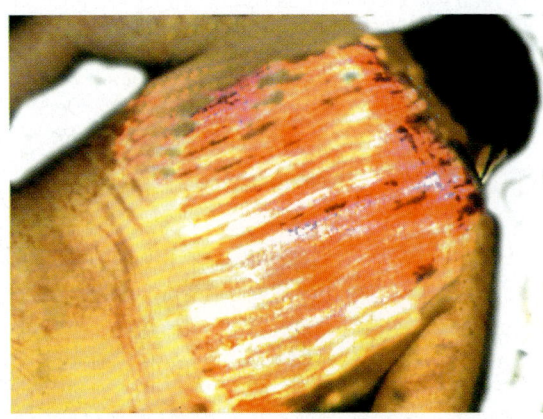

**Fig. 10.3:** Graze abrasions

### Pressure/Friction Abrasions

These are caused by crushing of the skin by a rough or hard object. The epithelium is crushed due to pressure and friction. There may be associated contusions of the area, if more force is applied. Then it is called an **abraded contusion**. The best example is a ligature mark caused by a coir or any other rough object. The abrasion having the same pattern of the agent which caused it, is called a **patterned/imprint abrasion**. In traffic accidents, the parts of the motor car which hit the victim may leave patterned abrasions/abraded contusions. A rough coir ligature can produce a patterned ligature mark. In a run over accident, tread marks of the tyres of the vehicle will be sometimes found (Fig.10.4). If the tyre is one with worn out treads, there will be pressure abrasion without any pattern. Fingernail

marks are seen as crescentic abrasions in throttling. If any patterns are detected, the exact shape and size should be recorded.

### Age of an Abrasion

A fresh abrasion will be red in colour due to oozing of blood from the injured capillaries in the exposed dermis of the skin. Over an abraded area, lymph and blood dry up and a red scab is formed within 12–24 hours. The red scab will change to brown after 2 days and will remain for 7 days unless it is removed forcibly. The colour of the scab may change from brown to black during the last phase. In the normal course, it will fall off by itself in 7–10 days time, leaving a pale area, which will become normal in a month's time. No scar is produced.

### Postmortem Abrasions

Abrasions sustained after death lack the characteristic vital reactions. They will be dark in colour and the texture will be leather like. There will not be any scab formation. If the superficial layer of skin is absent, the dermis will be pale. This type of postmortem injuries are sustained when a dead body is dragged on a rough surface.

### Medicolegal Importance

Abrasions are usually seen in accidents and assaults. Abrasions indicate that the area had come into contact with a rough object or surface. If they are patterned, the nature of the object can be deduced. Site of abrasion is very important especially in case of throttling, sexual offences, etc.

Scratch abrasions having crescentic shapes in the neck region may be indicative of throttling. Similarly abrasions on the face, breasts, genitalia or thighs may be indicative of sexual assault. Restraining a person can produce similar abrasions on wrists or ankles.

In case of an assault, it is necessary to examine the fingernails of the victim and the accused. Nail marks may be present both on the victim and the accused. There is a possibility of retaining the epithelium under the nails. The nails should be carefully clipped with a clean nail cutter and preserved in clean bottles or polythene bags. Extreme caution should be exercised to prevent injury to the finger as bleeding will vitiate the results. Fingernailbeds can be scraped or swabbed to collect foreign DNA material. The swab used for scraping should also be sent for examination. Microscopy and DNA typing can be done to find out the nature and origin of the material.

Ant erosions, skin lesions like scabies, psoriasis, etc. may simulate abrasions. Scratching of skin by self can produce scratch abrasions if the person is having long fingernails. These should not be mistaken as signs of violence.

### Contusion (Bruise)

Contusion is an injury in which the force of a blunt impact is transmitted through the skin to the underlying tissues with sufficient intensity to disrupt the walls of blood vessels and to cause interstitial bleeding (Figs 10.5 and 10.6). There will not be destruction of epidermis, if the object which caused the injury is smooth and blunt. But if the object is rough and the force applied is more, apart from the contusion, the skin will be abraded also. This is an abraded contusion. The interstitial bleeding is superficial and is visible through the skin and so a fresh contusion will be reddish in colour. Bruises may also be deep seated. An external force can cause bruising of internal organs. A kick or blow on the abdomen need not cause contusion of abdominal wall, but contusions of liver, spleen or intestines can occur. Vascular and lax areas bruise easily. Women, children and the elderly bruise easily even by minor force due to increased adiposity and fragility of blood vessels.

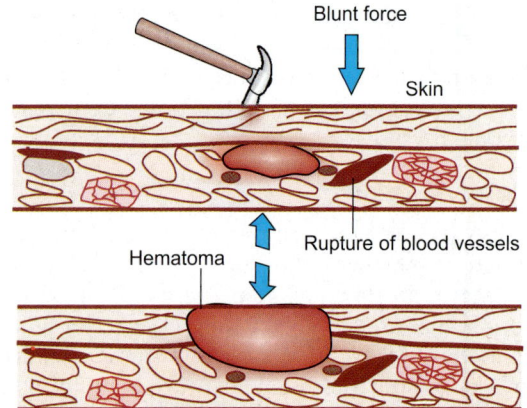

**Fig. 10.5:** Mechanism of bruising. Blunt impact ruptures blood vessels and extravasated blood forms a hematoma

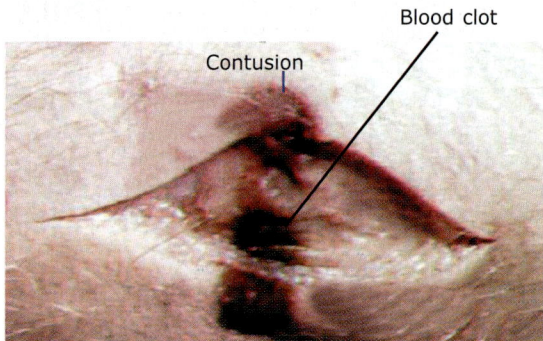

**Fig. 10.6:** Contusion — The area is incised to demonstrate the blood clot in the tissues

### Patterned Bruises

Sometimes the shape and extent of a bruise will correspond to the shape of the object which caused it. A hit with a shoe can produce an imprint of the sole of the shoe. Study of the pattern will be helpful in identifying the object which caused it. In blunt assaults, nature of the weapon can be inferred from the shape of the bruise. Reconstruction of a traffic accident is possible where a number of patterned injuries are likely to be present on the body of the victim (Figs 10.7 and 10.8).

**Bite mark** is either a patterned abrasion or a contusion. Sometimes a bite may cause laceration

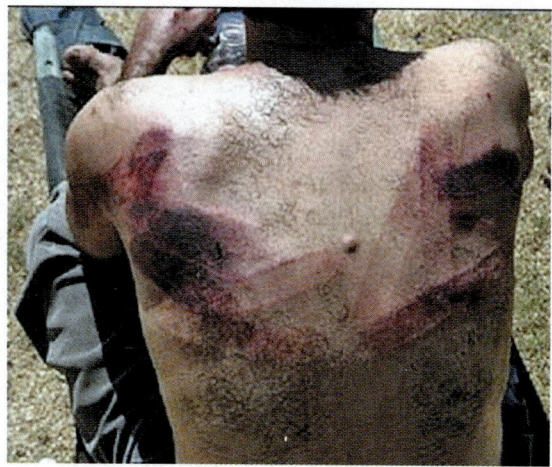

Fig. 10.7: Patterned contusions (Tramline bruises)

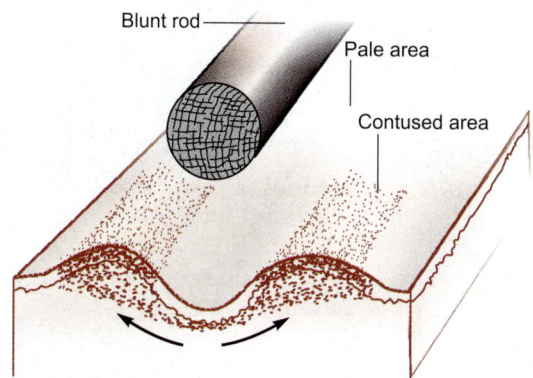

Fig. 10.8: Mechanism of production of Tramline bruises. (When contusions are inflicted by a blunt rod, the area of contact with the rod is dented inwards. Extravasated blood is displaced sideways. The gap between the bruised lines corresponds to the width of the weapon)

and loss of tissue at regions like fingers, nose or ears. Bite marks are inflicted during an assault offensively by the accused on the victim or defensively by the victim on the accused. Bite marks may be seen on inanimate objects like fruits, cheese, etc., left at the scene by the perpetrator. Bite mark will provide evidence to identify the accused.

Bite mark can be photographed with a scale (Fig. 10.9), enlarged to actual size and compared with the biting pattern of the dental cast impression

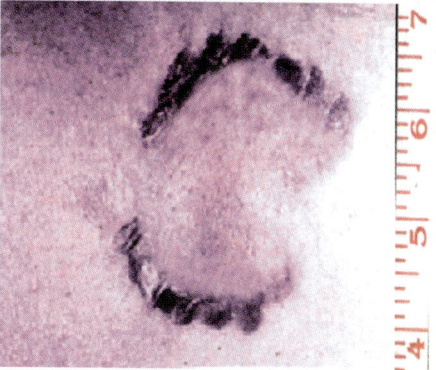

Fig. 10.9: Bite mark photographed with a scale

of the suspect. The diapositive transparent photo of the biting pattern of the dental impression is superimposed on the photograph of the bite mark pattern and compared. Recently, digital imaging of the bite marks and rendering it as a 3D data set is possible. The image is measurable to high precision and accuracy in three dimensions. This can be accurately compared with the measurements of the cast of the dentition of the suspect. Sterile swabs are to be applied to the bite mark and the swabs tested for ABO grouping or DNA analysis.

Blow to the head may result in the seepage of blood into the left eyelids. This condition is called **black eye** (Fig.10.10). Other causes for a black eye include a direct blow to the orbit or fracture of skull with leakage of blood from the coverings of brain through the orbital roof.

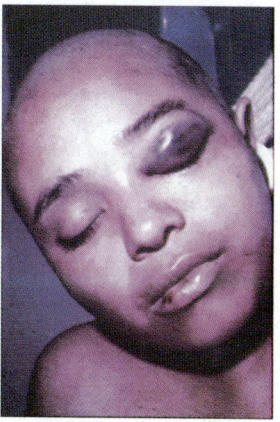

Fig. 10.10: Black eye

## Age of a Contusion

The extravasated blood in a contusion will disintegrate. The haemoglobin will undergo conversion to several pigments. A fresh contusion will be red in colour. The colour will change to blue in a day (reduced hemoglobin). It becomes blue black to brown (hemosiderin) in 2 to 3 days, green (hematoidin) in 5–7 days and yellow (bilirubin) in 8–10 days. The tissue can also be examined microscopically to note the changes for assessing the age.

## Artificial Bruises

These are produced by applying vesicating fluids like the juice of marking nut. This can be differentiated by the presence of vesicles in the margin of the false bruise. Some creepers having spinous processes in their stem are also used to produce artificial bruises. This is done by people for incriminating others or to charge a counter-case in serious crimes.

## Lacerated Wounds

Laceration is a split or tear caused by the effect of excessive stretching, crushing, grinding or compressing of the tissues (Fig. 10.11). A hard and rough object can cause laceration. A blunt object (Figs 10.12A to C) can also cause a split laceration especially in an area where the bone is superficial as in the head, shin or knee. Here the split injury will look like an incised wound. Hence it is called **apparent incised wound**. It is often possible to go wrong in distinguishing it. The edges will be irregular and on close scrutiny, bridges of tissues can be seen in the floor of the wound. Moreover, there will be bruising surrounding the edges. Beating on the head with a baton (lathi) can produce a split laceration which will look like an incised wound caused by a chopper (Figs 10.13 and 10.14). A hand lens may be used while examining the injury.

Lacerated wounds are liable to infection especially by anaerobic organisms because of the presence of crushed and dead tissues in the edges of the wound. Therefore, a lacerated wound should be kept clean and dead tissues should be removed (defibribridement). Prophy-

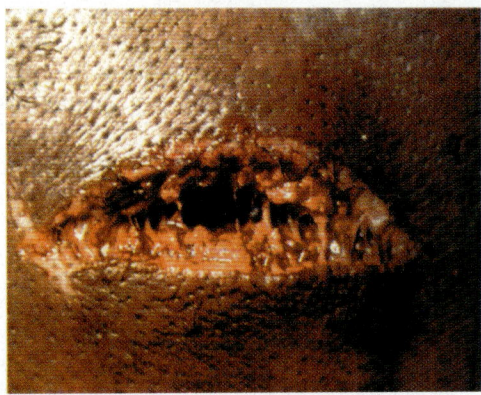

**Fig. 10.11:** Lacerated wound (The injury is caused by a blunt and rough force. The edges of the wound are irregular. Bridges of tissues are seen acrosss the edges)

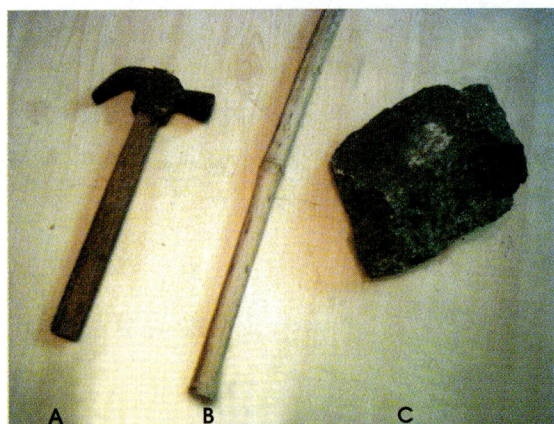

**Figs 10.12A to C:** Blunt weapons: A. Hammer, B. Baton, C. Stone

laxis against tetanus (injection of tetanus toxoid) and gas gangrene (antigas gangrene serum) should be given. When they heal, prominent scars are produced.

## Stretch Lacerations/Grinding Compressions (Tears)

When the force is of the nature of a grinding compression, the skin is torn due to over stretching (Fig. 10.15). Skin of one margin of the wound is relatively clean split, while there will be fraying and avulsion of skin of the other edge. Skin is ripped free from the subcutaneous tissues (Fig. 10.16). This

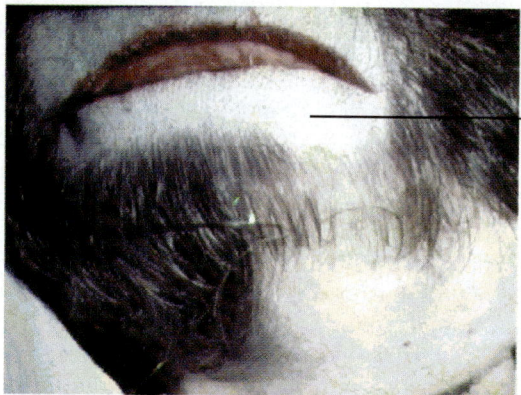

**Fig.10.13:** Split laceration of scalp (apparent incised wound. It looks like an incised wound caused by a heavy cutting weapon. But a close scrutiny will reveal irregular edges and bridges of tissues in the floor of the wound)

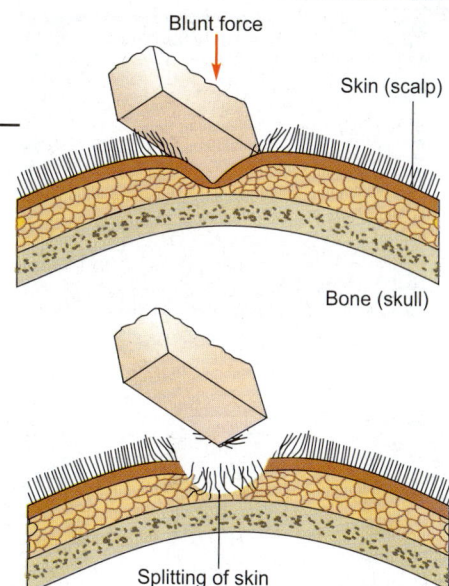

**Fig. 10.14:** Mechanism of production of split laceration (Blunt force causes splitting of the skin between the weapon and bone)

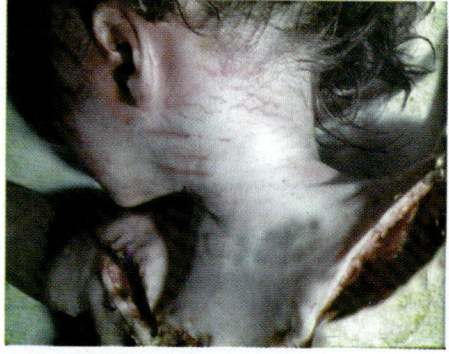

**Fig.10.15:** Stretch laceration—vehicle run over— tyre marks can also be seen

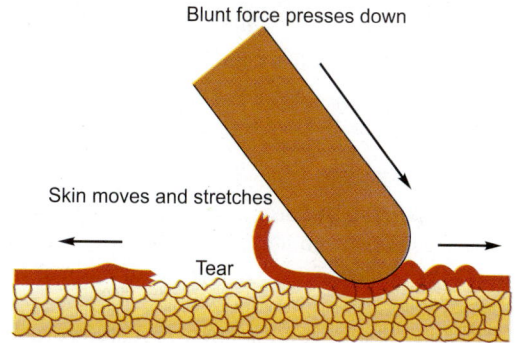

**Fig. 10.16:** Mechanism of tearing/stretch laceration

type of lacerations is seen in bodies run over by a heavy vehicle.

### Laceration of Internal Organs

A blunt force on the chest and abdomen can cause laceration of internal organs because of compressive force propagated internally. Even in severe blunt impacts, external injuries may be absent or minimal. Kicking or fisting on the abdomen can result in the rupture of liver (Fig. 10.17), spleen or intestine. Needless to say that these injuries can result in serious internal bleeding and death.

### Fracture

A fracture is a mechanically produced disruption of the continuity of a bone. The fracture is called *simple* or closed (Fig. 10.18B), if it is not visible on the surface. It is called *compound* or open, if the fractured bone is exposed by penetrating the tissues and skin(Fig. 10.18C). A minor force can cause a fracture. External force can be transmitted (Figs 10.18A to C) to a distant point and produce a fracture. For example, falling from a height and

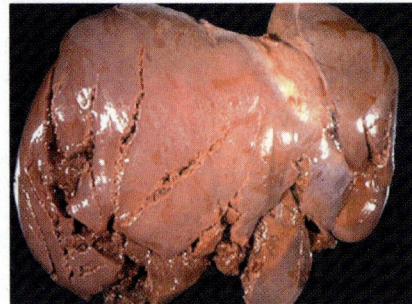

**Fig. 10.17:** Lacerations of liver

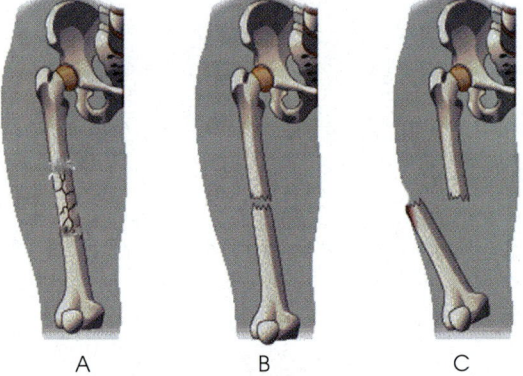

A                    B                    C

**Figs 10.18A to C:** Different types of fractures: A. Comminuted, B. Simple, C. Compound

landing on the heels can cause ring fracture of the base of skull as the force is transmitted through the vertebral column. A fall on the outstretched hands can cause fracture of the distal ends of the bones of forearm. Spontaneous fractures can occur in diseases of the bones such as osteoporosis, osteomalacia, Paget's disease, etc. *Greenstick fracture* is an incomplete fracture involving only part of the distance across a bone shaft, with bending or crushing of the bone. Incomplete fractures are found mostly in young children, whose bones are resilient. If the bone breaks into fragments due to dissipation of a large amount of force, it is called *comminuted fracture* (Fig.10.18).

Common symptoms of a fracture are severe pain in the fracture site, tenderness, and swelling with some degree of deformity. Fracture can be detected by taking an X-ray of the affected area. Compound fractures are liable to infection. If the

broken segments are not displaced, they are aligned by external manipulation.

This procedure is called closed reduction. If proper alignment cannot be achieved in this way, an operation is usually performed, and the fragments are joined with screws, nuts, nails, wires or metal plates. This is called open reduction. Once aligned, the fractured limb is immobilised by applying a plaster cast. New bone tissue is formed between the fractured ends and union takes place. Complete union will take place in 30 to 45 days.

A fracture of long bones such as femur can cause excessive haemorrhage and death. Even 2 liters of blood can collect in the thigh from a fracture of the shaft of femur and the diameter of the thigh will increase only by 2 cm. A fracture sustained during life can be distinguished easily by the presence of bleeding, infiltration of blood into the fractured ends and surrounding tissues. If the person survives, evidence of repair like callus formation, etc. will also be seen. Fracture of bones can result in fatal complications like pulmonary embolism, fat embolism, etc.

## SHARP FORCE INJURIES

### Incised Wounds

An incised wound is a clean division of tissues by a sharp cutting instrument like a knife, razor, dagger, etc. (Figs 10.19A and B). The wound is spindle-shaped with clean cut edges (Fig. 10.20). The spindle shape is due to the retraction of the edges as the elastic fibres in the skin are divided. This is an antemortem feature as the elasticity of skin is lost after death. In the neck and scrotal regions, edges of an incised wound will appear to be irregular due to the retraction of special type of muscles in those regions (platysma and dartos muscles, respectively).

The mode of infliction of an incised wound is by striking, drawing or sawing action of the sharp edges of the weapon against the tissues. An incised wound has two clean cut edges and two ends. Sometimes one end may show a tailing superficial linear incised wound or a linear abrasion. This will indicate the direction of withdrawal of the weapon. The breadth has no relation to the size of the blade of the weapon. Incised wound caused

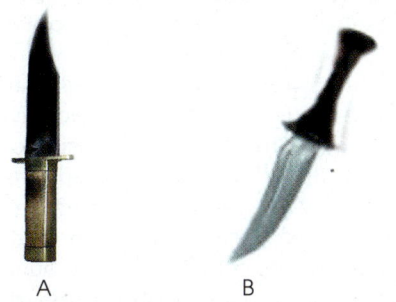

**Figs 10.19A and B:** Light cutting weapons: A. Single-edged knife, B. Dagger

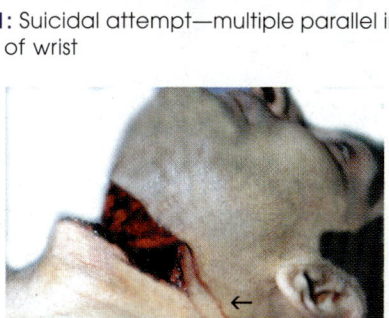

**Fig.10.21:** Suicidal attempt—multiple parallel incised wounds of wrist

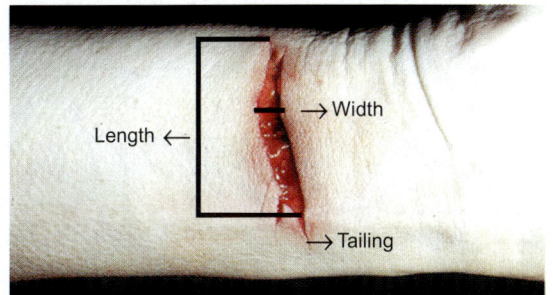

**Fig. 10. 20:** Incised wound caused by a sharp weapon

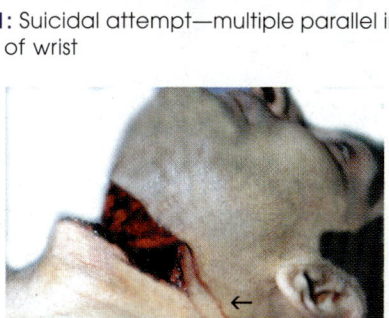

**Fig.10.22:** Suicidal cut throat injury—note the two hesitation cuts (arrows)

by a heavy cutting weapon like chopper/axe/sword may have a bevelled edge (over hanging or undermined). They are usually called **chop wounds**. These incised wounds may be deeper and can cause injury to deeper structures like bones. Most often they are homicidal.

Self-inflicted incised wounds are usually seen on the wrists (Fig. 10.21), throat (Fig. 10.22), chest and abdomen. There will be multiple, parallel, superficial cuts in those regions. They are called **hesitation cuts or tentative cuts**. The knife is used in a sawing manner. There will be several tentative incisions at the same location. In the neck, the several incisions will coalesce to form a single large wound ultimately. But the ends of the wound will show tentative cuts indicating repeated inflictions. Blood vessels and trachea will be severed. Deeper blood vessels may be spared. Death is often due to air embolism caused by entry of air through the severed jugular veins.

Following the negative pressure in the veins, air is sucked into the veins. Air reaches the right side of the heart, where it forms a foam and blocks the pulmonary arterial flow. Blood will also be inhaled, if the trachea is cut and death is caused by asphyxiation. The weapon will be present in the scene or it will be sometimes held in the hand of the deceased due to cadaveric spasm.

Homicidal cut throat injuries are usually caused by heavy cutting weapons like a chopper, sword or butcher's knife (Figs 10.23A to C). The infliction will be in a cutting manner. Homicidal cut throat injuries are also caused by sharp weapons like a razor or knife. Then the manner of infliction will be a slashing or sawing fashion. Homicidal injuries of the neck could be often single and deep (Fig. 10.24). Deeper structures may be involved. If a heavy cutting weapon is used, nicks or cuts may be seen in the neck vertebrae.

## Punctured Wounds

These are caused by a sharp-pointed object like a knife, spear, arrow, nail, etc. The skin and underlying tissues are punctured. If the depth of an incised

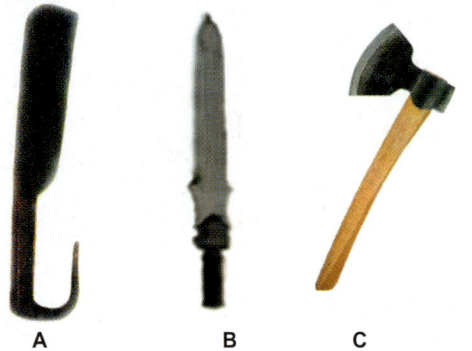

**Figs 10.23A to C:** Heavy cutting weapons A. Chopper, B. Sword C. Axe

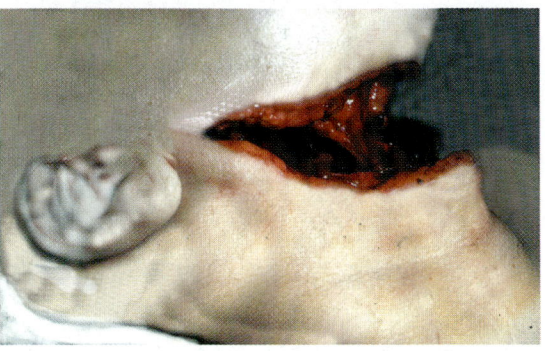

**Fig. 10.24:** Homicidal cut throat injury

correspond to the minimum depth of the wound. However, in yielding areas like abdomen, the depth of the wound can sometimes be more than the length of the blade. If a double-edged weapon is used, both ends of the wound will be clean cut (Fig.10.25). But one end will show splitting of skin, if the weapon is a single-edged one (Fig.10.26). A single-edged weapon with a pointed tip can sometimes cause a spindle-shaped wound resembling a wound caused by a double-edged weapon. A rubber tapper's knife will cause a bracket-shaped wound. A sickle can produce a stab and an adjacent incised wound.

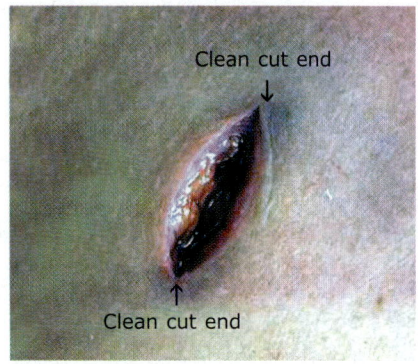

**Fig. 10.25:** Stab wound caused by double-edged knife

wound is more than its length, it is commonly termed as a stab wound or incised punctured wound.

The mode of infliction is by thrusting the weapon into the tissues. When the stab is into a body cavity, it is called incised penetrating wound. If an organ, limb or trunk is pierced through, the wound is an incised perforating wound. From an incised punctured wound, clues regarding thenature of weapon can be obtained.

The length of a stab wound can be more than the width of the blade due to a drawing action either during the initial thrust or during withdrawal, but will not be less. But owing to the retraction of muscle fibres, sometimes the length will be 2 to 3 mm less than the width of weapon. Width of the injury has no relation to the shape of the weapon as it is caused by retraction of edges. The length of the blade of the weapon will

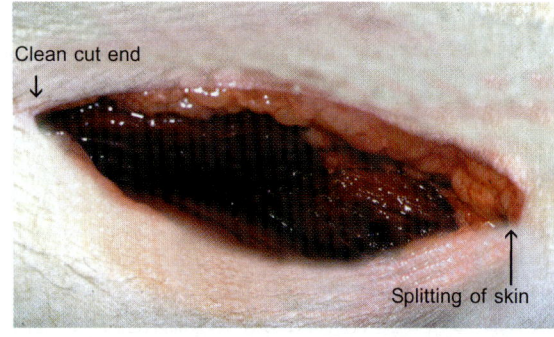

**Fig. 10.26:** Stab wound caused by single-edged knife

## Defence Wounds

Incised wounds found on the upper limbs of the victims of murder are produced during warding off an attack (Fig. 10.27) or grabbing the weapon (Fig. 10.28). These injuries are called 'defence wounds'. If the victim is in a lying posture during

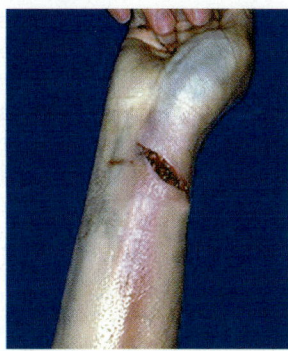

**Fig. 10.27:** Defence wound due to warding of the attack

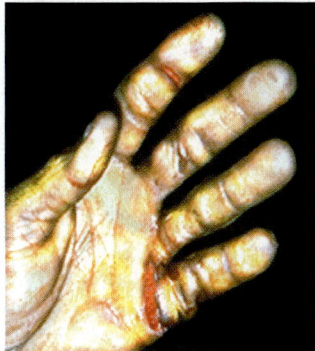

**Fig. 10.28:** Defence wounds due to grabbing the weapon

the attack, defense injuries could be seen on the lower limbs also. Besides defense injuries, superficial injuries on other parts of the body could indicate that a struggle had taken place between the victim and the assailant. Defence wounds are fabricated to substantiate a charge of homicidal assault. Usually these injuries will be accessible areas and may not be serious.

An incised penetrating wound will have a track inside the body. The track extends from the external wound to the inside of the body and will have a direction. This direction depends on the manner in which the blade of the weapon has entered the body cavity. For example, the external wound is on the middle of abdomen near umbilicus and the inferior border of right lobe of liver is injured. Now, the track of the wound is directed backwards, upwards and to the right

(Fig.10.29). This means that, the blade of the weapon on entering the abdominal cavity has travelled in this particular direction. This gives an idea as to the mode of inflicting the stab. External wound may be oblique, horizontal or vertical in placement (Fig.10.30). From this finding, the position of the plane of the blade at the time of stabbing, as well as the relative position of the accused and victim can be inferred. These findings taken together will be helpful in deducing how the weapon was held by the accused and in which way he has wielded it.

The depth of the stab wound can be more than the length of the weapon in the case of penetrating wounds into abdominal and chest cavities as these

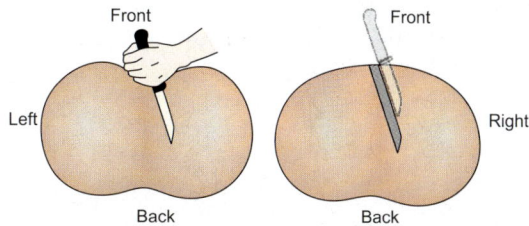

**Fig. 10.29:** Penetrating wounds into abdominal and chest cavities. Cross-section of abdomen (injury in the diagram is directed downwards, backwards and to the right)

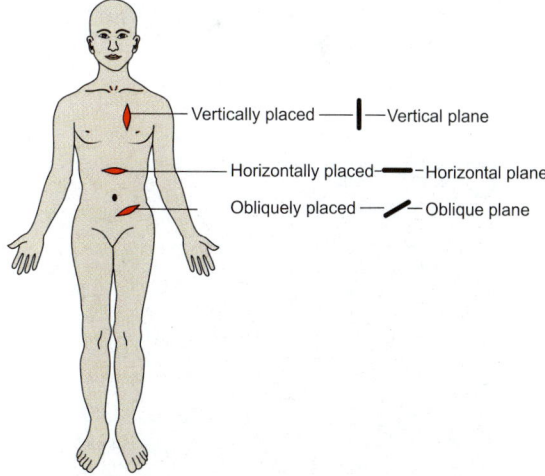

**Fig.10.30:** External injuries are described in relation to the plane of the body

are compressible areas. Ordinarily, the measurements of the wounds in the lung, pericardium and heart are not taken. When measurement is taken at the time of postmortem, the length of the injury in the collapsed lung will be less than actual. Moreover, the heart and lungs are moving organs and hence the length of the wounds will vary.

### Homicide/Suicide/Accident

Homicidal stabs can be anywhere in the body (Fig.10.31), but suicidal stabs will be in the accessible areas and usually there will be multiple ineffective hesitation stabs. Majority of the suicidal stabs are superficial and grouped together (Fig.10.32). Suicidal stabs are not uncommon. Regarding the stab wounds, an opinion as to whether it is suicidal or homicidal cannot be formed always. Medical officer should be very

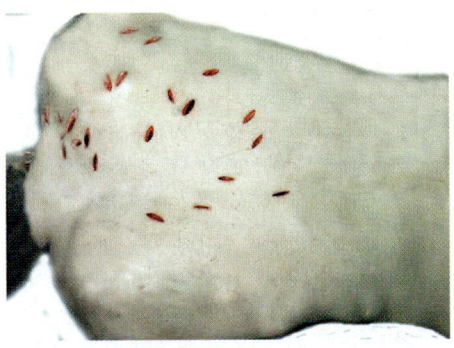

**Fig.10.31:** Homicidal stabs

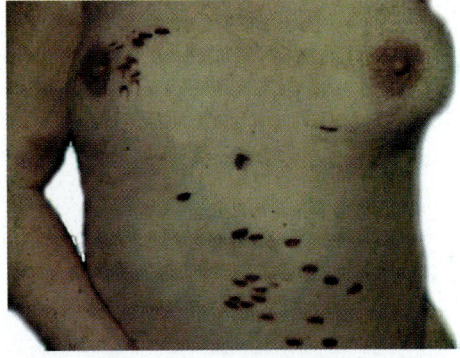

**Fig. 10.32:** Suicidal stabs

careful in forming an opinion. All stab wounds have to be considered as homicidal, unless otherwise proved. Possibility of stab wounds occurring during a scuffle between persons holding weapons cannot be excluded; but these stabs will not be deep and may have tailing ends. A deep stab wound is always caused as a result of a forcible thrust.

Accidental punctured wounds can occur by falling over sharp-pointed fixed objects; but in those cases, there will be other injuries like abrasions, contusions, etc. indicating a fall. In a murder trial very often, defence counsel will point out such possibility during cross-examination. Technical possibility of fixing a knife firmly and the victim falling over it and sustaining a stab injury is remote, the theoretical possibility, however, cannot be excluded !!

*Description of a stab wound from an autopsy certificate:*

"Incised penetrating wound 3×1 cm, horizontally placed on the right side of front of chest, 5 cm to the left of right nipple in the 3'o clock position. The inner end of the wound showed splitting of skin and outer end was cleanly cut. The chest wall was penetrated through the right 4th intercostal space. Underneath the upper lobe of right lung was penetrated through. Pericardium and wall of right ventricle were cut. Pericardial cavity contained 200 ml of blood and clots. Right chest cavity contained 1800 ml of blood. Right lung was collapsed. The direction of the track was backwards and to the left. Minimum depth was 12 cm."

From this description, the following deductions can be made:

1. Weapon used was a single-edged one.
2. Maximum width of the blade will not be more than 3 cm or 3.2 cm.
3. The blade of the weapon will have a minimum length of 12 cm.
4. A left-handed assailant could inflict this injury, if the victim is standing and facing the assailant. A right-handed assailant can inflict this injury from behind the victim.
5. The blade of the weapon was held horizontal to the body plane, it has entered the right side of

the chest, traversed backwards and to the left inside the body cavity and injured the heart.

6. It is a deep and forcible thrust and sustaining the wound in a scuffle is unlikely.
7. Injury is sufficient in the ordinary course of nature to cause death.
8. Death was not instantaneous (blood clots in pericardial sac).

## Dismemberment

The body of a victim of murder is dismembered and disposed at different places. Sometimes dismembering is done for easy transportation in a vehicle to a distant destination for disposal (Fig.10.33). Very often the aim of the accused may be to prevent the remains from being discovered and identified. In some instances, the head is severed and disposed of leaving the torso in the scene of crime, or both disposed off at different places. When one part of a dead body is received for medicolegal examination, it should be preserved anticipating the detection and recovery of other parts.

When other parts are received, the severed ends of limbs or torso should be placed in apposition and anatomical contiguity should be studied. The stature can be found out by this. Age should be estimated by examining the teeth, closure of sutures of skull and ossification data. Samples of hair, blood and other trace evidences should be collected apart from the collection of viscera for chemical analysis. In unidentified bodies, tissues, bones, teeth, hair roots, etc.

should be preserved for DNA typing. Skull and mandible should be preserved for dental identification, superimposition and reconstruction of face. Fingertips should be preserved for fingerprinting.

Postmortem dismemberment can be easily recognised. The edges of the wound will be lacking antemortem features such as bleeding, infiltration of blood into the edges of the wound and cut ends of the bones. The limbs are sometimes cut through the joints, disarticulating them. A little anatomical knowledge is needed for this manoeuvre. Butchers (and doctors!) have been involved in similar crimes. Cutting weapons like choppers, axes and swords are used for severing the limbs. Hand saws, hacksaws and electric saws have been used for cutting the bones.

## DIRECTIONS TO THE INVESTIGATING OFFICER

In the case of murder by assault with blunt or sharp weapons, the following steps may be taken during inquest:

- Photographing the body, scene, weapons and foreign materials in the scene. Close up pictures of the injuries may be taken by keeping a scale by the side.
- Record detailed description and measurement of injuries in relation to the nearest anatomical landmarks.
- Examination of the clothing in detail in the case of stab injuries. Look for corresponding tears and cuts on the clothes. Detailed description and measurements are to be recorded.
- Dry the blood-stained clothes in the shade and pack them in polythene bags.
- Loose trace materials are to be collected separately after noting the location and nature.
- Fingerprinting the dead body and the weapons.
- Preservation and photographing of foot-prints and palm-prints.
- Collection of blood stains from the scene. If there are stains in different areas in the scene, each stain should be collected and packed separately for determining the group. (It is possible that the accused also might have sustained injuries and bled in the scene.)

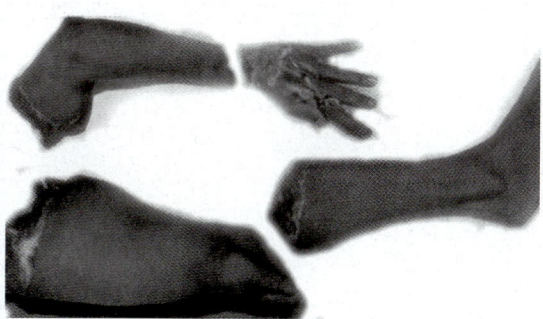

**Fig. 10.33:** Dismemberment

- Collection of all possible trace materials and foreign bodies from the scene. If there is delay in getting the service of the police sniffer dogs, the foreign materials may be kept in clean, wide mouthed glass bottles with caps, so that the scent will not be diminished or lost.
- Request the doctor to collect a sample of blood from the dead body and determine the blood group.
- Request the doctor to collect appropriate samples like blood, vaginal aspirations, tissues, hair roots, bone marrow, etc. and preserve them for DNA typing at a later date if necessary.

- Record a statement u/s 161 CrPC from the doctor regarding the nature of injuries, cause of death, mechanism of death, possible nature of weapons, probable time of death, nature of last meal, evidence of sexual intercourse (in female dead bodies), etc.
- Question the doctor again after receiving the autopsy report and recovery of the murder weapon. The investigating officer should try to correlate the medical evidence with the versions of the witnesses regarding the nature of weapon and infliction of injuries.

# 11

# Firearm and Explosion Injuries

## BALLISTICS

The study of firearms and ammunition is called ballistics. Exterior ballistics deals with the physical laws concerning the projectile. Interior ballistics is pure gunnery. Study of fire effects is known as terminal ballistics. Investigating officers should possess basic knowledge in all the branches of ballistics including the fire effects on a human body.

## FIREARMS

Firearms are generally of two types; smooth-bored and rifled, depending on the nature of the barrel. When the inside of the barrel is smooth, it is called smooth-bored. When the barrel is cut into a number of longitudinal spiral grooves, it is a rifled weapon (Figs 11.1A and B). Country guns, shot guns, etc. are smooth-bored weapons. Smooth-bored firearms fire pellets while rifled firearms fire bullets. Rifling will impart a spin to the fired bullet so that it attains stability in its path, unaffected by the resistance of air. Pellets from a smooth-bored weapon disperse after travelling together for a small distance. In some guns, the barrel is tapered **(choking)** to prevent early dispersion. This type of barrel is called a choked barrel.

Rifled weapons may be long- or short-barrelled. Most of the rifled weapons possess magazines or chambers to store a number of cartridges so that they can be fired in quick succession. In automatic weapons like machine gun, cartridges are automatically fed into the firing chamber. By keeping the trigger pressed, all the cartridges in the chamber are fired one after the other in quick succession and empty cases are thrown out.

The rifled weapons are designated according to the diameter of the calibre. It is the distance between two opposite lands between the grooves. The calibre of a 303 rifle is 0.303 of an inch. Metric system is employed in continental countries. Shot guns are classified in a different way like 12 bore/16 bore. The diameter of a 12 bore weapon is equal to the diameter of a spherical lead ball weighing $1^{1/3}$ ounce. Weight of 12 balls is equal to one pound (16 ounce).

## Cartridges

A cartridge is a ready-made ammunition. In country guns, the ingredients are to be loaded through the muzzle end of the barrel. First of all, gun powder is filled, followed by pellets and then a wad made of coconut husk is pushed in. The gun powder is ignited by detonating a percussion cap by the hammering action of the firing pin connected to the trigger by levers and springs. In a breech loading shot gun, ready-made cartridges are

**Figs 11.1 A and B:** Bore of fire arm: A. Smooth bore, B. Rifled,

loaded through the breech end of the barrel. The guns are hinged at the level of the breech end. They are called breech loaders, while country guns are muzzle loaders.

Cartridge has a case made up of metal or card board with a metallic base (Fig.11.2). The percussion cap is fitted on to the base. The percussion cap contains detonating chemicals such as lead azide or mercury fulminate. Above the percussion cap, gun powder is filled and to keep the powder intact a felt or card board wad is fixed. Above it, the pellets are loaded. On top, there is again a wad made up of card board. The gun powder may be either black or smokeless. Black powder consists of charcoal, sulphur and potassium nitrite. Smokeless powder consists of nitrocellulose or nitroglycerine. Many cartridges contain the same propellant in the form of **cordite stick**, which has got high explosive power. The number of pellets in a shot gun cartridge varies from a single one to three thousand or more.

Rifle cartridge has a metal case and a single projectile, the bullet (Fig.11.3). Bullet has a lead core and a cupronickel covering.

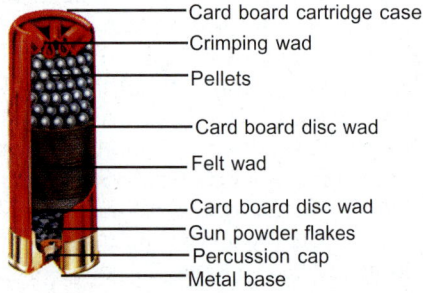

Card board cartridge case
Crimping wad
Pellets
Card board disc wad
Felt wad
Card board disc wad
Gun powder flakes
Percussion cap
Metal base

**Fig. 11.2:** Basic structure of a shot gun cartridge

Bullets are of different shapes conical, blunt-nosed, etc. Cartridges of revolvers have a rim at the base, while pistol cartridges are grooved at the base. The pistol being a semiautomatic weapon, the empty case is ejected out through the ejector hole after firing a cartridge (Figs 11.8 and 11.9). In order to catch hold of the empty case by the ejector mechanism of the gun, a groove is provided at the base of the cartridges. Cartridges of fully automatic

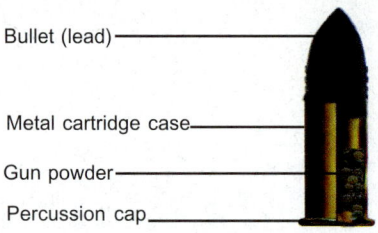

Bullet (lead)
Metal cartridge case
Gun powder
Percussion cap

**Fig. 11.3:** Basic structure of a Rifle cartridge

weapons like machine guns are also grooved. The empty cases of these cartridges are often recovered from the crime scene and can be thus identified. Different types of cartridges are shown in Figs 11.4 A to G.

## Mechanism of Firing

The cartridge is loaded in the firing chamber which will be the breech end of the barrel of a shotgun (Fig. 11.5). In the case of revolvers, the cartridge is loaded in the revolving chamber adjacent to the breech end of the barrel (Figs. 11.6 and 11.7). The trigger is connected to a metallic pin called firing pin by means of springs and levers. When the trigger is pulled, the firing pin strikes at the base of the cartridge case where the percussion cap is fitted. The percussion cap contains a detonating substance like mercury

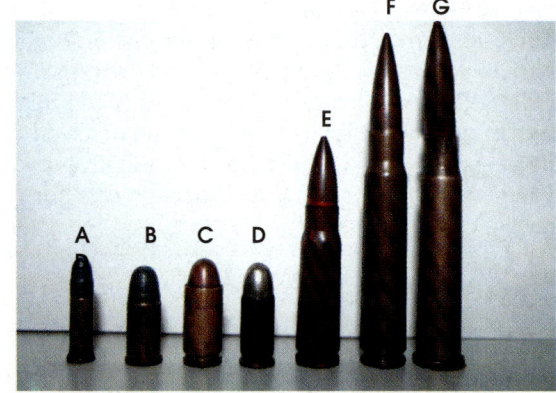

**Figs 11.4A to G:** Different types of cartridges: A. 0.22 rifle cartridge, B. 0.32 revolver, C. 9 mm pistol, D. 0.32 pistol, E. AK 47 Machine gun, F. AK 56 Machine gun, G. 0.303 rifle

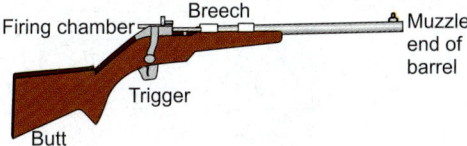

**Fig. 11.5:** Basic parts of a gun

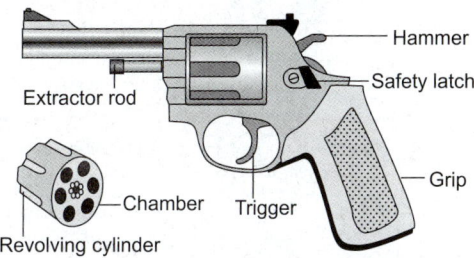

**Fig. 11.6:** Basic parts of a revolver

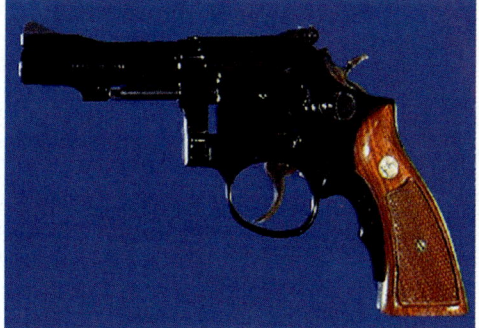

**Fig. 11.7:** Revolver

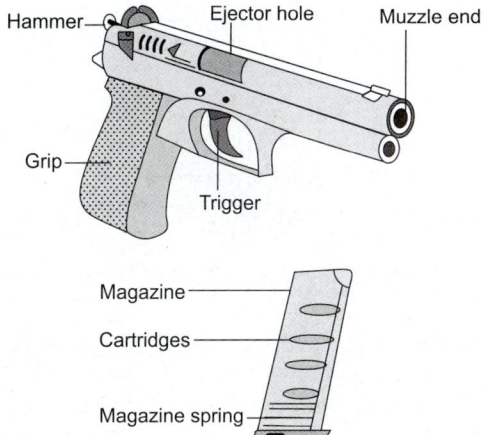

**Fig. 11.8:** Basic parts of a semiautomatic pistol

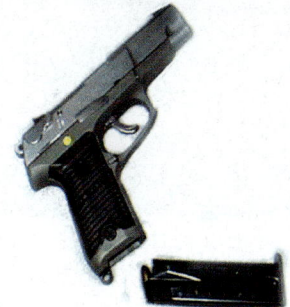

**Fig. 11.9:** Semiautomatic pistol and magazine

fulminate or lead azide. Due to the impact of the firing pin, the substance detonates and the sparks generated will ignite the gun powder. The large volume of gas produced will push the projectile out through the barrel.

In a rifled weapon, the projectile is a single bullet. This will get detached from the cartridge case and is propelled through the rifled barrel with high velocity. The velocity of a rifle bullet is about 800 metres/second and the range is 1000–3000 metres. Range of a revolver/pistol is up to 400–600 metres. Due to the rifling, the bullet acquires a gyrational motion in its flight which will help to overcome the air resistance. In a shot gun, the mechanism of firing is the same as that of a rifled weapon. The shot gun projectile may be a single lead pellet or multiple pellets. Multiple pellets travel as a single mass for only a short distance. At a distance of 3–4 metres, the pellets start dispersing. The effective range is 30–40 metres.

### Fire Effects

Apart from the projectile, other products of combustion also escape from the muzzle end of the barrel when the fire arm is discharged (Fig.11.10). They will travel for varying distances. Highly compressed hot gases escape along with the flame, which will travel up to a distance of 6 to 8 cm. Smoke will travel about 15 cm, while unburned powder particles travel up to 60 to 70 cm. The bullet will be smeared with dirt or grease present in the barrel.

The fire effects are important as they will produce various changes in the areas surrounding

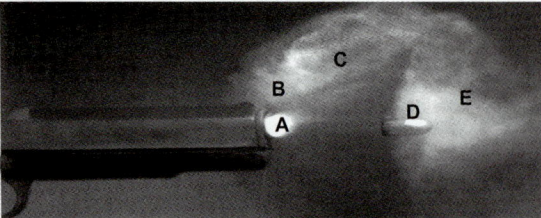

**Fig. 11. 10:** Fire effects: A. Flame, B. Explosive gases, C. Smoke, D. Bullet, E. Unburnt powder particles

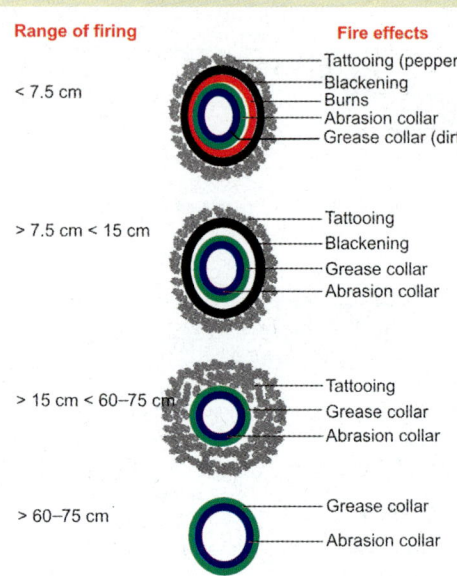

**Fig. 11.11:** Characteristics of entry wound of a rifled firearm

the entry wound. Explosive gases can enter the tissues in contact firing and will cause splitting of skin. This will produce a large stellate entrance wound or sometimes gross destruction of tissues. Flame will produce burns surrounding the entrance wound with singeing of hairs. Smoke can produce a halo of blackening. Unburned powder particles can produce peppering or tattooing effect around the entrance wound. Grease can cause a collar around the margin of the wound.

Entrance wounds will have a collar of abrasion produced by the impact of the bullet, grazing the skin. These effects are seen only around the entrance wound (Fig.11.11). In clothed areas, the clothes may show the evidence of fire effects. If the effects on the clothes are not seen by naked eyes, the clothes may be sent to forensic science laboratory where special techniques are employed to detect them.

Abrasion collar is produced by the bullet grazing the skin (Figs 11.12 and 11.13). When the bullet passes through the barrel of the gun, it is smeared with grease and dirt present inside the barrel; the same is deposited around the entry wound in the shape of a collar. Burns are produced by the effect of flames escaping through the muzzle end. Smoke escaping through the barrel will cause a black halo around the entry wound. Unburned powder particles will be deposited in the skin resembling peppering in an egg fry.

When a bullet penetrates and traverses the body, the kinetic energy is expended in the tissues causing destruction of tissues in its flight path. It causes crushing and laceration of tissues due to the transfer of energy. Bullets from low velocity weapons like revolver or pistol will produce low energy transfer wounds. Injury to the tissues will

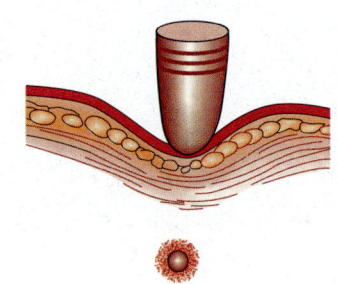

**Fig. 11.12:** Abrasion collar-m echanism of production

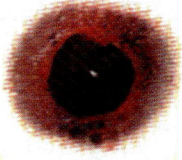

**Fig. 11.13:** Entrance wound with abrasion collar

be confined to the wound track. In the case of high velocity weapons like rifles, machine guns, etc. high energy transfer wounds are produced. Apart from the local laceration and crushing, injuries remote from the wound track are also caused. This phenomenon is known as temporary cavitation (Fig.11.14).

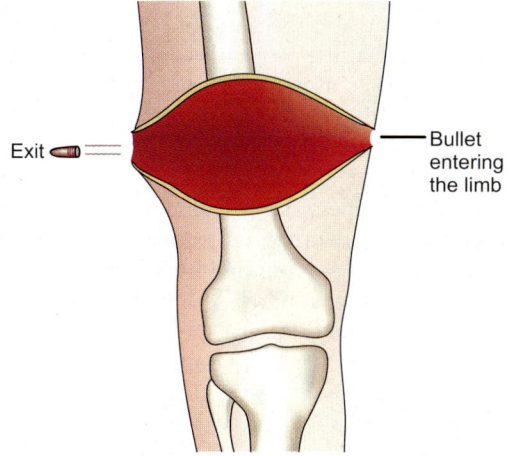

Fig. 11.14: Phenomenon of temporary cavitation

The extent of cavitation depends upon the nature of tissues such as density and elasticity. Solid organs like liver, spleen or kidneys will be shattered or extensively lacerated. Cavitation will be less in the lungs having elastic tissues. Bone will be shattered and the bone splinters will produce further injuries. When a missile penetrates the skull, there may be bevelling of the edges of the entrance and exit wounds. Inside the closed skull cavity, a high pressure shock wave may be produced causing widespread disruption. The entire brain matter may be destroyed. In contact firing, the explosive gases will also enter the skull cavity causing bursting of skull.

Wounding capacity of a bullet is more than that of a pellet because of its gyrating flight. Bullets often cause perforating wounds, especially in near ranges. There will be entrance and exit wounds. Except in contact firing, the entrance wound will be small and the exit wound will be large and irregular. If a low velocity bullet strikes against bone or any tough tissues, the momentum is lost and will be retained in the body. In long range firing or in ricochet bullet, exit wounds may not be present.

## Entrance Wounds

### Contact Firing

When the muzzle of the gun is pressed firmly against the body, all the fire effects are discharged into the track of the wound. In that case, the expanding gases will produce enlargement of the entrance wound. It will be star-shaped or irregular (Fig.11.15). Sometimes, an impression of the muzzle end is stamped on the skin as a patterned contusion or abrasion.

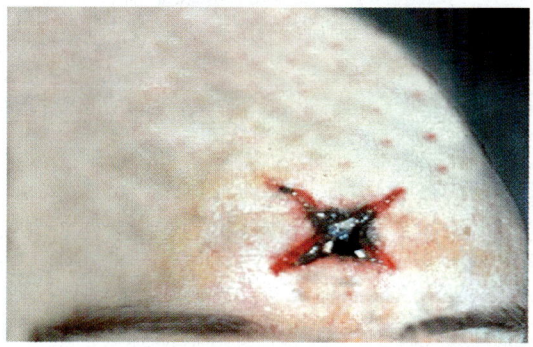

Fig. 11.15: Contact firing

### Close Range (up to 15 cm)

The entrance wound will be circular with inverted margins and surrounded by a collar of abrasion. This is produced by the impact of the high velocity bullet before it actually penetrates the skin. There will be grease collar, burning, and a halo of blackening and tattooing (Fig. 11.16). Beyond 15 cm, there will not be burning and blackening. There will be only tattooing apart from the abrasion collar and grease collar. Tattooing will be present up to arms length, i.e. about 60–75 cm.

When the bullet penetrates the skin, the sides of the bullet scrape the skin of the edges of the perforation and a collar of abrasion will be seen around the entrance wound (Figs 11.11 and 11.12). The shape of the abrasion collar will be circular, if the bullet strikes the body perpendicularly. If the bullet hits in a tangential manner, the shape of the abrasion collar will be oval. This shape will vary according to the angle at which the bullet strikes the body. Presence of an abrasion collar around an

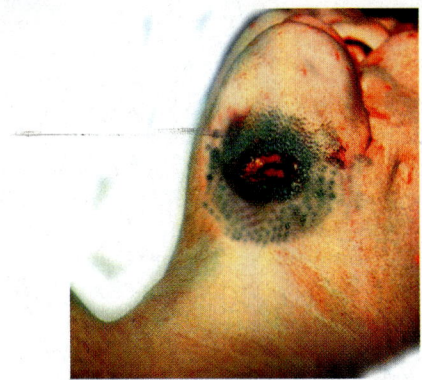

**Fig. 11.16:** Blackening and tattooing around the wound of entry

entrance wound definitely proves that the wound is due to the entry of the bullet.

### Distant Range

In distant shots, there will be only abrasion collar and grease collar around the entry wound. Suicide can be excluded in this range as it is beyond arms reach.

### Exit Wounds

When a bullet leaves the body, the velocity is low and usually produces an irregular large wound with everted margins. Bullet injuries on the head can cause inward bevelling of the entry and outward bevelling of the exit wounds of the skull. There will not be any other effects. The entrance and exit wounds are usually in a straight line, provided the path of the bullet was not obstructed within the body. From this, the direction of firing can be inferred. The elliptical or oval shape of the

entrance wound will also give a clue regarding the direction of fire.

### Shot Gun Injuries

Shot guns have also the same fire effects, the only difference is that the projectiles are pellets instead of a single bullet, as in a rifled firearm. These pellets travel as a single mass for a very short distance, maximum of 2 meters. Hence up to that range, a single irregular entrance wound will be seen. Beyond that, pellets start dispersing and at about 3 meters, the entrance wound will be a large irregular wound surrounded by a few individual 'satellite' entrance wounds. As the range increases, dispersion also increases and there will be multiple entrance wounds (Figs 11.17 and 11.18).

Contact firing with a shot gun can cause explosive type of injuries with gross destruction of tissues. In the head region, a contact firing can cause blasting of the skull and brain. Up to a range of 75 cm, fire effects are marked in shot gun injuries, because, in most of the cartridges, black powder is used.

Abrasion collar is not seen around entrance wounds, but sometimes the margins of the wound may show infiltration of blood in individual pellet wounds. In shot gun injuries, exit wounds are rare because the pellets on entering the body lose momentum and do not exit. But in close range firing using large grain cartridge, some pellets may exit.

From the dispersion of pellets, range of firing can be estimated roughly. The diameter of dispersion measured in centimeters and divided by two will give the approximate range in meters in the

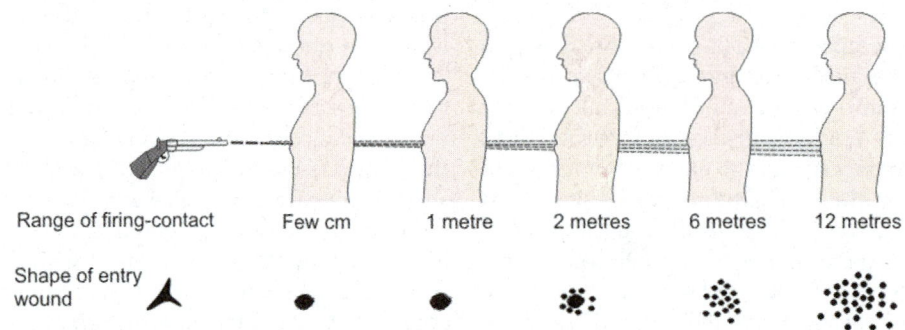

Range of firing-contact    Few cm    1 metre    2 metres    6 metres    12 metres

Shape of entry wound

**Fig. 11.17:** Characteristics of shot gun entry wounds

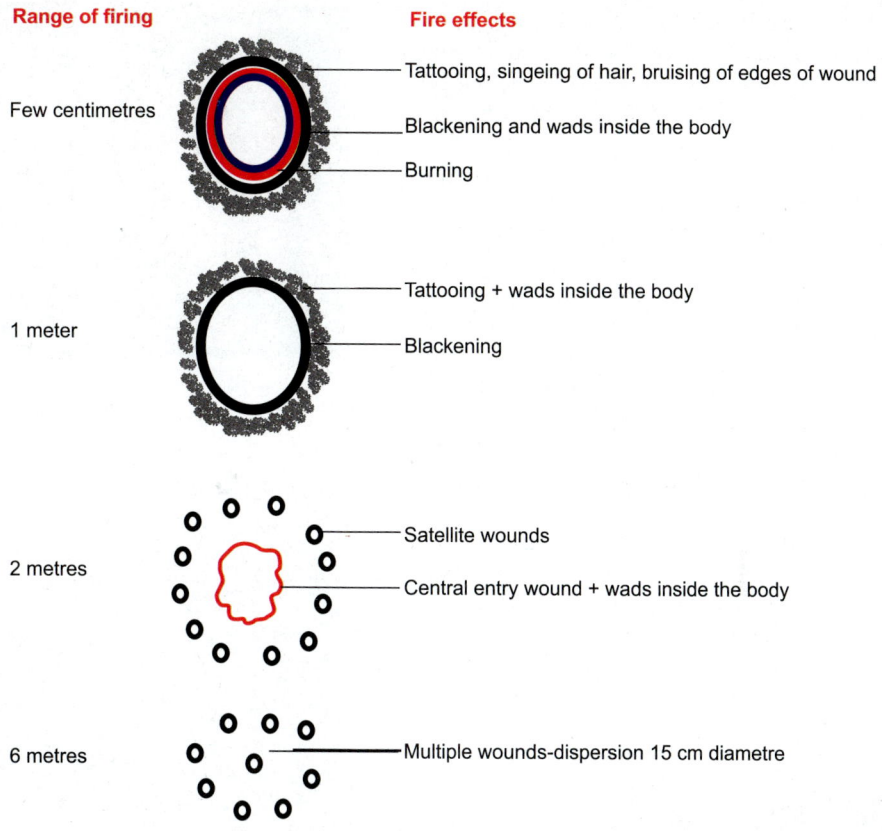

**Range of firing**

**Fire effects**

Few centimetres
— Tattooing, singeing of hair, bruising of edges of wound
— Blackening and wads inside the body
— Burning

1 meter
— Tattooing + wads inside the body
— Blackening

2 metres
— Satellite wounds
— Central entry wound + wads inside the body

6 metres
— Multiple wounds-dispersion 15 cm diametre

**Fig. 11.18:** Characteristics of shot gun entry wounds

case of fully choked weapons. In non-choked weapons (true cylinder), the dispersion will have double the diameter and hence the diameter is divided by 4 to get the range. Wads will also be projected along with the pellets and will be found inside the body. Wads can travel up to 2–3 meters. Wad of a shot gun is made of card board or felt while a piece of coconut husk or clothes is used as wad in country guns.

## Autopsy on Victims of Gun Shot Injuries

The medical officer should examine the scene of crime along with the police officers. Empty cases, wads and projectiles may be recovered from the crime scene. Careful examination of the scene can reveal so many clues regarding the range of firing, mode of firing, etc. The clothes should be exami-

ned and fire effects surrounding the entrance hole noted. The clothes shall be dried in shade, packed, and sealed for transmission to the forensic science laboratory. If there are no exit wounds, the projectile(s) will be present in the body and is a material evidence. The projectiles should be recovered carefully. X-ray examination prior to autopsy is very helpful to locate the projectile (Fig.11.23). When the projectile is located, it should be taken out by hand or with insulated forceps. When a bullet passes through the rifled barrel of a weapon, the marking of the lands will be imprinted on it and use of a metallic forceps can tamper it.

A weapon will have some peculiarities in the lands and all the bullets passing through the same barrel will acquire the same type of impressions

(Fig. 11.19). This is made use of in the identification of the murder weapon. **Test bullets** are fired using the suspect weapon into boxes filled with cotton wool. Those are recovered and the rifling impressions are compared with those found on the crime bullet with the help of a comparison microscope (Figs 11.20 to 11.22). When a bullet is dissected out of the body, care should be taken to prevent alterations to the rifling impressions. The bullets recovered are wrapped in cotton, placed in a card board box, sealed and forwarded to the expert. No markings shall be made on the bullet for the purpose of identification; instead, labels are affixed on the box containing them. A probe can be passed through the entrance wound up to the position of the projectile in the body or to the exit wound if there is one. The direction of firing can be thus found out. But sometimes the bullet will be deflected within the body if it strikes a hard organ or bone and will be located in unusual positions.

The entrance wound is described first, the internal injuries are noted and finally the exit wound is described. So the course of the projectile

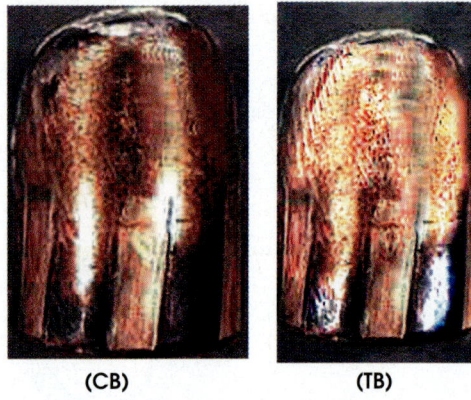

**(CB)**                **(TB)**

**Fig. 11.21:** Crime bullet (CB) and test bullet (TB)

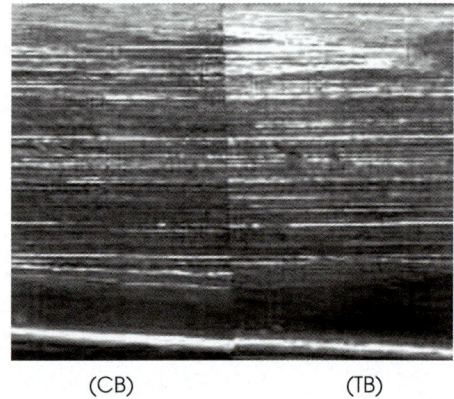

(CB)                (TB)

**Fig. 11.22:** Photomicrograph — comparison of the grooves on the crime bullet (CB) and test bullet (TB)

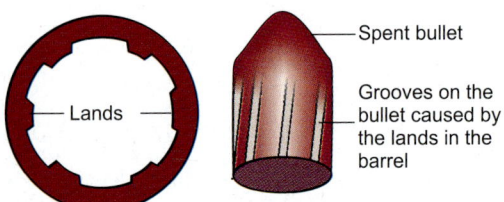

**Fig. 11.19:** Lands and grooves in the rifled barrel of a firearm

Spent bullet

Lands

Grooves on the bullet caused by the lands in the barrel

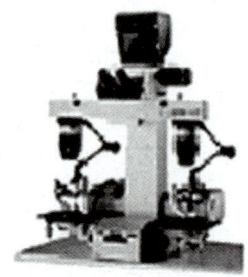

**Fig. 11.20:** Bullet comparison microscope

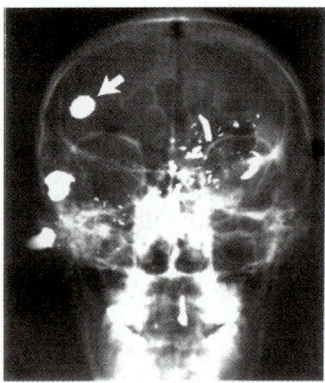

**Fig. 11.23:** X-ray skull showing images of bullets

and the damage done can be narrated in a single passage. If possible, photographs of the wounds are to be taken. Even though a medical officer is competent to make inference regarding the range from fire effects, it is better not to form any dogmatic opinion. Ballistic expert is the competent person to draw conclusions based on scientific experiments.

The medical officer who conducts the autopsy shall collect and forward the clothes of the victim, skin and tissues around the gun shot wounds, along with the recovered projectiles to the ballistic expert. The skin and tissues are to be preserved in rectified spirit.

## Air Guns

Air pistols and air rifles use compressed air or some inert gas to propel a small lead or steel projectile. In ordinary air guns, there will be a cylinder with a piston. By moving a lever, the piston is moved and the cylinder is filled with compressed air. In some type of guns, the lever is connected to the barrel. Bending the barrel will activate the lever (Fig.11.24). The lead slug is placed in the breech end of the barrel. When the trigger is pressed air is released through a small vent and the slug is projected through the barrel. In modern air rifles, a gas cylinder fitted in the gun will provide compressed air. These guns are more powerful and the effective range will be higher than the ordinary air weapons. In some air guns, the barrel will be rifled also.

Even though the air weapons do not require a licence for possession, these can produce fatal injuries at close ranges. Energy of the projectile depends upon the type of weapon and the pressure generated by the compressed air/gas. Projectile of a sophisticated air gun (Fig.11.25) can attain the same muzzle velocity of a revolver. Entrance wound caused by an air gun may be similar to that caused by a 0.22 rifle bullet. The wound will have an abrasion collar too. There will not be any fire effects. Usually, there will not be any exit wound due to the low power of the weapon. But in the case of high power rifled air guns, the slug may exit producing a wound with everted margins.

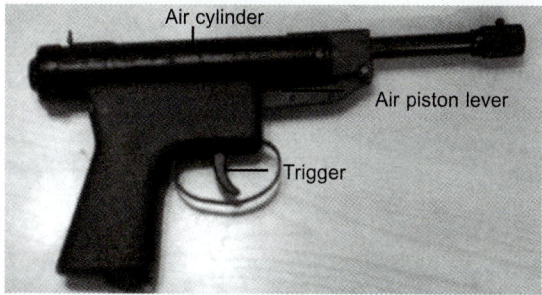

**Fig. 11.24:** Air pistol

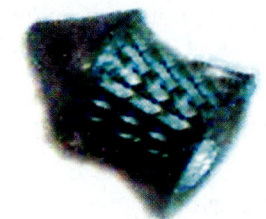

**Fig. 11.25:** Pellet of air pistol (5.5 mm)

## Rubber/Plastic Bullets

Police fire rubber/plastic bullets using special type of guns to control a riotous mob. Common rubber/plastic bullets are about 10 cm long, 3.5 cm in diameter and weigh about 100–150 gm. Usually these bullets will not produce serious injuries if fired from a distant range. They should not be fired at ranges less than 20 meters. At close range, fracture of ribs, fracture of skull, injuries to eyes and fatal internal injuries may be sustained.

## Stud Guns

Stud guns fire rivets, studs or steel pins to metal or wood by means of an explosive charge. These guns have been used for homicide or suicide.

Accidental injuries are commonly seen. The entry wound will be similar to that of a small caliber rifled firearm. Detection of the rivet or stud from the body will help in identifying the weapon.

## Examination of Gun Shot Residue

When a gun is discharged, the powder and primer of the cartridge undergo combustion. The residue of the combustion products, unburned powder and primer will be deposited around the entrance wound of the victim or on the clothes or body of the accused. The residue may even be deposited on the persons nearby the accused or victim.

Black powder consists of potassium nitrate (75%), charcoal (15%), and sulphur (10%). Modern smokeless gun powder contains nitrocellulose and/or nitroglycerine. The primer may consist of lead azide/lead styphnate/mercury fulminate/barium nitrate/potassium chlorate/antimony sulphide. Smokeless gun powder residue contains up to 23 organic compounds. Major primer residues are lead, barium and antimony. Along with these, traces of aluminium, sulphur, tin, calcium, potassium, etc. are also present.

### Paraffin Test (Dermal Nitrate Test)

When a person fires a gun, due to gas leakage from the breech end, gun powder residues will be deposited in the hands. If the accused in a gun shot injury case is apprehended 'dermal nitrate test' can be done to prove that he has fired a weapon recently. In suspected cases of suicides also, this test has to be performed on the hands of the deceased. A gauze cloth dipped in molten paraffin is wound round the hands. Later, it is cut and removed. Diphenylamine reagent is added to the inner surface of the cloth and a positive reaction is indicated by the appearance of blue colour. False positive results will be obtained if there is contamination with tobacco, urine, etc. Therefore, a negative test is of more value.

### Gunshot Residues on Clothes

Detection of the gunshot residues on the clothes or entrance wound will provide valuable information regarding the range of firing. Gun Shot residues from the muzzle can travel to one meter in most of the firearms. Beyond this, sometimes traces of particles may be detected by special tests. At a distance of 45 to 60 cm, there will be considerable deposit of residues which may or may not be visible to the eye. But below 30 cm heavy deposit of residues will be seen. Gun Shot residue is normally a combination of gun powder residues and lead residues. Gun powder residue will be in the form of nitrite compounds. Lead residues will

be in a particulate form. This can come from the primer and the projectile. There are simple chemical tests to detect the gun shot residues.

### Modified Griess Test

This test is performed to detect nitrite residues. It is a primary test to determine whether a wound is an entry wound and if so to find out the range of firing. A photographic paper is desensitised by exposing the paper to hypo-solution. It is then treated with solutions of sulfanilic acid in distilled water and alpha naphthol in methyl alcohol. This chemically treated paper will be reactive to nitrite residues. The cloth or material is placed face down against the treated photographic paper. The back of the cloth to be examined is steam ironed with a solution of dilute acetic acid. The electric steam iron is filled with dilute acetic acid instead of water. The acetic acid vapours will penetrate the cloth and a reaction takes place between nitrite residues on the clothe and chemicals in the photographic paper. The resulting colour change will appear as orange specks on the paper.

### Sodium Rhodizonate Test

This chemical test is designed to detect lead residues in an exhibit. A weak solution of sodium rhodizonate in distilled water is sprayed on the exhibit. The solution has dark yellow or orange colour. Then a buffer solution is sprayed; which causes the disappearance of the background colour. Sodium rhodizonate reacts with any lead that may be present and a positive reaction is indicated by the appearance of a bright pink colour. To confirm the presence of lead, the pink coloured area is treated with dilute hydrochloric acid. Presence of lead is confirmed if the pink colour turns blue.

### Other Modern Methods

Latest tests like neutron activation analysis, atomic absorption spectroscopy, scanning electron microscopy with energy dispersive analysis, etc. are employed. Propellant constituents are also identified by using gas chromatography and high performance liquid chromatography. Smokeless powder residue can be analysed by another method called "capillary electrophoresis".

These tests are used to detect gun shot residues on the surface of the body and clothes of the victim also. The investigating officer should despatch the clothes of the accused or victim, swabs from the entrance wounds/body or paraffin gauze to the forensic science laboratory for conducting the tests. Adhesive tapes can also be used for lifting the residues left on the surface of the body and clothing.

### Firing Distance

From the patterns of fire effects and gun shot residue found on the entry wound or clothes of the victim, the firing distance can be found out. This is necessary to find out the manner of death as well as the relative positions of the accused and victim at the time of firing. The fire effects and deposition of gun shot residues will vary from weapon to weapon. Different brands of ammunition will produce different effects even if the firing distance is the same. Even the wind and weather conditions can cause variations in the residue pattern. Therefore, to arrive at a near accurate opinion, firing experiments have to be conducted and standards have to be prepared.

The firing experiment is conducted using the same weapon and same brand of ammunition used in the actual case. Several panels are prepared with white pieces of cotton twill cloth fixed on a stand. Firing on to the panels is done at different firing distances. Usually the ranges will be contact, 7.5, 15, 30, 45, 60, 75 and 150 cm. Griess test and sodium rhodizonate tests are done on the panels. The results are compared with the actual residue pattern found on the victims clothing. From this, a minimum and maximum firing distance can be assessed. The patterns on the human skin are compared by conducting firing experiments conducted on panels made up of pig's skin. In terms of morphology, the pig skin and the human skin are much alike!!

### Accident/Suicide/Homicide

Position and direction of the wound are very important in arriving at an opinion as to the manner of death. Accessible sites such as temple, mouth, jaw, forehead, chest, etc. are usually selec-ted in suicidal attempts. Very often, the muzzle end of the barrel will be pressed firmly to the site so that effects of contact firing are seen. In long barreled weapons, the trigger is pulled by toes, by placing the stock of the gun on the ground. Fingers or a string attached to the trigger may be used for pulling the trigger. In hand gun shots, absence of fire effects surrounding the entrance wound generally indicates a range beyond arms reach and will exclude suicide. Multiple wounds are also possible in suicides, but the location, range and fatality of the injuries sustained in each firing, should be taken into account before forming an opinion. Homicidal gun shot injuries can be anywhere on the body and will be from any range. A close range does not exclude homicide, while a distant range is only in favour of homicide.

### EXPLOSION WOUNDS (BLAST INJURIES)

Blast injuries are caused by the explosive pressure which accompanies the bursting of explosive devices like bombs, shells, etc. Many of the explosive devices have metal casings containing the explosive material and the detonating substances. The explosive chemicals commonly used are nitroglycerine, trinitrotoluine (**TNT**), penta-erythritol tetranitrate (**PETN**), triacetone triperoxide (**TATP**), cyclomethylene trinitramine (**Cyclonite/RDX**), etc.

The explosive material is ignited due to the detonating substance. The explosive pressure which develops due to the bursting of bombs or shells ruptures their casing and imparts a high velocity to the resulting fragments. These fragments will cause devastating injury to the tissues. In home made bombs, the casing may be made up of metal, fibre or card board.

Different materials like metal pieces, glass fragments, nails, etc. are filled inside, enveloping the explosive material. Some of the bombs have wick fuses. The fuse wire is lit and thrown at the target. In some other type of country bombs, detonating substance is placed amidst small pebbles. When the bomb is thrown on the victim or on a hard surface, the detonator sparks and ignites the gun powder. The flying sharpnels tear through tissue at high speed. Modern bombs carry preformed munitions, such as notched wire or ball bearings, or have their casing etched to allow predictable fragmentation patterns resulting in a multitude of small, relatively low-energy fragments producing multiple low-energy transfer wounds. Grenade is an example of such a device.

All bomb explosions are accompanied by a complex blast wave. The two main components of this wave are a **blast pressure wave** and the **blast wind wave** due to mass movement of air. The blast pressure wave has a positive and negative phase. The positive pressure phase of the blast wave lasts for only a few milliseconds, but the effects on the human body will be devastating, especially in confined spaces. Extensive lacerations, traumatic amputation of limbs and lacerations of internal organs can be sustained (Fig. 11.26).

The blast pressure waves flow over and around an obstruction like a sound wave and affect anyone sheltering behind a wall or in a trench. A person standing in front of a wall or other vertical surface facing an explosion is subjected to the added effect of a reflected pressure also. The negative effect of a pressure wave is of low amplitude, lasts longer than the positive wave and will not produce any significant damage.

Rapid expansion of gases of explosion will displace air at supersonic speed. This fast movement of air at high pressure is known as blast wind wave and disrupts the environment, hurling debris and people. The blast wind can cause total body disruption. The mass movement of air may disrupt buildings and can cause crush injuries to persons entrapped inside. The pressure waves travel at the speed of sound in the medium being traversed. In water, velocity and distance are greater and injuries tend to be more complex and severe. For example, blast pressure waves in air rarely affect the gastrointestinal tract to any clinically significant extent in survivors; however, in water, the blast wave exerts a 'water hammer' effect with gross damage to internal orgns.

When the body is impacted by a blast pressure wave, it sets up a series of stress waves which are capable of injury, particularly at air-fluid interfaces. Injuries to the ear, lungs, heart and to the gastrointestinal tract are caused. Usually extensive lacerated injuries with great disruption of tissues are seen. They are often associated with burns, abrasions, contusions and puncture — lacerations **(injury triad)**. Ruptures of organs and tearing of clothes due to air blasts may also be seen. Sharpnels in the devices such as nails, stones, glass pieces and metallic fragments are driven into the body causing multiple injuries (Fig.11.27). The clothes, tissues and debris have to be collected and sent to the forensic science laboratory. Tissues are to be preserved in rectified spirit for detection of explosive chemicals and their residues.

## DIRECTIONS TO THE INVESTIGATING OFFICER

Death due to gun shot injuries are rare in our country. Therefore, the investigating officers do not possess sufficient practical experience in handling such cases. Doctors are also not aware

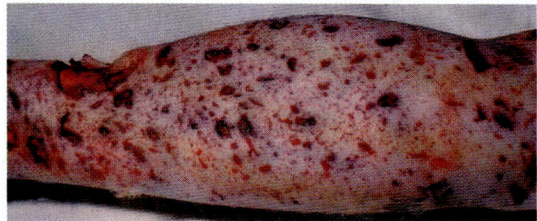

**Fig. 11.27:** Lower limb of a victim of bomb explosion, (The victim was standing away from the seat of an explosion. Characteristic 'injury triad' of abrasions, contusions and small irregular lacerations are seen. The lacerations will contain sharpnels and their fragments. Residue of the explosive material will also be present. These should be collected and sent for forensic analysis)

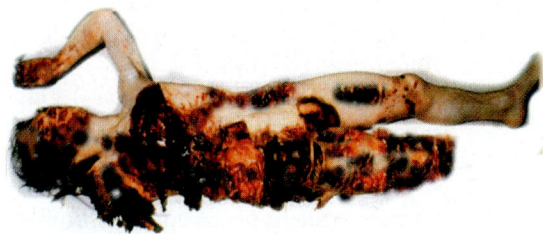

**Fig. 11.26:** Victim of a bomb explosion, (As injuries are mostly on the right side of the body, the inference is that the seat of explosion was on the right side of the victim)

of the importance of collecting evidence. While treating a victim of gun shot injury, inadvertently, trace evidences are destroyed and the wounds are altered. Sometimes, investigation goes astray as the findings are misinterpreted.

The most common error is in identifying the entrance wound. The general assumption is that the entrance wound is smaller than the exit. The size and nature of the entrance and exit wounds depend upon many factors such as the nature of the projectile, its velocity, the site of impact, etc. It is always better to seek the help of forensic experts in all the stages of investigation. The following crucial questions are to be answered:

- Are the injuries due to a gun shot?
- What is the nature of the firearm?
- Which is the entrance wound? (if there are two injuries)
- What is the range and direction of fire?
- What are the fire effects found on the body/clothes?
- What is the nature of the projectile recovered from the body/surroundings?
- Was there any empty cartridge case in the scene? What is its nature?
- What is the cause of death?

### Specific Tasks

- Photograph the dead body and the scene with close up pictures of injuries.
- Photographing the fire effects around the wounds.
- When injuries are measured, distance from the feet and nearest anatomical landmarks should be noted for reconstructing the shooting incident.
- Fingerprinting the dead body and the firearm (if recovered).

- Detailed description and measurements of fire effects.
- Remove all clothes carefully, dry and pack in paper bags.
- Cover the tears on the clothes with cellophane sheets to prevent loss of residues.
- Search for bullets/pellets/wads/empty cases in the scene (if exit wounds are present).
- Cover the recovered projectiles with cotton wool and packed in wide mouthed containers.
- Collect the fragments of the explosive device, debris of tissues, clothes, etc. in the case of bomb explosion and preserve them separately.
- Human tissues should be put in glass bottles with rectified spirit as the preservative.
- Cover the hands of the victim with paper bags (polythene bags will cause sweating).
- Request the forensic scientist to collect residues/trace evidence from the hands of the victim as well as the suspect (if any).
- Request the doctor who treats the victim of gunshot to preserve tissues removed from the margin of a wound.
- Request the forensic doctor to take X-rays/CT scan before autopsy if the projectile is lodged inside the body.
- Request the forensic doctor to preserve tissues around the entrance and exit wounds separately after photographing and noting down the findings.
- Request the forensic doctor to recover and preserve the projectile(s) without causing scratches on them.
- Use metal detectors for locating projectiles from the putrefied dead bodies and scenes.
- Despatch the firearm to the forensic science laboratory after closing the muzzle end of the barrel.

# 12

# Regional Injuries

## HEAD INJURY

Various types of injuries can occur to the head depending upon the nature of force applied. Scalp, skull and brain can be affected in varying degrees. Brain will be affected without any injury to scalp or skull. Persons who sustain injury to the head may develop symptoms of brain damage only later. They will be apparently normal for a considerable time. Therefore, when any person complains of a hit or fall involving the head to the police officer, he should be sent to the hospital and kept under observation for a minimum period of 24 hours.

## Scalp

Contusion, abrasion and lacerations can occur to scalp due to blunt force. Contusions may not be visible externally due to thick scalp hair. But on dissection of the scalp, a hematoma will be detected. A split laceration of scalp will be mistaken as an incised wound. Scalp injuries bleed profusely. Collection of blood under the scalp can be misinterpreted as a depressed fracture on palpation. Avulsion of scalp can occur, if scalp hair is entangled in some moving or rotary machinery.

## Fracture of Skull

*Due to direct impact:* A blow on the head or a fall from a height striking the head can cause fracture of skull.

*Fissured fracture:* Linear fractures are called fissured fractures (Fig. 12.1). Temporal and parietal bones are easily fractured than the occipital bone.

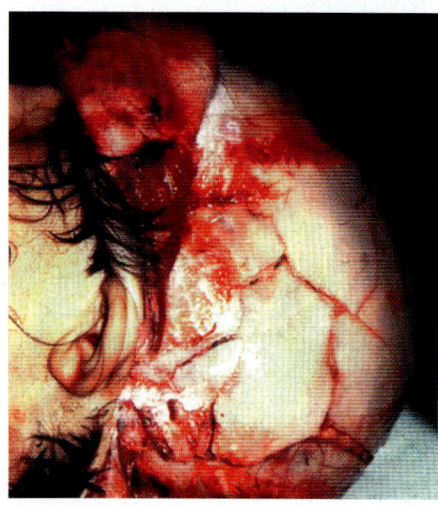

**Fig. 12.1:** Multiple fissured fractures of skull (Fracture lines do not cross)

The fracture line need not always be at the site of impact. A fissured fracture may extend to the base of skull (Fig. 12.3).

*Comminuted (complex) fracture:* The bone is fractured into fragments. This is due to a heavy blunt impact or violent fall. This is as a result of multiple adjacent fissured fractures.

*Depressed fracture:* The fractured segment of the bone is displaced inwards. This is called **signature fracture** because very often the shape of the fracture will correspond to the shape of the striking surface of the object (Fig. 12.2). This helps in identifying the weapon.

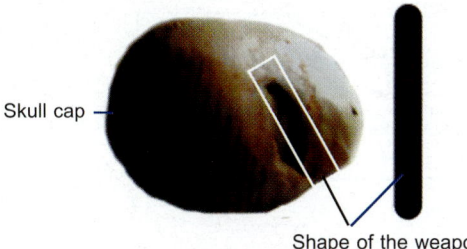

Skull cap

Shape of the weapon

**Fig. 12.2:** Depressed fracture skull and shape of the weapon which caused the fracture

*Pond fracture:* They are seen in the elastic skulls of children. The inner table of skull is not fractured. The fracture appears as an indentation of the outer table.

*Gutter fracture:* The outer table of the skull is removed in the shape of a gutter as in the case of a bullet glancing the head.

*Suture separation:* Separation of sutures occurs in direct impact to skull of young persons.

*Ring fracture (indirect impact):* This is a circular fissured fracture surrounding the foramen magnum. When a person falls from a height landing on his feet or buttocks, the force is transmitted upwards through the vertebral column causing a ring fracture of the base of the skull (Fig. 12.3).

## INJURIES TO BRAIN

Injuries to brain depend upon factors such as the site, severity of force, position of head, etc. Brain is not compressible and can glide within the skull

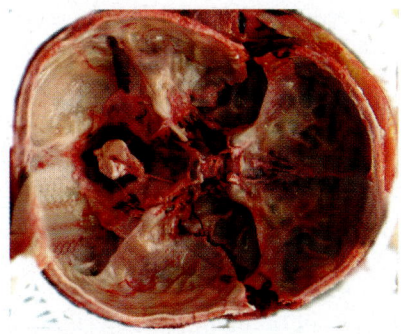

**Fig. 12.3:** Fracture of the base of skull involving the middle cranial fossa

to which it is attached by membranes and meninges. When the head is resting, a blow on the head will produce an injury of the brain corresponding to the site of impact (coup injury). But when the head is not fixed, injury is sustained to the opposite pole of brain, as it will strike the fixed structures of the vault of skull (contrecoup). From this, we can infer the position of head at the time of sustaining the impact. When the victim is sitting, standing or falling, contrecoup injuries are sustained.

### Cerebral Concussion

This is the mild form of cerebral injury. Following an impact on the head, temporary unconsciousness occurs the duration of which may vary. This is due to a temporary derangement of neurons and there will not be any permnent damage. The person may recover if concussion is not associated with cerebral contusion or laceration. The recovery is followed by symptoms like confusion, headache, convulsions, amnesia, etc. Severe concussion can rarely cause death.

### Cerebral Contusion and Lacerations

They vary in severity depending upon the force of impact and are usually seen on the frontal, temporoparietal and occipital poles of brain. These occur as a result of coup or contrecoup injuries. They are associated with bleeding in the brain, swelling and the increased tension inside the skull cavity can result in death. These injuries can be sustained with or without a fracture of skull. The person will be unconscious in almost all cases of brain laceration and bleeding. Formation of brain abscess is a complication of this type of injury.

### Intracranial Haemorrhages

#### Extradural Haemorrhage

Bleeding occurs outside the dural covering of brain and the clots formed will exert pressure on the brain. They are often associated with fracture of skull. There may be a lucid interval between the time of injury and onset of symptoms. Unless the blood clot is removed by a burr hole operation, the person will die of increased intracranial tension (Fig.12.4).

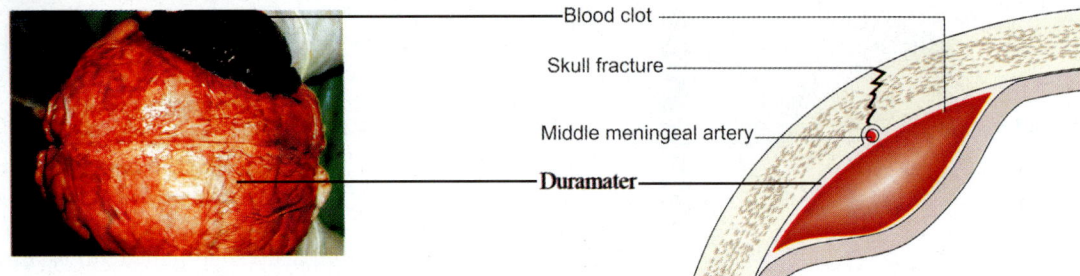

**Fig. 12.4:** Extradural haemorrhage

## Subdural Haemorrhage

Bleeding occurs under the dural covering. This usually appears as a thin film or clot (Fig.12.5). Subdural bleeding is almost always due to injury and if the subdural blood clot is large, it can cause death due to compression of brain. If it is small, it will get organised into a chronic subdural hematoma causing neurological symptoms simulating a brain tumour.

## Subarachnoid Haemorrhage

Bleeding is seen underneath the arachnoid covering of brain. This is either due to injury or natural causes like sclerosis of blood vessels, congenital aneurysms, etc. The bleeding occurs from cerebral vessels. Brain contusion and lacerations are associated with subarachnoid bleeding. Person will lose consciousness following the bleeding. Slight subarachnoid bleeding is seen in fracture of the cervical vertebrae also.

## Intracerebral Haemorrhage

Bleeding in the substance of the brain can be like spots or massive (Fig.12.6). They are either due to

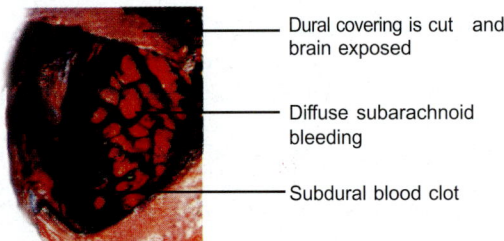

**Fig. 12.5:** Subdural and subarachnoid haemorrhages

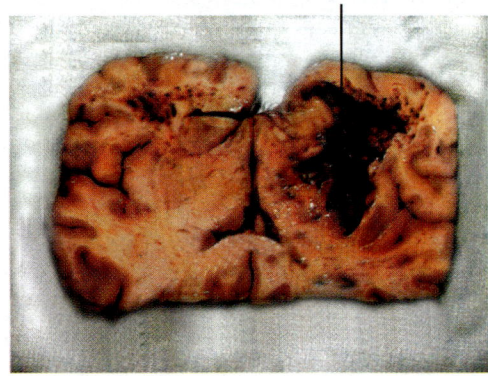

**Fig. 12.6:** Section of brain showing an area of intracerebral haemorrhage

injury or natural causes. The medicolegal problem is to distinguish these two varieties during autopsy. The most common natural cause is cerebral arteriosclerosis complicated by high blood pressure. Bleeding due to head injury is often spot like in nature. It will be often associated with evidence of other injuries such as fracture of skull, contusion of brain, etc.

A person becoming unconscious due to spontaneous intracerebral bleeding may fall down and sustain head injury also. In that case, the condition of cerebral arteries and site of bleeding will give a clue. Bleeding can occur inside the ventricles of brain also.

In all types of brain injuries, swelling (edema) of the brain develops soon after the injury. The exact mechanism of the development of edema is not fully understood. Following edema, brain swells within the rigid skull cavity and intracranial tension increases. This can cause death.

### Head Injuries in Boxing

Acute brain injuries are not uncommon in boxers. Death can occur due to subdural or subarachnoid haemorrhages. Skull fracture and extradural bleeding are rare. Boxers develop a condition known as **punch drunk syndrome** as a result of chronic changes occurring in the brain due to repeated injuries. The affected persons may develop Parkinsonian symptoms and Alzheimer's like condition.

## INJURIES TO NECK

Neck is a prominent and vital part of the body. Neck contains arteries supplying blood to the brain, veins draining the brain, pharynx, larynx, spinal cord, spinal nerve roots and important nerves like vagus. Trivial injuries can have a fatal outcome. Neck can be easily compressed by hands or ligatures resulting in the obstruction of blood vessels and airway. If the carotid arteries are occluded on both sides, the victim will become unconscious immediately. Sustained pressure can cause death. Pressure or blows to the neck region will result in **vagal inhibition** causing reflex cardiac arrest. Heart will stop suddenly following minor or trivial trauma or pressure to the neck. In such deaths, there will not be any specific autopsy findings.

In such deaths, there will not be any specific autopsy findings. The trauma may be so trivial that there will not be any evidence in the neck. In death due to vagal inhibition, it is difficult to form an opinion as to the cause of death for want of specific morbid anatomical changes. Specific autopsy findings will be absent in death due to vagal inhibition.

Various types of injuries are seen in the region of neck in cases of asphyxial deaths like hanging, strangulation, etc. These are described elsewhere. Sharp force injuries to the neck are found in cases of suicide and homicide. Cut throat injuries are of medicolegal importance. The forensic doctor will be able to distinguish suicidal cut throat injuries from homicidal ones. In suicidal attempts, the weapon used will be usually a light cutting knife or a razor. The injury will be on the side of the neck or in the front. The ends of the wound will show **'hesitation nicks'**. These hesitation nicks/cuts indicate the number of times the weapon was drawn against the skin. Usually cut throat injuries will not be deep. Air will be sucked in through the cut jugular veins. This air reaches the right side of the heart and with blood forms a froth. This will block the flow of blood into the major artery to the lungs, thereby causing death. If the injury is on the front of neck and wind pipe is cut, death may be due to aspiration of blood into air passages.

Homicidal wounds are usually inflicted by heavy cutting weapons like chopper, axe, sword, etc. They are deep and without any hesitation nicks. Deeper structures are affected. Homicidal wounds are also inflicted by a slash with a razor or knife.

## INJURIES TO VERTEBRAL COLUMN AND SPINAL CORD

Fractures and/or dislocation can occur to the vertebral column. Both can cause injury to the spinal cord (Fig. 12.7). Fractures and dislocation can be caused by direct or indirect force. Falling from a height hitting the buttocks or feet, falling of a weight on the back, etc. can cause these injuries. Fracture dislocation of cervical vertebra can occur due to sudden bending of spine forwards or backwards. These injuries are common in the occupants of a vehicle involved in an accident.

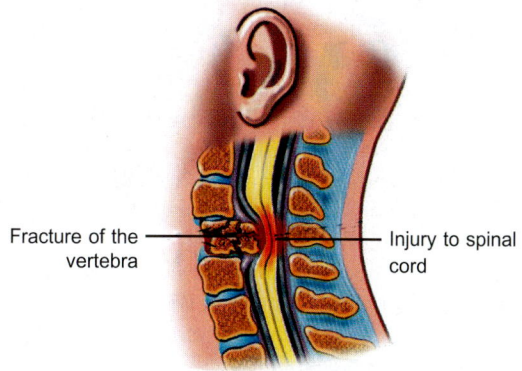

Fracture of the vertebra — Injury to spinal cord

**Fig. 12.7:** Fracture of cervical vertebra and injury to spinal cord

Injury to muscles and ligaments of neck will also be sustained. These injuries called **whiplash** are due to sudden deceleration of the vehicle in the event of a head on collision.

Fracture above the 3rd cervical vertebra with injury to spinal cord can be instantly fatal because of the involvement of phrenic nerve originating from the corresponding area of the spinal cord. Phrenic nerve supplies the diaphragm and hence death is due to the paralysis of diaphragm and respiratory arrest. Cord involvement below that level will produce quadriplegia (paralysis of all the four limbs), paraplegia (paralysis of lower limbs), urinary incontinence, etc. Fracture of 1st lumbar vertebra will involve the sacral segments and impotence can result. Similar to the cerebral injuries, spinal cord may be concussed, contused or lacerated. Bleeding will also occur in the coverings or in the substance. Symptoms will depend on the site of injury.

## INJURIES TO CHEST

Chest can sustain a variety of injuries. The injuries of the chest may be penetrating or non-penetrating. Non-penetrating wounds are as a result of blunt impacts. Blunt impacts to the chest can cause abrasions and contusions to chest wall, fractures of ribs and sternum, contusion or laceration of lungs, heart etc. Blunt impacts need not cause any external injury. Fall from a height and run over accidents can cause multiple fractures of ribs on both sides. Direct hit will also cause fracture of the ribs and sometimes the fractured ends may penetrate the lung or heart. Sternum is usually fractured in direct impacts. Driver of an automobile in a collision accident will strike his chest against the steering column and can sustain sternal fracture, or contusion and laceration of heart (Figs 12.8A and B). Heart is ruptured during diastole when it is filled with blood.

Myocardial infarction can also cause softening of the heart muscle and spontaneous rupture. Traumatic rupture is associated with contusion of heart muscle. Microscopical examination will confirm the diagnosis. Penetrating injuries of the chest can produce pneumothorax (air in the pleural cavity), hemothorax (blood in the pleural cavity),

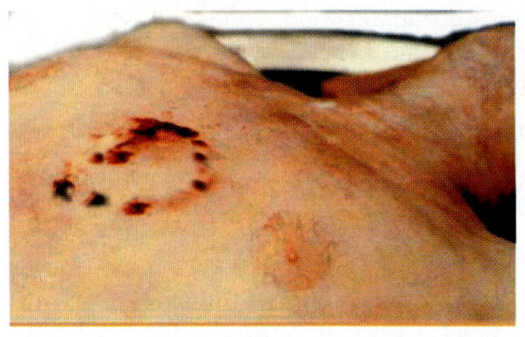

A

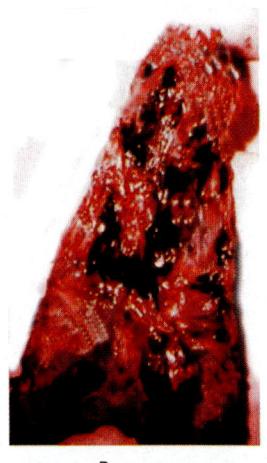

B

**Figs 12.8A and B:** Steering wheel impact—blunt impact injuries on chest (The deceased, driver of a motor vehicle sustained steering wheel impact on the chest: A. Patterned contusion caused by the hornboss. Sternum and ribs show extensive fractures, B. Multiple contusions and lacerations of heart and lungs)

chylothorax, etc. It can also cause sudden death due to pleural shock. Hemothorax is usually as a result of injury to the intercostal blood vessels, and the bleeding can be fatal as these arteries are the direct branches of aorta. Lung injuries bleed very little as the pressure of the pulmonary circulation is less, but tension pneumothorax can develop easily in lung injuries and will be fatal quickly.

Penetrating injuries of the heart can cause collection of blood in the pericardial cavity and subsequent compression of heart (**cardiac tamponade**).

If the injury is in the ventricle and across the muscle fibres, the wound will gape and bleeding will be profuse. Wound tends to close as the heart contracts, if it is in the direction of muscle fibres. All injuries of heart need not be necessarily fatal. But injuries to the auricles can bleed profusely and can be imminently fatal.

## INJURIES TO ABDOMEN

Injuries to abdomen can also be classified into penetrating or non-penetrating. Blunt trauma to abdomen can produce abrasions and contusions of abdominal wall and injuries to internal organs like stomach, intestines, liver, spleen and kidneys (Figs 12.9 and 12.10). Injuries may vary from contusions to lacerations. Lacerations can produce bleeding in the abdominal cavity. Rupture of intestines will lead to infection (peritonitis). Purulent peritonitis can develop within 36 hours. Blunt impacts to abdomen need not always produce external injuries, as the abdomen is yielding and the force will be dissipated internally injuring the internal organs.

Penetrating injuries can cause intraperitoneal bleeding and peritonitis. Penetrating injury involving the peritoneum can cause sudden death due to peritoneal shock or delayed death due to peritonitis. Hence it can also be considered as sufficient in the ordinary course of nature to cause death.

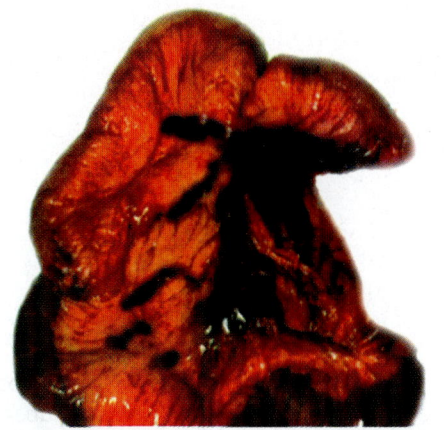

**Fig. 12.9:** Contusions of mesentery and intestines

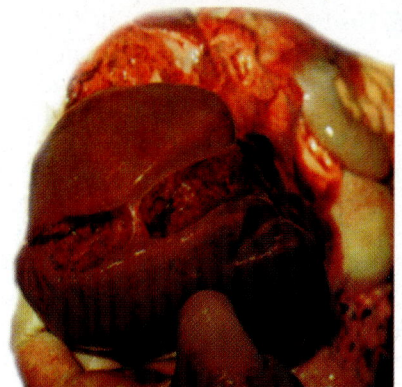

**Fig. 12.10:** Laceration of spleen

## INJURIES TO LIMBS

All types of injuries can be sustained to limbs due to blunt and sharp forces. Most of the injuries are sustained in accidents. Surface injuries like abrasions, contusions and lacerations are usually not serious unless they are infected by bacteriae like *Clostridium tetani* and *Clostridium welchii*. Such infections are common in crush injuries. Injuries to blood vessels, fractures of long bones and crush injuries are possible in vehicular, industrial and domestic accidents. Fractures sustained to the leg and thigh bones can be open, displaced, comminuted or complicated. Vascular and nerve injuries are also possible in this type of trauma. Old people sustain fracture of the neck of femur in trivial domestic accidents.

Injuries to the major blood vessels of limbs, especially femoral vessels sustained due to blunt trauma are of medicolegal significance. Fatal bleeding can occur and often it goes undetected. There will not be any external bleeding. The extravasated blood will collect in the fascial compartments of the thigh. Several persons have died following minor trauma of the thighs. Autopsy will reveal rupture of femoral vessels and large collection of blood inside the thigh. Externally there may be trivial abrasions or slight bruising.

This type of fatal injury to the blood vessels of the thigh is possible in a type of torture known as 'rolling' practised sometimes on the detainees

a bench. His hands and feet are tied. A metal or wooden rod is rolled over his legs and thighs by men standing on either side of the victim. This type of torture will produce excruciating pain. Muscles will be crushed and blood vessels may be ruptured. Delayed deaths are also possible due to renal failure caused by the crushing of muscles. Myoglobin, a muscle protein is liberated from the crushed muscles into the bloodstream. This will dissociate into globin and ferrihemate moities. Ferrihemate is toxic to the kidneys. Death can occur due to failure of the function of kidneys.

## DIRECTIONS TO THE INVESTIGATING OFFICER

Usually, external injury may be an indication of an internal injury. But it is quite possible for a person to sustain fatal internal injuries without any external injury. Sometimes the external injury may be very trivial and the injured will be apparently normal for a long time. For example, blunt impact on the abdomen can result in serious injuries like rupture of mesentery and intestines, lacerations of spleen, liver and kidneys. Death may be delayed due to slow internal bleeding or infection. Similarly, a blunt impact on the chest can fracture a rib. The fractured rib can injure the lung and cause fatal pneumothorax. There need not be any external injury and the victim will not have any serious symptoms till death. Head injuries can also result in delayed death.

Taking these factors into account, investigting oficers should not ignore a victim of assault with trivial external injuries. The injured should be sent to the nearest hospital and should be kept under medical observation for at least 24 hours.

During inquest, all the external injuries on the dead body shall be examined and recorded under column 7 and 8 of the report. These injuries shall be entered in the requisiton for autopsy to bring them to the notice of the forensic surgeon. Trivial contusions on the face may be indicative of smothering. Small abrasions or contusions on the neck region may be due to throttling.

When the doctor is examined u/s 161 CrPC, his opinion as to the nature and mode of causation of all injuries may be elicited and recorded. It is better to mark the injuries in a diagram.

# Injuries due to Fall

All types of injuries can be sustained from falls. Falls can be from a standing/walking posture, from the cot to the floor during sleep, or from a height. Of these, death due to fall from height are common. The majority of the cases are falls from high rise buildings and tall trees. The pattern of injuries varies depending upon the site of impact, nature of landing surface and the height of fall. Most of the cases will be accidental falls and there might be eye witnesses. When there is no reliable history or eye witness evidence, it will be difficult to determine the manner of death. The medicolegal expert should be able to analyse the nature and pattern of injury sustained by the victim for making scientific deductions. In case of fall from height, the part of the body which first hits the landing surface is termed the site of **primary impact** (Figs 13.1A and B). The injuries are not confined to the site of primary impact alone. The force is transmitted through the skeletal system and injuries will be sustained along the line of transmission of force. The anatomical configuration of the vertebral column plays a significant role in causing injuries by transmission of force of impact to the other areas of the body.

When there is suspicion of an assault prior to the fall, meticulous examination must be made to detect injuries which are due to assault and not due to fall. But there are very few injuries which cannot be ascribed to a fall from height. However, it may not be difficult to distinguish injuries due to a fall from height. But death due to fall from bed, fall from standing/walking position, fall

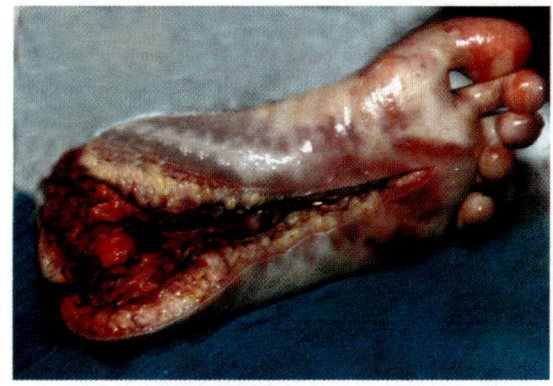

A

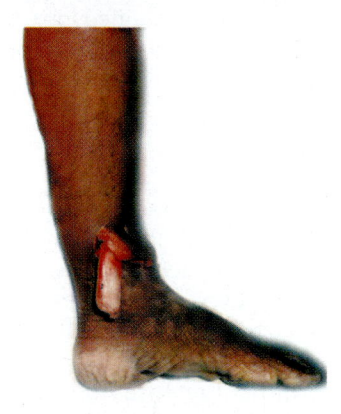

B

**Figs 13.1 A and B:** Primary leg impact: A. Lacerated wound of the heel with fracture of heel bone (calcaneum), B. Compound fracture of Leg bone (tibia) (*Courtesy:* Dr. V. Prathapan)

within a house, etc. may pose problems in identifying the manner of death. Examination of the scene of occurrence, collection of trace evidence and thorough medicolegal investigation may be necessary in such cases.

In the case of a voluntary jumping from a height, feet may be the primary site of impact. But if the body strikes any intervening object, the direction will be changed and the primary site will be some other part of the body. Similarly, if the fall is from a considerable height, the body may turn or twist during flight and any part of the body may strike the landing surface. When a person falls or jumps from a height, the distance from where the body strikes the ground to the jumping point will be variable. It will not be possible to differentiate an active jump from a passive fall. In a case of fall from height, the primary sites of impact are feet/leg, buttocks, trunk and head.

## FEET/LEG IMPACT

In primary leg impact, the feet may be the first site of impact. Lacerated wounds, compound fracture of calcaneum and other tarsal bones will be seen (Fig. 13.1). The force will be transmitted to the leg bones, hip, vertebral column and to the skull. When the impact is transmitted to the skull through the spine, a ring fracture of the base of skull can also occur.

In leg impacts, leg bones can be fractured at any point. Because of the transmitted force through the thigh bone (femur), the pelvis may be fractured. Fracture of the neck of thigh bone may also be sustained.

## BUTTOCK IMPACT

Buttock impact is characterised by extensive fractures of the pelvis/lumbar spine and visceral injuries. Buttock impact is also associated with head injury due to secondary impact. In buttock impacts also, the force is transmitted through the vertebral column to the base of skull causing ring fracture around the foramen magnum and dislocation of atlanto-occipital joint.

## TRUNK IMPACT

Trunk impact can be on the front, back or sides of the trunk. Extensive lacerations, multiple fractures of the ribs, sternum, spine and pelvis are seen in primary trunk impact. Sometimes, associated head injuries are also seen. Usually thoracic and lumbar spines are fractured. Various visceral injuries will also occur in trunk impacts.

## HEAD IMPACT

The injuries sustained to the head are very serious in nature in a primary head impact. Lacerations of the scalp, fracture of the skull, laceration of brain and all types of intracranial haemorrhages will be seen. Secondary head impact is a common feature in all types of primary impacts. In cases of fall from erect posture or from cot, fatal injuries to the head may be sustained.

## FALL FROM A STANDING POSTURE

Fall from a standing or walking position can occur due to accidental tripping, assault, intoxication, or unconsciousness due to diseases. In most of these cases, death will be due to head injury and injury to spinal cord of the upper cervical segments from sudden bending of the vertebral column (hyperflexion or extension).

Erect posture of a person is maintained by the extensor muscles of the back and legs. When a person becomes unconscious, the muscle tone is lost, body will flex at the groins and knees, and the person will fall forwards as the line of centre of gravity of a human body is in the front of the vertebral column. If the unconsciousness was not sudden, the person may stagger for sometime trying to regain his balance and then fall forwards or to one side. When a person is pushed or assaulted from the back, he is likely to fall forwards. Similarly a forcible impact from the front can cause a person to fall on his back.

When a person develops brain stroke like hemiplegia, there will be paralysis of muscles of one side of the body and he may fall to the side of the paralysed side. In epileptiform convulsions, the person falls backwards due to the spasm of muscles on the back. Death due to head injury is not uncommon in cases of fall from a cot during sleep especially in young children and old people. Old people will sustain fractures of the femur and arm bones even in trivial falls. Osteoporosis is the main reason for such injuries.

## DIRECTIONS TO THE INVESTIGATING OFFICER

Investigation of death due to fall from height can pose many problems. It may be difficult to find out the manner of death. Allegation of foul play may be raised even in a case of suicidal jump or accidental fall from height. Homicide may be masqueraded as an accidental fall from height. Sometimes the body of the fallen victim may be shifted to hospital. It may be difficult to identify the exact place where he had fallen from the height. Evidence of witnesses may not be correct also. The following points may be considered.

- Request the forensic surgeon and scientists to visit thescene of occurrence to collect trace evidences and help in reconstruction of the incident.
- When the doctor is examined U/S 161 CrPC, elicit his opinion regarding the nature and causation of all injuries found on the body.
- With the help of the doctor, try to identify the primary impact injuries.
- Request the doctor to collect viscera and body fluids for chemical analysis with special reference to alcohol, narcotic drugs and psychotropic substances.
- Collect and preserve all trace evidences from the dead body and scene.
- Conduct a thorough field investigation to arrive at the manner of death.

# 14

# Traffic Accidents

Incidence of vehicular accidents are on the increase. Every year more than 50,000 vehicular accidents are reported in our state. Nearly 3500 persons die. Actual number of injured will be manyfold. The victims may be pedestrians, cyclists, motor cyclists, drivers or occupants. Detailed investigation may be necessary for the reconstruction of the accident. From the nature of injuries, inferences can be drawn regarding the relative positions of the victim and the vehicle at the time of the accident. Moreover, in hit and run cases, analysis of the injuries and collection of trace evidence may help to connect the suspect vehicle with the crime. It is also possible to give an opinion as to whether the vehicle had run over the victim or not.

## INJURIES TO THE PEDESTRIANS

Mainly three types of injuries are sustained by the pedestrians.

### Primary Impact Injuries

When a person is hit by a moving vehicle, the various parts of the vehicle may come into contact with the body during the impact producing patterned injuries (Fig. 14.1). The pedestrian can be hit from the front, behind or sides. The parts of the vehicle which usually produce patterned injuries are the bumper, grill, head lights, etc. A bumper hit can produce fracture of the bones of leg commonly known as 'bumper fracture'. In a hit and run case, the height of the bumper can be found out, if measurements are taken from the heel to the fracture site in the dead body. Grill

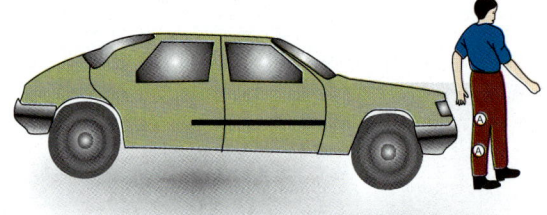

**Fig. 14.1:** Primary impact injuries at sites marked 'A'

and head light rims may produce patterned abrasions and contusions. Glass pieces and particles of paint recovered from the body will help to connect the vehicle with the crime. The detection of a primary impact injury will help to find out the relative position of the pedestrian and the vehicle. This is very important either to corroborate or to refute the versions of the eye witnesses of the incident.

### Secondary Impact Injuries

After the primary impact, the feet of the victim slide and the whole body is lifted off the ground and thrown on to the vehicle. The head may strike the windshield and torso may strike the bonnet or other parts of the car. Some times, he may even land on the roof of the car. During this impact, a set of injuries can be produced (Fig. 14.2).

The particle of the broken windshield, flag post of the bonnet, etc. can produce contusions, lacerations, etc. After the secondary impact, the victim may be forcibly thrown on the ground.

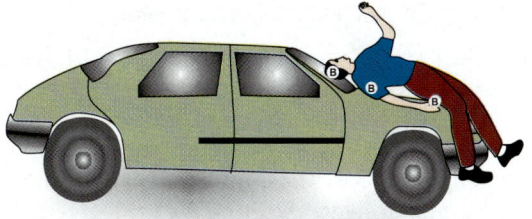

**Fig. 14.2:** Secondary impact injuries marked 'B'

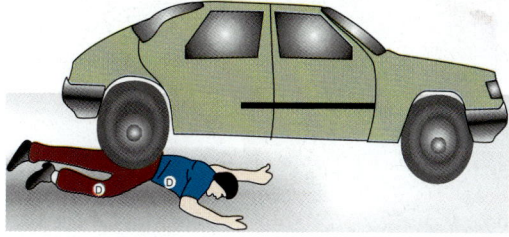

**Fig. 14.4:** Run over by the vehicle

## Tertiary Impact Injuries

These injuries are caused by the victim striking the ground (Fig. 14.3). The victim may sustain graze abrasions, lacerations, fractures of long bones and pelvis, thoracic and abdominal injuries. Head injury is the most common injury of this group. Victim may be thrown on the side railings, fencing and trees. Very often death will be as a result of tertiary impact injuries. The victim can fall on the ground in the flight path of the same vehicle or another vehicle. Then he may be run over by any of the vehicles. In secondary impact, if the victim lands on the roof of the vehicle, he may be thrown behind the vehicle. In that case, he may be run over by a vehicle coming from behind the vehicle which hit him.

## Run Over Injuries

The victim may be sometimes run over by the vehicle causing crush injuries (Fig. 14.4). Tyre marks may be seen on the body, if the tyres are not worn out. If tyre marks are seen, the exact measurements and pattern have to be noted. Photograph of the tyre mark with a scale included is to be taken and it will help in future comparison. The clothing of the victim will be soiled with grease, oil and dirt from the under surface of the vehicle. The edges of the wound will also be

stained. In **hit and run** cases, if the suspect vehicle is apprehended, it should be subjected to forensic examination for the detection of trace evidences transferred from the victim. These include blood, hair, skin, tissues, etc. Paint flakes, glass pieces, oil, grease, etc. will be transferred from the vehicle to the body or clothes of the victim.

## Injuries Sustained to the Cyclists/Motor Cyclists

The injuries will be similar to those sustained by the pedestrian. The primary impact will be usually against some part of the cycle/motorcycle. Secondary and tertiary impact injuries can be more severe. Examination of the cycle/motor cycle is also necessary for the reconstruction of the accident. Trace evidences should be collected from the cycle and from the body of the victim.

## Injuries Sustained to the Occupants of the Vehicle

During collision, the occupants of a speeding vehicle will sustain different types of injuries on various parts of the body depending upon the type of vehicle, speed of the vehicle, direction of impact, degree of deceleration, position of the occupants, use of seat belts, provision of air bags, etc. (Fig. 14.5). These injuries are caused by the impact of the occupants against some portion of the car. Sometimes the occupants may be partially or completely ejected out of the vehicle. Following collision, the vehicle may catch fire and the occupants will sustain burns. They can be trapped inside the burning car and can die due to burns and asphyxiation. After the accident, the car can go out of control and may fall into a canal or river nearby. The trapped occupants may die due to drowning.

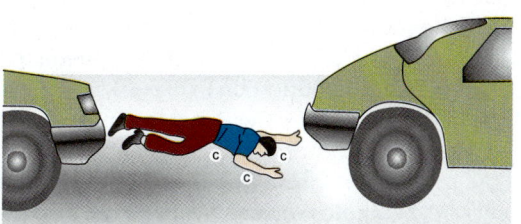

**Fig. 14.3:** Tertiary impact injuries (C)

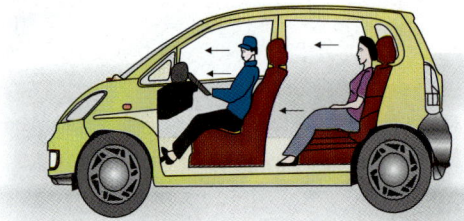

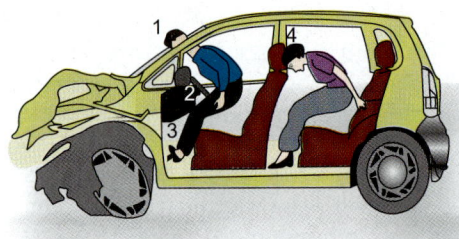

**Fig. 14.5:** Injuries to the occupants in a head on collision: A. Arrows indicate the probable sites of impact, B. Bullets nos 1–4 indicate sites of deceleration injuries

### Injuries to the Driver

The driver may get an impact on the chest by the steering column, especially the horn boss resulting in fracture of ribs and sternum, contusions and lacerations of lungs, heart, etc. His head may strike against the windshield producing head injury. Force will be transmitted from the pedals causing fracture of leg and thigh bones.

Sometimes he may be thrown out, if the door of the vehicle opens during the collision. Seat belts and air bags can prevent gross injuries. However, air bag and seat belts can produce injuries.

### Injuries to Other Occupants

The front seat occupants can sustain head and chest injuries by striking against the windshield and dash board (Fig. 14.5). As a result of the sudden deceleration, acute flexion or extension of the neck can occur resulting in the injury to muscles and ligaments of neck, dislocation of cervical vertebrae and injury to spinal cord (whiplash injury). The back seat passengers will sustain head and chest injuries by striking against the front seat. Whiplash injuries are also possible. The passengers can also be thrown out of the car.

### EFFECTS OF ALCOHOL ON DRIVING

Alcohol impairs driving related skills to a considerable extent. Drunken driving is a major factor contributing to severe traffic accidents. Alcohol produces impairment of judgement, muscular incoordination, diminished visual acuity, impairment of hearing, slowing of reflexes and reaction time, drowsiness, etc. The most important driving skills are vigil and judgement. These may be impaired by even at blood alcohol concentration of 20–30 mg%. Another feature is the tendency of a drunken driver to take risks. Overspeeding, reckless overtaking, cornering, etc. are some of the rash and negligent ways of driving seen in intoxicated drivers. In order to curb the practice of drunken driving, most of the countries have passed laws. In India, maximum permissible blood alcohol concentration (**BAC**) is 30 mg%. Permissible BAC level in UK is 80 mg%, and in USA, it is 100 mg%.

### Driving by a Drunken Person or by a Person Under the Influence of Drugs

As per the provisions of Section 185 of Motor Vehicles Act of India, whoever, while driving or attempting to drive, a motor vehicle (a) has, in his blood, **alcohol exceeding 30 mg per 100 ml of blood** detected in a test by a breath analyser, or (b) is under the influence of a drug to such an extent as to be incapable of exercising proper control over the vehicle shall be punishable for the first offence with imprisonment for a term which may extend to 6 months, or with fine which may extend to 2 thousand rupees, or with both. For a second or subsequent offence, if committed within 3 years of the commission of the previous similar offence, with imprisonment for a term which may extend to 2 years, or with fine which may extend to 3 thousand rupees, or with both.

*Explanation:* For the purposes of this section, the drug or drugs, specified by the central government on this behalf, by notification in the official gazette, shall be deemed to render a person incapable of exercising proper control over a motor vehicle.

As per Section 202, a police officer in uniform may arrest without warrant any person who in his presence commits an offence described above. He should be subjected to a medical examination as per Section 203/204, by a registered medical practitioner within 2 hours of his arrest, failing which he shall be released from custody.

## Section 203 Breath Tests (using breath analyser/drunkometer/alcometer)

1. A police officer in uniform or an officer of the motor vehicle department, may require any person driving or attempting to drive a motor vehicle in a public place to provide one or more specimens of breath for breath test there or nearby, if such police officer or officer has any reasonable cause to suspect him of having committed an offence under Section 185, provided that requirement for breath test shall be made (unless it is made) as soon as reasonably practicable after the commission of such offence.

2. If a motor vehicle is involved in an accident in a public place and a police officer in uniform has any reasonable cause to suspect that the person who was driving the motor vehicle at the time of the accident had alcohol in his blood or that he was driving under the influence of a drug referred to in Section 185, he may require the person so driving the motor vehicle, to provide a specimen of his breath for a breath test (a) in the case of a person who is at a hospital as an indoor patient (b). In the case of any other person, either at or near the place where the requirement is made, or if the Police officer thinks fit at a police station specified by the police officer: Provided that a person shall not be required to provide such a specimen while at a hospital as an indoor patient, if the registered medical practitioner in immediate charge of his case is not first notified of the proposal to make the requirement or objects to the provision of specimen on the ground that its provision or the requirement to provide it would be prejudicial to the proper care or treatment of the patient.

3. If it appears to a police officer in uniform, in consequence of a breath test carried out by him on any person under subsection 1 or subsection 2 that the device by means of which the test

has been carried out indicates the presence of alcohol in the person's blood, the police officer may arrest that person without warrant except that person is at a hospital as an indoor patient.

4. If a person, required by a police officer under subsections 1 or 2 to provide a specimen of breath for a breath test, refuses or fails to do so and the police officer has reasonable cause to suspect him of having alcohol in his blood, the police officer may arrest him without warrant except while he is at a hospital as an indoor patient.

5. A person arrested under this section shall while at a police station, be given an opportunity to provide a specimen of breath for a breath test there.

6. The result of a breath test made in pursuance of the provisions of this section shall be admissible in evidence.

*Explanation:* For the purposes of this section, "breath test" means a test for the purpose of obtaining an indication of the presence of alcohol in a person's blood carried out, one or more specimen of breath provided by that person, by means of a device of a type approved by the central government, by notification in the official gazette, for the purpose of such a test Section 204 laboratory test (testing of blood for alcohol).

1. A person, who has been arrested under Section 203 may, while at a police station, be required by a police officer to provide to such registered medical practitioner a specimen of his blood for a laboratory test, if (a) it appears to the police officer that, the device, by means of which breath test was taken in relation to such person, indicates the presence of alcohol in the blood of such person, or (b) such person, when given the opportunity to submit to a breath test, has refused, omitted or failed to do so: Provided that where the person required to provide such specimen is a female and registered medical practitioner is a male medical practitioner, the specimen shall be taken only in the presence of a female, whether a medical practitioner or not.

2. A person while at a hospital as an indoor patient may be required by a police officer to provide at

the hospital a specimen of his blood for a laboratory test, (a) if it appears to the police officer that the device by means of which test is carried out in relation to the breath of such person indicates the presence of alcohol in the blood of such person, or (b) if the person having been required, whether at the hospital or elsewhere to provide a specimen of breath for a breath test, has refused, omitted or failed to do so and a police officer has reasonable cause to suspect him of having alcohol in his blood; provided that person shall not be required to provide a specimen of his blood for a laboratory test under this subsection, if the registered medical practitioner in immediate charge of his case is not first notified of the proposal to make the requirement or objects to the provision of such specimen on the ground that its provision or the requirements to provide it would be prejudicial to the proper care or treatment of the patient.

3. The results of a laboratory test made in pursuance of this section shall be admissible in evidence.

*Explanation:* For the purpose of this section, laboratory test means the analysis of a specimen of blood made at a laboratory established, maintained or recognized by the central government or a state government.

## Drugs and Driving

Driving motor vehicles after consuming drugs may result in accidents. Consumption of narcotic drugs and psychotropic substances also affect the driving-related skills of a person. A wide variety of substances can impair the driving performance. According to motor vehicle laws, driving under the influence of drugs is also an offence punishable like drunken driving. The common drugs used by the drivers are benzodiazepines, opioids, cannabis, amphetamines, heroin, cocaine and other stimulants. Traffic safety is considerably affected by the consumption, especially of a higher dose of benzodiazepines and related sedatives and hypnotics. Cannabis can cause serious impairment of driving skills for the first few hours after consumption. Amphetamines and related drugs make the driver 'high' and accident prone.

Anihistamines can make a driver drowsy. Unlike drunken driving, 'drugged driving' is difficult to detect. Screening tests like breathalysers are not yet available. But rapid testing of urine, saliva and sweat by immunologic techniques have been developed. Immunoassay devices for common drugs like cannabis, cocaine, amphetamines, opioids, benzodiazepines are available. Road side testing of saliva for drugs using these devices are becoming popular.

## NATURAL DISEASES AND TRAFFIC ACCIDENTS

Natural diseases cause or contribute to traffic accidents. Ischemic heart disease, cerebrovascular accidents, epilepsy, hypoglycemic episodes, encephalitis, brain tumours, AV malformations etc. can cause fatal accidents. Sometimes the driver dies 'at the wheel' and the vehicle goes out of control and results in accidents involving other vehicles or pedestrians. A detailed autopsy, examination of the scene of occurrence and evidence from the eye witnesses can provide clues to the cause and manner of death.

## Autocide

Committing suicide by driving a vehicle at high speed and wilfully crashing it against a wall or a tree or another vehicle is not uncommon. This method of committing suicide is known as autocide. It is difficult to prove a car crash as autocide without evidences like a suicide note and other circumstantial evidence.

## Auto-homicide

Homicide using a motor vehicle is also not uncommon. Death of the victim is caused by hitting him with the vehicle when he is walking along the road or riding a cycle/motor cycle. Heavy vehicles like trucks are used to kill a victim travelling in a small car. Similarly victims are rendered unconscious or killed in the vehicle and a vehicular accident is simulated. A careful autopsy and investigation can reveal the truth.

## Railway Accidents

A careful autopsy has to be conducted on a body recovered from the railway track to determine whether the injuries are antemortem or not. The majority of the cases may be accidents or suicides, but murdered victims may be placed on the rails to simulate suicide. A clean decapitation may be suggestive of suicide. As death is instantaneous in run over cases, the vital reaction in the injuries will be minimal. However, postmortem injuries can be differentiated by the absence of staining of the edges and profuse bleeding. As in the case of automobile accidents, patterned injuries can be discernible due to the primary and secondary impact, but they will be of a very serious nature.

### Hit by a Speeding Train

The victim will be hit by a speeding train while crossing the line, walking along the railway line or jumping in front of it. The engine of the train has got a bumper known as cattle guard. During the primary impact, the victim will sustain injuries caused by the contact with the cattle guard and other parts on the front of the engine. These injuries will be similar to those seen in an automobile accident. During autopsy, the distance from the heel to each injury is to be measured for future reconstruction. Immediately after the secondary impact, the victim will be thrown forward and sometimes run over. In such cases, the injuries sustained will be of a dismembering nature.

If decapitation and amputation of torso or limbs are seen, the distance between those two are also to be measured and compared with the breadth of the railway track. In the absence of other injuries, this indicates that the victim was lying across the track. In all cases, the body has to be examined for signs of violence, intoxication, natural disease, etc. Persons standing or walking by the side of a railway track can sustain fatal injuries by impact with the side of the engine or bogies.

### Falling from a Speeding Train

The victim may sustain multiple injuries of different types to various parts of the body. The body will be recovered from the outside of the track unless the victim fell in between the carriages. Homicides are possible by pushing the victim out of a speeding train.

### Collision and Derailment

The victim may show injuries to head, spine and legs similar to those found in automobile accidents. Persons sleeping on the bunks may be thrown on to the floor can sustain dislocation or fractures of vertebral column and injury to the spinal cord. Broken fragments of the carriage may produce penetrating injuries as well. A derailed or crashed compartment can catch fire and the trapped passengers can sustain fatal burns.

## AVIATION ACCIDENTS

Even though aircraft accidents are rare in our country, the forensic expert should possess sufficient knowledge and skills to conduct a medicolegal investigation in such a mass disaster. The main task is to identify the dead bodies of the victims. This is the most difficult task, as majority of the bodies will be mutilated, fragmented and charred. Physical characteristics, dental peculiarities, personal articles, fingerprints and DNA typing will be helpful in establishing identity of the victims. Medicolegal expert should obtain the help of forensic odontologists, radiologists, anthropologists, fingerprint experts and forensic scientists. Autopsies should be conducted at site.

When modern jet planes crash there will be total disintegration of the aircraft with fragmentation of the bodies of the passengers. Sometimes extensive fire causes charring of the body fragments. It may be difficult to find out the cause of death in majority of cases. When an aircraft catches fire during flight, the polyurethane insulation materials and furnishings of the cabin will emit noxious fumes and gases. Many of the deaths will be due to asphyxiation and inhalation of irrespirable gases. Modern toxicological analysis is required to establish the cause of death.

Each body fragment is examined, information recorded and then stored separately. Matching of the information collected is done to match the fragments. In this way, several fragments can be shown to have derived from the same body. Detailed autopsy and toxicological analysis of the bodies of the crew members will sometimes yield clues to the cause of the accident.

## DIRECTIONS TO THE INVESTIGATING OFFICER

Many factors are responsible for the increasing incidence of vehicular accidents in our country. One of the main causes is the dearth of properly constructed and maintained motorable roads. Planning and construction of the roads are not done scientifically. The surface of the road becomes slippery during rains. The existing roads are absolutely inadequate to cope up with the increase in number of motor vehicles. Lack of driving skills, disobeying the traffic rules, driving under the influence of alcohol and/or drugs, deficient eyesight and hearing, etc. are some of the driver-related factors in the causation of accidents. Pedestrians also contribute to the accidents by violating the traffic rules and carelessl trekking on the roads, etc. Majority of the motor cyclists overspeed and do not obey the traffic rules. They are involved in the majority of vehicular accidents.

The investigating officer has to conduct detailed investigation in cases where pedestrians and occupants either die or sustain serious injuries. If it is a case of "hit and run"the offending vehicle and the driver have to be traced. This is not an easy task. Detailed field investigation and application of scientific methods are essential for the detection of the case.

## The following Steps of Investigation may be Conducted

- Record detailed description of all injuries both in the case of living and dead victims.
- Look out for patterned injuries including tyre marks.
- Note the height of the patterned injuries from the heels of the victim.
- Note the direction of injuries.
- Collect all trace evidences such as glass, grease, paint, etc. from the dead body.
- Examination of the clothing for tears and trace evidences.
- Request the doctor to collect viscera and body fluids of all the deceased persons (victim/occupants/pedestrian) for chemical anlysis with reference to alcohol and drugs.
- Look out for blood, hair, tissues, remnants of clothings, etc. on the vehicle.
- Conduct an examination of the scene of occurrence to look out for skid marks and trace evidences.
- With the help of the forensic surgeon and scientists, try to reconstruct the accident.
- Conduct a deep and thorough field investigation especially in cases of 'hit and run'.

# 15

# Medicolegal Aspects of Injuries

## ANTEMORTEM INJURIES

Inuries can be sustained during life (antemortem) or after death (postmortem). Bleeding is the most important sign of an injury inflicted during life. The extravasated blood will be infiltrated into the tissue interspace in the vicinity of the wound resulting in the staining of its edges. The effused blood will clot normally in 5 to 10 minutes. Because of the elasticity of the skin, the edges of wound will be retracted. This feature will not be seen in a postmortem injury as the elasticity of the skin is lost after death. If the person survives, signs of inflammation and repair process will be evident in an antemortem wound. This can be demonstrated conclusively by histological and histochemical examination of the tissues around the wound. Antemortem fractures also will show staining of the fractured ends due to the infiltration of blood. Injuries sustained during or just after death also may show antemortem features to a lesser extent. It is very difficult to distinguish these perimortem injuries from antemortem injuries. Antemortem features will be obliterated in decomposed bodies especially those recovered from water.

## Cause of Death from Injuries

### Bleeding and Shock

The main cause of death from injuries is bleeding. Bleeding can be external through open injuries like lacerations and incised wounds or from body orifices. Internal bleeding is from contusions, internal organs and major blood vessels. Total volume of blood present in the body of an adult is about 5 to 6 liters. Rapid loss of approximately one-third of total blood volume is sufficient to cause death. When a person loses blood, the arterial blood pressure will be lowered and the condition is called shock. This is characterised by cold and clammy skin, sweating, thready rapid pulse and pallor. Shock secondary to bleeding, loss of fluids as in the case of burns, etc. are termed secondary shock. Shock can also develop due to a reflex neurovascular disturbance which may result in death. This is called primary or neurogenic shock. This condition is seen in severe pain, injuries to vital organs, circulating toxins or poisons, hypersensitivity reactions, etc. Death will be sudden in primary shock, while it is delayed in secondary shock. There will not be any specific autopsy findings in death due to primary shock.

### Infection

Open injuries are liable to infection by various microorganisms. Crush injuries and lacerations are more susceptible to infection. Many types of bacteria are responsible for wound infection. The most common are staphylococci, streptococci, *Coliforms, Pseudomonas aeruginosa* and the anaerobes such as *Clostridium tetani, Cl. perfringens,* etc.

With the advent of powerful antibiotics, incidence of death due to infections is becoming less. However, even infected minor wounds can be fatal, if adequate treatment is not given in time.

135

A criminal assault that ends in death because of neglected or inadequate treatment will not exonerate the accused from all responsibility.

### Pulmonary Thromboembolism

Forced bedridden state will have pressure effect on the calf muscles which in turn will reduce the flow of blood in the veins. This will lead to the formation of blood clots (thrombosis) in the deep veins. This condition is called deep vein thrombosis (DVT). This is also seen in passengers of long distance air travel or old people who sit for a long time on hard chairs. Injury to the tissues of legs and pelvis can also lead to local venous thrombosis. Contused muscles, fractures of leg bones and pelvis are some of the causative injuries. Pelvic vein thrombosis is also associated with pregnancy, abortion and delivery. The thrombus in the calf veins spread proximally to the saphenous, femoral and iliac veins. Many thrombi detach and form a mass which is carried to the right side of the heart. They reach the pulmonary circulation and cause obstruction to the pulmonary blood flow and cause death. This condition is called pulmonry thromboembolism.

The medicolegal significance is that even trivial trauma can lead to fatal pulmonary thromboembolism. The victim develops pulmonary embolism several days after the trauma during the recovery period. Death is sudden and clinical diagnosis and treatment may not be possible. Prophylactic steps to prevent deep vein thrombosis should be taken to prevent pulmonary embolism in bedridden victims of trauma, especially in old people.

### Air Embolism

Air embolism can occur in injuries to the neck veins, induced abortion, etc. When a considerable volume of air reaches the right side of the heart, the air mixes with blood to form a froth which obstructs the pulmonary flow like an air lock. To cause death, 100–150 ml of air is sufficient.

### Fat Embolism

Fat embolism develops as a complication of fractures of long bones, injury to fatty tissue/fatty liver and burns. The mobilised fat globules appear in the small blood vessels of the lungs. Pulmonary fat embolism is not significant unless it is so gross as to produce hypoxia. Pulmonary capillaries can only retain a certain amount of fat and when the threshold increases, fat will appear in the systemic circulation. In fat embolism syndrome, fat in the systemic circulation will reach many organs like brain, kidneys or myocardium. Systemic fat embolism will produce punctate haemorrhages in the organs. Obstruction of arterioles can cause death of tissues. In brain stem, it can cause sudden death.

### Acute Tubular Necrosis

Run over by vehicles, torture by rolling a rod over the thighs, etc. can cause crushing of muscles and other tissues. Cellular debris and metabolic products will affect the kidneys. The condition is called acute tubular necrosis. Renal failure due to acute tubular necrosis can cause death. This condition is called **crush syndrome**.

### Disseminated Intravascular Coagulation (DIC)

There are several factors responsible for DIC. It is an abnormal activation of the clotting process of blood. Damaged tissue from injuries and burns can trigger clotting of blood. In DIC, clots are formed throughout the vascular system. When clotting factors are depleted, widespread bleeding occurs. Autopsy will reveal fibrin clots in vessels and evidence of internal bleeding.

### Adrenal Haemorrhage

Few days after severe trauma or infection, bleeding can occur in the adrenal glands. Sometimes the bleeding will be massive. Meningococcal infection can produce adrenal bleeding on both sides. This condition is known as Waterhouse-Friderichsen syndrome. Any type of shock can cause adrenal bleeding.

### Trauma and Pre-existing Disease

Injuries can precipitate death due to acceleration of a pre-existing disease. For example, physical and mental stress and strains following even a minor injury can precipitate heart attack and sudden death especially in a person with pre-existing heart disease. Many diseases can be aggravated by injuries.

## Trauma and Tumour/Diseases

It has been reported that tumours develop at the site of a previous injury. Brain tumours have developed following focal head injury. The causal connection has not been established. If a tumour develops on the site of the focal injury within a reasonable time interval, it can be presumed that injury was responsible for its development. Skin cancers are found to develop at the site of injuries and burns. Head injury is also considered as the exciting factor in the development of diseases like multiple sclerosis, Parkinsonism, epilepsy, psychoses and neuroses.

## Acute Respiratory Distress Syndrome

Severe lung injury, blast injuries, aspiration of stomach contents, infections, shock, poisons and inhalation of irrespirable gases can produce damage to the alveolar epithelium. Clinically, the victim will develop difficulty in breathing and progressive respiratory failure. Autopsy will reveal stiff lungs with bleeding and swelling.

## MANNER OF CAUSATION OF INJURIES

Conclusions can be drawn as to whether injuries are suicidal, homicidal or accidental by observing the site, number, extent and nature of injuries. Suicidal injuries will be in accessible areas. They will be multiple, parallel or close to each other and superficial in nature. The usual sites are neck, chest, abdomen, wrist or genitalia. For example, there may be a number of superficial parallel incised wounds on the front of wrist in the case of a person committing suicide by cutting his wrist. Similarly in a suicidal cut throat injury, there may be a number of parallel, superficial cuts coalescing into a single wound with notches or tags of skin at its ends. These notches are called **hesitation cuts**. This finding indicates the hesitation of a person who inflicts injury by himself. Multiple superficial punctured wounds on chest or abdomen in a group are suggestive of self-infliction. One or a few of them may be penetrating and fatal. Even in suicidal gun shot injuries, it is not uncommon to find more than one entry wound. If one attempt does not result in imminent death, it is natural that a person determined to die will inflict subsequent injuries until he dies.

Homicidal injuries will be usually severe and found widely distributed. Inference can be drawn from non-accessibility of the site, direction of the track of wounds, absence of hesitation cuts, etc. Injuries inflicted by heavy cutting weapons are almost always homicidal. Presence of **defence wounds** sustained due to warding of the infliction or grabbing the weapon may be seen in the forearms and hands. Injuries through the clothing of the victims are generally indicative of homicide. The fatality of each injury must be ascertained before drawing conclusions as to the manner of infliction. This will also help in finding out which of the several injuries had caused death.

## VOLITIONAL ACTIVITIES FOLLOWING FATAL INJURY

Persons who sustain fatal injuries may be able to perform voluntary activities like speaking, walking, etc. It depends upon many factors like the severity of the injury, regions affected, etc. For example, an injury of neck involving the windpipe below the level of vocal cords may render a victim speechless. The victim may be able to speak or produce sounds, if the injury is above the level of the vocal cords. Fractures and severe injuries of the lower limbs and spine can render a person immobile. Severe injuries to the brain can result in immediate unconsciousness. Even after sustaining imminently fatal injuries, some times the victim may be able to perform volitional activities.

## WOUND CERTIFICATION

All injury cases brought to the hospital are examined by the casualty medical officer/duty medical officer. Seriously injured are admitted immediately and necessary treatment given. The necessary first aid and resuscitation treatment are given in the casualty itself. If the person has lost blood or body fluids, arrangement for transfusion is made. If the person needs admission, the casualty, medical officer alerts the doctors concerned for further management.

For want of adequate facilities in a hospital, the injured person can be referred to another hospital. But before transferring such cases, necessary first aid should be given. Supreme Court has given directions that it is mandatory on the part of every medical practitioner to render first aid and life saving measures in all types of medicolegal cases brought to them. Therefore private hospitals and private practitioners are also bound to attend medicolegal cases. If facilities are not available for managing the case, the patient can be referred to another hospital after giving first aid and other measures to save the life.

Apart from the medical duties, a doctor has certain legal duties to perform. Details of the injuries found on the person are recorded in the accident register cum wound certificate by the doctor who attends the patient first.

This register is kept in the casualty under safe custody by the duty doctor. The forms in the register are arranged in duplicates to facilitate taking a carbon copy. The original is the wound certificate, which is to be detached and issued to the police officer. The carbon copy will remain in the register and serve as a permanent record with the medical officer. Private hospitals and nursing homes also maintain Accident register and other records. The format of the register is given in Proforma 15.1 (G.O Ms 44/71/Health dt 4-2-71). This method is highly satisfactory as it will ensure that the wound certificate is written immediately after the doctor has examined the injured. Injuries of persons relating to non-police cases should also be entered in the same register. Entries regarding the injured persons who come to hospitals with police requisition and cases which appear prima facie as medicolegal cases should be specially marked in the register by writing the capital letter *P at the right hand on top of the form.

## Informing the Police

Under Section 39 of Criminal Procedure Code, medical officers are legally bound to inform the police all cases of homicide/homicidal attempt, crimes of treason, dacoity, robbery, etc. In a case of poisoning, if the victim is conscious and coherently gives a history of accidental or

---

**Proforma 15.1:** Accident Register Cum Wound Certificate

### Accident Register Cum Wound Certificate

*P

1. Serial no.
2. Date and hour of examination
3. Name
4. Age
5. Sex
6. Address
7. Marks of identification 1. ...................................2. ......................................
8. History and alleged cause of injury
9. Details of injuries/clinical features
10. No. of additional sheets if any
11. Is dying declaration required?
12. If yes, whether police/magistrate is informed
13. Investigation results, if any
14. Date of admission as inpatient and IP no.
15. Date of discharge
16. Condition on discharge
17. Opinion as to the cause of injury

Name of institution                                  Signature of M.O................................
Station                                              Name of M.O....................................
Date                                                 Designation......................................
                                                     Regn: Number..................................

Issued to ................... of police as per his requisition no. ....................................
Dated ........................ Signature of issuing Medical Officer................................

voluntary consumption of poison, police need not be informed but entries should be made in the accident register. But later, if the condition of the victim deteriorates, then police should be intimated. At the time of admission, if the victim is unconscious, police should be informed. All cases of homicidal poisoning should be invariably intimated.

When the injured person comes first to the hospital without informing the police, the medical officer should inform the local police station over telephone or otherwise about the arrival of the case. This is followed by a letter of intimation the station house officer. Copy of the intimation is filed. The police officer in charge of the station gives a written requisition to the medical officer for treating the patient and issuing the wound certificate. When the injured person is directed to the hospital by the police officer, he should send the requisition through a constable with a local delivery register along with the patient. The medical officer will acknowledge the receipt of the requisition in the local delivery book brought by the constable. He also maintains a register of requisitions from police in which he will note the particulars of the police requisitions received.

### Recording the Injuries

The medical officer records the preliminary particulars including the identification marks, general condition of the injured, history of the alleged cause of injury/injuries and the opinion as to the cause of injury.

Under the caption, history and alleged cause of injury, information given by the injured regarding the causation of injury is included. The doctor has to record verbatim the information given by the injured if he is conscious and coherent. It is not the duty of the doctor to ascertain the identity of the assailant. However, if the injured volunteers such information, he shall record it. In a criminal appeal **(1985 SCC-Cri-464)** Supreme Court has made the following observation that failure of a witness to disclose the name of the assailant to the doctor would not discredit him as an eye witness (In the said case, this witness had taken the injured to the hospital).

"A doctor is not at all concerned as to who committed the offence or whether the person brought to him is a criminal or an ordinary person, his primary effort is to save the life of the person brought to him and inform the police in medicolegal cases. Doctors before whom dead bodies are produced or injured persons are brought, either themselves take the dying declaration or hold the postmortem immediately and if they start examining the informants, they are likely to become witnesses of the occurrence which is not permissible...."

In another case, **2005(1) KLJ 743,** the Hon:High Court of Kerala has held as follows:

"...The mention or non-mention in the wound certificate about the names of the assailants is also not decisive. The duty of the doctor is to save the patient. He is not concerned about who committed the offence. He is not expected to elicit from the injured or from those who brought him there about the identity of the actual assailants. His enquiry would be confined to the ascertainment of the manner in which the injured or the deceased received the injuries and the weapons if any, used...."

From these observations, it is clear that if the injured or the accompanying persons do not give a history regarding the occurrence and identity of the assailant, the doctor need not elicit the information from the persons concerned. But if the injured gives a coherent version, he may record it. At the same time, apart from the history of the incident, the alleged cause of injury should be described in the exact words of the injured. Hence it is preferable to record it in vernacular. For example, 'stabbing with a knife' 'beating with an iron rod'.

If the victim is unconscious, the information is obtained from the accompanying policemen/relatives/witness. In such cases, the name and relationship of the person who gives the information are also be recorded. The injuries and clinical features are to be recorded under column no. 10. The clinical features shall include the general condition of the person such as his level of consciousness, ability to speak, mental status, pulse rate, blood pressure, etc.

## Recording of Dying Declaration (Sec 32 of Evidence Act)

Dying declaration is a statement of a dying person, relating to the cause and circumstance of his death. The principle behind recording a dying statement is that a dying man will tell only the truth. Therefore, a dying statement is relevant and admissible in evidence. Dying declaration can be made before any person including magistrate, doctor or police. But it is always better to have it recorded by a magistrate.

If the duty medical officer, after examining a seriously injured person, feels that the person is dying and there is no hope of recovery, he should arrange for the recording of a dying declaration. Judicial First Class Magistrates having jurisdiction should be requested to record the declaration. Police can make necessary arrangements for this. Before recording, the doctor should ascertain that the deponent is conscious and his mental faculties are normal. This fact should be recorded.

After recording the statement, the same will be read over to the dying person by the magistrate. When the deponent admits it as correct, the magistrate signs the statement. If possible, the signature or thumb impression of the deponent is obtained. The doctor should also sign the statement after certifying that the deponent is conscious and is in a fit condition to give the statement and affix his signature or thumb impression.

If the condition of the injured is very serious and if there is no time to inform the magistrate, the doctor himself can record his statement in the presence of two witnesses. If the person is able to write, he can do it himself. Otherwise, the statement is taken down by the doctor, copying the same words of the dying person without any alterations. Then it is read over to him and his signature or thumb impression is taken. The doctor and two witnesses should also sign the statement. This declaration is then sent to the magistrate in a sealed envelope with a covering letter. A copy of the same may be kept as an office copy.

If the duty doctor conducts special investigations such as X-rays, CT scans, etc. the results are to be recorded under column 14 of the wound certificate.

If the person is admitted, the date, inpatient number, date of discharge and condition on discharge should be noted in columns 15,16 and 17. Column no.18 is very important. Medical officer, after carefully examining the injuries, should express his opinion as to the causation of the injuries.

## Discharge Certificate

In the case of injured persons who are treated as inpatients, a discharge certificate is issued in continuation with the wound certificate. The discharge certificate will be issued by the duty doctor who had attended the patient first and issued the wound certificate. If investigations are done or if any further injury is noticed subsequently, the fact along with the name of doctors who dealt with it should also be mentioned in the discharge certificate. If the injured is referred to another hospital, the attending physician in the second hospital has to issue the discharge certificate (Proforma 15.2).

## Referring an Injury Case (Government Order No.GO Ms 131/72 dated 26th June 1972)

All medicolegal cases brought to a hospital should be examined by the medical officer who sees the case first and necessary treatment should be given. For want of adequate facilities, the person can be referred to another hospital. However, before transferring a seriously injured case to another hospital due to want of adequate facilities for treatment in the first hospital, necessary first aid should be given by the medical officer who examined the patient first. A copy of the accident register/wound certificate and referral letter shall be sent to the referral institution along with the patient. Local police should be informed about the referral.

The Supreme Court has also given general directions in this regard. The doctor of the first hospital is legally bound to give all life saving measures before referring the patient. If the injured needs any life support system during transit, it should be provided. If medical attention is necessary during transportation, medical personnel may accompany the injured to the referral centre. These measures can save the life of the injured and prevent unnecessary litigations against the first hospital.

**Proforma 15.2:** Discharge Certificate for Police Cases

No.                                                                    Date ..............................
From:

    Name of Medical Officer.................................
    Designation..................................................
    Name of Institution......................................
To
    The S.I of the police ....................................

Sir,
    In continuation of wound certificate No...................dated ..............-................ I have to inform you that Sri./
Smt...............................................aged.....admitted on ................ as IP No...................was discharged/cured/relieved
on .........................
    Given below are further remarks of the case:
1.  X-ray and other special investigations
    a...............................................................
    b...............................................................
    c...............................................................
2.  The following surgeons and specialities were concerned
    a. Dr.........................................................
    b. Dr.........................................................
3.  Other relevant information

                        Yours faithfully,
                        Sd/-
                        Name ..........................................................
                        Designation ................................................
                        Regn: Number............................................

If the injured is admitted and treated in the first hospital and later referred to a second hospital for further treatment, the medical officer of the first hospital should issue the wound certificate immediately to the police officer so that it can be produced before the medical officer in the second hospital who continues the treatment of the injured. In that case, the discharge certificate is issued by the attending doctor of the referral hospital.

## DIRECTIONS TO THE INVESTIGATING OFFICER

Sometimes the injured will come to the police station and lodge a complaint. In that case after registering the complaint, the injured should be sent to the nearest hospital with a requisition to treat the person and issue a wound certificate. Wound certificate is a document prepared by the doctor who sees the injured for the first time. It is generated at the time when the doctor enters the details in the accident cum wound certificate register using a carbon sheet. Wound cerificate is the original copy which is detached and issued to the police officer. Therefore, the wound certificate should be obtained without delay.

The doctor who issued the wound certificate should be examined u/s 161 of Cr.PC after obtaining the wound certificate and record his statement regarding the nature of injuries and opinion as to the alleged cause. This will be helpful in corroborating the versions of the witnesses to the incident of assault.

# 16

# Asphyxial Deaths

The term 'asphyxia' has originated from a Greek word *"asphuxia"* meaning loss of heart beat. It is a condition characterised by the lack of oxygen in the blood. When asphyxia is brought about by mechanical means, it is called mechanical asphyxia. Common asphyxial deaths are hanging, strangulation, drowning, suffocation, traumatic asphyxia, etc. Asphyxia is also caused by the inhalation of irrespirable gases like carbon dioxide/carbon monoxide which affect the mechanism of respiration; poisons which affect the respiratory muscles, high altitudes, hypothermia, etc. In almost all types of death, respiratory failure is the terminal event and the body will show some asphyxial changes.

## GENERAL FEATURES OF ASPHYXIA

### Cyanosis

If the body is examined within a few hours of death, presence of cyanosis is of significance, because by about 24 hours, oxygen will be dissociated from the blood and cyanosis will appear in any dead body. On the contrary, cyanosis need not be present in asphyxial deaths, if the dead body is exposed to cold atmosphere. When there is cyanosis, the lips, nails and sometimes, the face or other parts of the body will assume a bluish discolouration.

### Petechial Haemorrhage

Minute haemorrhages are seen under the conjunctivae, skin, mucus membranes, meninges, pleura, pericardium and internal organs in asphyxial deaths (Fig.16.1). The haemorrhaging occurs as a result of increased pressure in the small blood vessels (capillaries) as well as increased permeability of the vessel walls due to lack of oxygen (hypoxia). Even though these haemorrhages are seen in asphyxia, they are seen in other conditions like blood dyscrasia, exanthematous fevers, poisoning, etc.

## Pharyngeal and Laryngeal Haemorrhages

Bleeding under the mucus membrane (submucosal) seen in the pharynx and larynx in asphyxial deaths, especially hanging, stran-

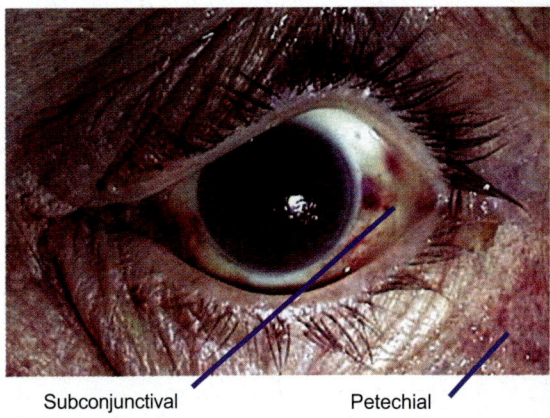

Subconjunctival          Petechial
haemorrhages             haemorrhages

**Fig.16.1:** Subconjunctival and petechial haemorrhages of facial skin

gulation, suffocation, etc. This is sometimes ascribed to direct pressure in this region which occurs in the above mentioned cases.

## Congestion

Pooling of blood in the internal organs ( venous congestion) is a common finding in asphyxial deaths. But it is seen in other types of death also. The lungs will also be congested (pulmonary congestion).

## Pulmonary Edema

Pulmonary congestion is associated with escape of fluid from the capillaries the air sacs of lungs (pulmonary oedema). Minor amount of pulmonary edema is a common finding in many types of deaths. But severe oedema is diagnostic of asphyxia along with the other features.

## Fluidity of Blood

In all sudden deaths and asphyxial deaths, a lot of fibrinolysin (a factor which dissolves blood cots) is liberated into the blood from the cells lining the blood vessels (endothelial cells) and blood remains fluid in the blood vessels after death.

## HANGING

Hanging is a form of mechanical asphyxial death in which the body is suspended by means of a ligature tied around the neck, the constricting force being the weight of the body.

## Examination of the Dead Body and Scene

Usually in a typical case of hanging, the body will be in a suspended posture with one end of the ligature tied around the neck and the other end tied to a suspension point. The suspension point may be indoors or outdoors. The ususal suspension point indoors are beams, rafters, fan hooks, etc. Tree branches are the usually chosen sites outdoors. There may be a stepping device like a chair or ladder to reach the suspension point. The stepping device like chair may be found toppled. The following examinations are to be conducted. They are:
- The scene
- The dead body

- The ligature
- The suspension point
- The ligature mark
- The stepping device
- The external signs.

## Examination of the Scene

It is always better to conduct an examination of the scene before the body is removed from the suspension point. The main point to be noted in a scene examination is the accessibility of the suspension point. When the ligature is tied around a rafter or beam in a room, there may a stepping device like a chair or table ( Fig. 16.2 ). It is advantageous to reconstruct the occurrence by attempting to tie the ligature at the suspension point by a person having the same height as that of the deceased. Presence of faeces, urine or blood detected just beneath the dead body is suggestive of antemortem suspension. Faeces, urine and semen are voided due to relaxation of sphincters in violent asphyxial deaths. Bleeding can occur from hemorrhoids (piles), urethra, uterus, or from

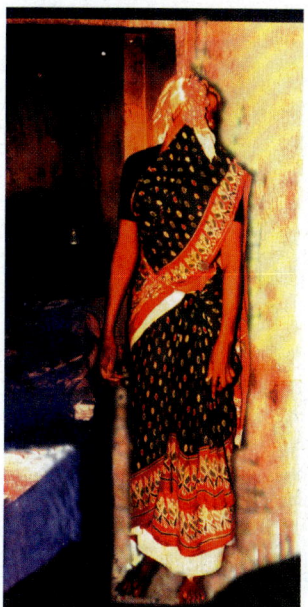

**Fig. 16.2:** Typical hanging — the box on the left side of the picture could be the stepping device. Both feet are above the floor level (Photo: Dr. Kurian Kuriakose)

injuries if any sustained during the act of suspension. All these discharges will produce vertical stains in the case of antemortem suspension. Disturbance in the scene is suspicious. But sometimes the stepping device will be found toppled as a result of the victim jumping from it.

In a hanging body, the upper limbs will be kept by the side of the body and will be fixed in rigor. Any abnormal position of the limbs fixed in rigor is suspicious. Postmortem staining is also seen in the lower part of limbs. Any contrary finding is also inconsistent with antemortem suspension. It is worthwhile to examine the hands of the deceased for fibres if he/she has handled the ligature material. Adhesive cellotapes applied over the palms are removed and despatched to the forensic scientist for detection of fibres if any and comparison of the same with those of the ligature **(cellophane test)**.

Sometimes the body is seen in a partially suspended position **(partial hanging)**. The body may be seen in a position with knees flexed and the toes or feet touching the ground (Fig. 16.3). Kneeling, sitting and even reclining positions can also be assumed in a case of partial hanging. Very

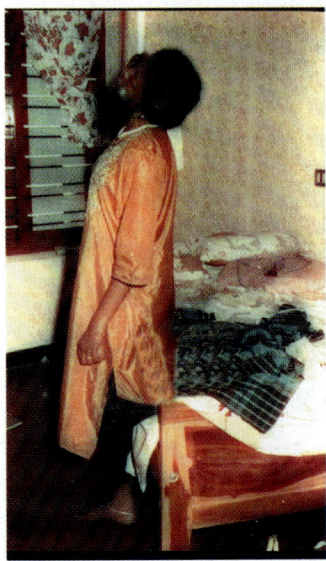

**Fig. 16.3:** Partial hanging — the cot might be the stepping device. One leg is touching the floor; the other leg (not visible) is resting on the cot (Photo: Dr. Kurian Kuriakose)

often this is due to a long ligature. When the person jumps from the stepping device after applying the knots around the neck and at the suspension point, he may land on his feet, knees or buttocks if the ligature is very long. The mechanism of death is cardiac arrest or cerebral congestion and asphyxial features may be absent or rare. This type of hanging will always induce suspension in the minds of the public. But partial hanging is almost always suicidal.

When the drop is long as in the case of judicial hanging, fracture dislocation of the neck vertebrae and damage to spinal cord can occur resulting in sudden death. Occasionally, spinal injuries are seen in short drops also. Severe injuries to the neck and even decapitation can occur if the ligature used is a narrow nylon rope or metal string with great tensile strength. The causative factors are the tensile strength of the ligature, a long drop and heavy weight of the body. The force is concentrated on the narrow ligature which will sever the delicate tissues of the neck including the spinal cord through the intervertebral disc. In a case of hanging, the ligature can break or the slip knot can become loose and the body may fall down. Sometimes postmortem injuries may also be seen on the dead body. A proper examination of the scene and forensic investigations can be helpful in drawing conclusions in such cases.

### Examination of the Ligature

The ligature may be of any material such as coir, nylon cord, dhothy, saree, etc. Usually, it is found tied around the neck with a slip knot. This knot may be seen anywhere in the neck, usually on one side of the neck. If the knot is on the back of neck, the hanging is called 'typical' and the body will show maximum asphyxial features (Fig.16.2). During inquest, the knot should not be disturbed. When the body is sent for autopsy, the ligature should be untied from the suspension point. The ligature with the slip knot kept in situ should be sent along with the dead body for autopsy. After autopsy, the ligature has to be obtained from the doctor as it is an important material object which may be required for further examination.

## Ligature Mark

The ligature mark is a pressure abrasion caused by the ligature material. If the material is soft, the mark will not be distinct. If the ligature is rough and patterned like a coir, the mark will be distinct and patterned similarly. Bruises and abrasions, especially in the margins of the ligature mark are important as they are of antemortem origin. Even if a dead body is suspended, a ligature mark will develop, but it will be devoid of vital reactions like bruising.

The ligature mark is usually above the level of thyroid cartilage, oblique on the sides of neck and non-continuous beneath the position of the knot. The length and average width of the mark should be measured. If a soft and broad ligature material like a dhothi or saree is used, the ligature mark need not be above the thyroid cartilage (Fig. 16.4).

Many variations are possible in a case of hanging with regard to the ligature and the ligature mark. Instead of a slip knot, sometimes a reef knot may be seen. There may not be a knot at all, the ligature material being simply wound round the neck once or twice. Ligature mark may be sometimes found below the level of thyroid cartilage and almost continuous. This is especially seen when a thin cord is used as a ligature material which will not slip upwards on suspension. Sometimes two ligatures-form the first position. This will normally appear suspicious, but one should look for abrasions and bruising in the skin between the two ligature marks. Strangulation of a victim by using a running noose with the force directed upwards can produce an oblique ligature mark similar to hanging, but internal examination of neck can reveal signs of violence indicative of strangulation.

## External Signs

The face may be livid with petechiae under the skin and conjunctiva. Tongue may be protruded and bitten. Blood stained froth may be present in the mouth and nostrils. The head is tilted to the opposite side of the knot and from the corner of the mouth saliva or blood-stained fluid may trickle down vertically. The salivary trickle marks will get dried and can be seen as a vertical streak on the side of the chin, front of chest or on the clothes. This is one of the signs of antemortem suspension. Lips and nails will be blue. Faecal and seminal discharges may be present.

In some cases of hanging, due to the pressure of the ligature on the sympathetic nerves, one eye

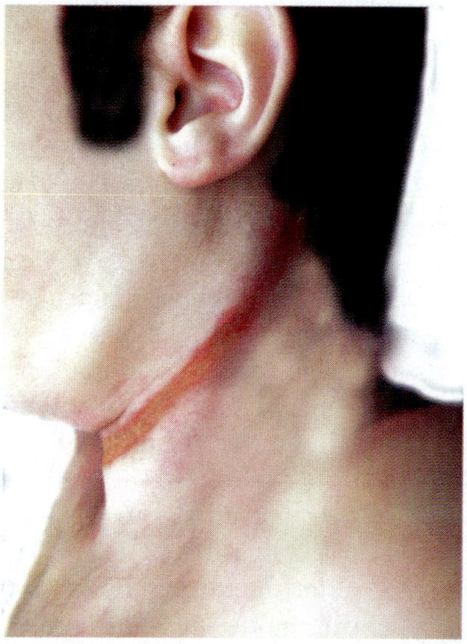

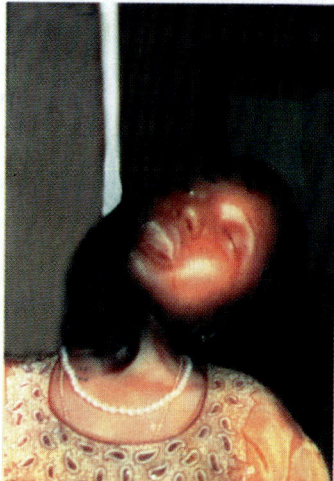

**Fig. 16.5:** Hanging facies — head is tilted towards the opposite side of the knot. Left eye closed, right open (la facies sympathique). Tongue protruded and bitten, saliva dribbling from the left corner of mouth

**Fig. 16.4:** Ligature mark—ligature mark is patterned, bruised and oblique on the sides of neck

will be open with its pupil dilated and the other eye will be closed. This appearance is called **La facies sympathique** (Fig.16.5).

## Findings in the Neck

When the doctor performs autopsy in a case of hanging, the dissection of the neck is postponed after removal of brain and internal organs. This will provide a bloodless field in the neck region devoid of artefacts. This is very important because artefacts can simulate violence.

The tissues of the neck will be pale. The tissues underneath the ligature mark will be dry and white in colour. Usually there will not be any bruising of the muscles or any damage of the midline structures like hyoid, thyroid, cricoid or tracheal rings. But if considerable force of constriction has occurred as in the case of judicial hanging, bruising of neck muscles may be seen. Partial rupture of sterno-mastoid muscles in their lower attachments to sternum and clavicle with infiltration of blood are also seen in some cases of hanging.

In old people, fractures of the cornua of hyoid bone and thyroid cartilage can occur as those will be calcified. Following traction of muscles of neck, avulsion fractures of these structures can occur. This finding can simulate local violence. Therefore, one should be cautious in interpreting the findings. When a suspended body is brought down shortly after suspension and the constriction of the neck is removed by loosening the ligature, there can be extravasation of blood into the tissues of neck due to rupture of capillaries. This finding can simulate violence at the region of neck. The intima of the carotid arteries may show rupture. In long drops, there could be fracture dislocation of the cervical vertebrae and laceration of spinal cord. In **judicial hanging**, this finding is usually seen. Bleeding into the outer layers of the intervertebral discs of lumbar vertebrae **(Simon's haemorrhage)** are seen in bodies suspended for a long time. They appear as red stripes in between the vertebral bodies. They cannot be considered as typical of antemortem hanging.

## Changes in the Internal Organs

The changes are variable, but mostly asphyxial changes like petechial haemorrhages on the surface of lungs/pericardium/meninges, pulmonary edema, generalised venous congestion, etc. are seen.

## Discussion

The findings described above are those seen in a case of typical hanging. All the findings need not be present in each and every case. For example, mechanism of death in partial hanging may be due to cardiac arrest by vagal inhibition. Asphyxial features need not be present. That is why even a person with a tracheostomy can commit suicide by hanging. When the autopsy surgeon gives an opinion as to the cause of death is as hanging, it implies that the suspension was antemortem. A medical officer cannot give an opinion regarding the manner of death such as accident, suicide or homicide. A detailed investigation is needed to find the manner of death.

To mask homicide, the victim may be suspended after death. Postmortem suspension can be easily identified. The actual cause of death can be found out by a careful autopsy. If a person is strangled to death and suspended afterwards, there will be two ligature marks, one antemortem mark caused by strangling and another post-mortem mark produced by suspension.

It is difficult to detect homicidal hanging, i.e. suspending a man alive. In the ordinary course, it is difficult to lynch a healthy, conscious, sober person by another man. Possibility of suspending an unconscious or intoxicated person by more than one person cannot be ruled out. Signs of violence and other evidences will be usually present in such a case.

The presence of findings which are abnormal or inconsistent can sometimes provide clues in support of foul play. Scene examination will be helpful in this regard. It is the duty of the investigating officer to find out the manner of death. It is very useful to apply cellophane tapes to the hands of the deceased to transfer the fibres, if any present, due to handling the ligature material. The tapes are examined under the microscope to detect the fibres. Nail clippings of the victim can also be examined for the presence of fibres. Presence of fibres of similar nature can also be looked for in the suspension point. If the ligature material is absent or has been found removed from the neck, cellophane tapes should be applied to the neck region also. Facts regarding the time of last meal, time when he was last seen alive, etc. are important to correlate with the postmortem findings.

### Directions to the Investigating Officer

- Ascertain cooling of the body, the extent of rigor mortis and position of postmortem staining.
- Phtograph the body and the scene from various angles—close up pictures of the ligature, slip knot, suspension point, salivary stains, faecal and seminal discharges if any and face.
- Cellophane test: Apply cellophane tapes to the palms of the deceased. Tapes having a breadth of 2 cm are ideal. Peel the tape from the roll, cut it into pieces of sufficient length and apply the gummed surface to the palms and fingers. Cover the entire surfce of the palm. Remove the strip and fold inwards. Repeat the process in the other palm. Pack the folded tapes in separate paper envelopes marked 'right palm and left palm'. Write on the envelopes, the deatils such as crime number, name of the deceased, date of collection, etc.
- Apply cellophane tapes to the neck of the deceased as well as the alleged suspension point, if the dead body is not found in a hanging posture due to a rescue attempt by the relatives.
- Take the following measurements in the scene:
  1. Distance from the ground to the suspenion point.
  2. Distance from the ground to the feet (in full suspension).
  3. Length of ligature from the suspension point to the knot in the neck.
  4. The circumference of the neck.
  5. Length of ligature in excess of the knot.
  6. Height of the stepping device, if any.
- The presence of a probable stepping device, if any in the scene has to be looked for. If there is no such device, look for possible method by which the deceased might have reached the suspension point to tie the ligature.
- Look for stains in the scene: Look for vertical salivary stains, discharge of semen, urine and faeces directly underneath the body. Bleeding from body orifices like nostrils, mouth, urethra, vagina and rectum is a common finding. In hanging (antemortem suspension), the blood stains from these orifices show a vertical track or found directly underneath the hanging body.

- Presence of injuries: Photograph the injuries, draw a diagram and mark the injuries in it.
- Request the doctor to collect vaginal swabs and smears, if the victim is a female.
- Reconstruction of the act: The mode of hanging has to be reconstructed. Find out whether it is possible for a person of the same height as that of the deceased to tie the same type and length of the ligature in the suspension point with or without a tepping device.
- Chemical analysis of viscera and body fluids: Request the doctor to collect viscera, blood and urine for chemical analysis. In homicidal hanging the victim could be rendered unconscious or incapacitated by administering alcohol or narcotics.
- Collect information regarding the time and nature of last meal.
- Collect information regarding the time the deceased was last seen alive.
- Preserve clothing for the detection of biological stains. Salivary and seminal stains may not be visible in normal light conditions. Therefore, even if stains are not visible, clothes are to be sent for forensic examination.
- Examine the autopsy surgeon U/S 161 CrPC and record salient findings and his opinion as to the cause and probable manner of death. If there are injuries on the hanging body, ascertain from the autopsy surgeon, the nature and probable cause for each injury. Opinion as to the age of each injury is to be obtained. Injuries could have been caused either before or during the act of hanging. It is also possible for the ligature to break and the victim may sustain injuries due to a fall.

### STRANGULATION

Strangulation is a form of death due to the construction of neck by a ligature or by any other means without suspension of the body.

Strangulation is almost always homicidal. Strangulation can be either by manual or by ligature. In both cases, there will be evidence of violence in the region of neck. There will not be suspension of the body. In some cases, body may be suspended after death. Death is due to asphyxia, cerebral ischemia and vagal inhibition.

## Ligature and Ligature Mark

Any type of ligature may be used in ligature strangulation. The ligature may be found tied around the neck usually below the Adam's apple or over it. The knot will be usually a reef knot either on the front or back of neck. Very often the ligature is retained in the neck by the assailant (Fig.16.6). The removal of the ligature is similar to the procedure adopted in a case of hanging. Ligature mark depends upon the nature of the ligature used. The mark will be completely encircling the neck and horizontal. Bruising and abrasion on the edges of the ligature may be more marked.

In manual strangulation, the neck is constricted by one or both hands. The skin of the neck may show crescentic abrasions caused by nails and contusions caused by fingers. They may be seen on the front, sides or back of the neck depending upon the nature of application of force (Fig. 16.6).

## External Features

The face will be severely congested with petechial haemorrhages under the skin and conjunctivae. Marked cyanosis will be seen with blood-stained froth coming through the mouth and nostrils. Salivary stains may also be seen as horizontal trickle marks, if the victim was in a lying position. Very often, discharges of faeces, semen, urine etc. may be seen. There may be other injuries on the body indicative of a struggle.

Rarely, cadaveric spasm has been found when the victim's hands may contain hair or torn fragments of clothes of the accused. The investigating officer should invariably examine the hands and finger nails of the victim as trace evidences may be found. Sometimes the nails of the victim may contain blood and skin of the accused. He should request the doctor to collect finger nail scrapings and clippings for forensic examination.

## Findings in the Neck

In a suspected case of strangulation, the forensic surgeon conducts dissection of the neck in a bloodless field. Unlike in hanging, the neck structures may show a variety of injuries. There

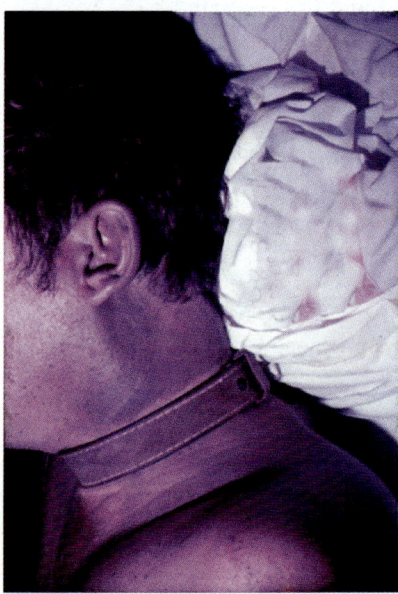

**Fig. 16.6:** Ligature strangulation—ligature used is a leather belt. Areas above the ligature is markedly livid

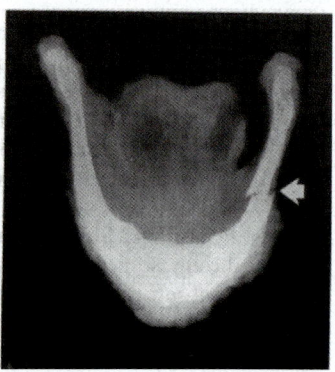

**Fig. 16.7:** Fracture of hyoid bone—X-ray showing inward fracture of the left cornua of the hyoid bone is indicative of violence due to strangulation

will be haemorrhages of varying size in the subcutaneous tissues, muscles, thyroid gland, etc. Fracture of the midline structures is a common finding especially in manual strangulation.

Any of the structures like hyoid (Fig. 16.7), thyroid, cricoid or trachea may show fractures with haemorrhages around the site of fracture. The fracture of these structures will depend upon the force applied. In cases of fall from a height, due to violent pull and jerking of the neck muscles, fracture of the cornua of hyoid bone and thyroid cartilage can occur. This finding will be mistaken as signs of violence. These fractures (**avulsion fracture**) will not be associated with external injuries as in the case of strangulation.

In ligature strangulation, the midline structures need not be fractured especially in young persons. But bruising is a common feature in both types of strangulation. The reason for this is the localised application of force without continuous constriction of neck as in the case of hanging. This will result in rupture of blood vessels and infiltration of blood into the tissues. Changes seen in the internal organs are mainly those of asphyxia. But in some cases of manual strangulation, death may be due to vagal inhibition and violence will be minimal.

## Discussion

Manual strangulation is always homicidal, but ligature strangulation can be rarely suicidal also. If the ligature is tied around the neck and kept in situ tightly, a person can die due to cerebral venous congestion. To keep the ligature tight, a stick or lever may be used in the form of a tourniquet. In some cases, self-retaining plastic or rubber banding devices have been used to sustain the constriction. Lack of evidence of any struggle on the body or in the scene may support a suicidal attempt.

Homicidal strangulation is usually associated with signs of general violence. There may be injuries on the hands sustained by restraining the victim. Sometimes, the assailant may exert pressure on the chest manually or sit on the chest of the victim (**burking**). But if the victim is weak or intoxicated, there need not be any signs of general violence. Similarly a sleeping victim will not offer much resistance and can be easily strangled.

The assailant may also sustain injuries during the scuffle. Nail marks and bite marks may be found on the accused. During the agonal frenzy, the victim may catch hold of the clothe or hair of the accused. Hair may be pulled or clothes may be torn. The hands and nails of the accused should be examined for the trace evidences from the victim. Epithelium found under the skin can be subjected to DNA typing.

## DIRECTIONS TO THE INVESTIGATING OFFICER

- Take photographs of the body and scene.
- Take close up photographs of the neck region.
- Ascertain cooling of the body, the extent of rigor mortis and position of postmortem staining.
- Do not disturb the ligature around the neck (if present).
- Preserve the ligature mark as a material object after the autopsy.
- If ligature is absent, take close up photographs of the ligature mark. If it is patterened, record the measurements and peculiarities of the pattern. Apply cellophane tapes to the palms and fingers and preserve the tapes for forensic examination. The cellophane tapes should also be applied to the neck region.
- Note the nature and direction of the salivary stains, if any. In strangulation, there may not be any vertical salivary stains.
- Look for trace evidence in the hands and finger nails of the deceased. Hair and remnants of the clothes of the accused may be found on the hands. The finger nails may contain skin and blood of the accused. DNA typing can be done for comparison with the DNA pattern of the suspect(s).
- Request the autopsy surgeon to collect finger nail scrapings and clippings from the dead body and forward them to Forensic Science laboratory.
- Request the autopsy surgeon to determine the grouping of blood of the deceased and collect a sample of blood for DNA typing.
- Collect samples of scalp hair —loose hairs are collected by running a comb through the hair. A sample of cut hair may also be colleceted.

- Collect foreign bodies and trace materials from the dead body and the scene.
- Look for signs of sexual violence on the clothing as well as the body.
- Collect and preserve all the clothing worn by the victim.
- Request the doctor to collect viscera and body fluids for chemical analysis.
- Request the doctor to collect vaginal swabs and smears in the case of female victims.
- Examine the doctor u/s 161 CrPC and ascertain from him the cause of death, time of death and manner of death.

## SUFFOCATION

Suffocation is a form of death due to prevention of air entering the lungs by means other than constriction of neck. The following types of suffocation are possible:
- Smothering
- Choking
- Traumatic asphyxia
- Inhalation of irrespirable gases
- Absence of oxygen in the surrounding atmosphere.

## Smothering

Suffocation is brought about by the occlusion of the mouth and nostrils either by the hands of the assailant or by any material like cloth or a pillow. In such cases, asphyxial signs will be prominent. Usually children and weak or unconscious victims are killed by this means.

The face will be extremely congested with petechial haemorrhages under the skin and conjunctiva. Blood-stained froth or even frank blood will come out of the mouth and nostrils. If hands are used for smothering, abrasions and bruises will be seen around the mouth and nostrils. Lacerations of lips and gums, loosening of the teeth, etc. may also be seen. There will be other injuries on the body indicative of a struggle. Smothering with cloth or a pillow may not produce gross injuries; but can cause injuries to lips and gums. An area of pallor around the mouth may be seen in some cases (**circumoral pallor**).

Another form of suffocation is by thrusting into the mouth, a piece of cloth or such other material. This is called **gagging.** If the gag is retained in the mouth and the victim is unconscious or unable to remove it, it may slowly pass into the oropharynx and cause occlusion of the air passage. This is highly possible especially if the victim is struggling. The gag becomes wet due to saliva and forms an effective plug to occlude the air passage. In such cases, injuries to the tongue, palate and pharynx are possible. The material used for gagging is not found in situ, but recovered from elsewhere, it should be preserved and sent for testing the presence of buccal epithelial cells and saliva.

### Directions to the Investigating Officer

Smothering is the commn mode of murdering infants and weak persons who cannot offer much resistance. There will be minimal injuries on the face and less evidence of struggle in the scene. The investigating officer shall:
- Take photogrphs of the scene and dead body.
- Take close up photographs of the face.
- Look for contusions and abrasions on the face, around the mouth and nostrils.
- Examine the inner aspects of cheeks and gums for contusions and lacerations.
- Examine the hands for foreign bodies, hair and other trace materials.
- Collect nail scrapings/clippings for the presence of trace materials.
- Examine the clothes and pillows for blood and salivary stains and preserve them.
- Look for signs of struggle in the scene.
- Request the doctor to collect viscera and body fluids for chemical analysis.
- Request the doctor to collect vaginal swabs and smears in the case of a female victim.

### Choking

Choking is usually due to accidental occlusion of the air passages by foreign bodies such as food particles, vomited matter, etc. A person while eating may inhale a piece of meat or food bolus and if the air passage is completely obstructed, death will be sudden (Fig. 16.8). This is quite often mistaken as death due to coronary occlusion

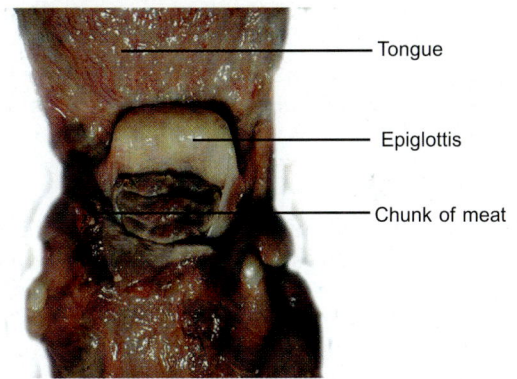

**Fig. 16.8:** Impacted chunk of meat in the air passage

— Tongue

— Epiglottis

— Chunk of meat

(**cafe coronary**). Edema, spasm of larynx and reflex vagal inhibition play a role in causing death. Children may accidentally swallow articles which may get impacted in the larynx.

Bleeding from a tumour or a tuberculous cavity in the lung can cause death due to choking. An unconscious person can choke to death by his vomitus aspirated into the air passages. In some accident victims, who had sustained injuries of the nose or mouth can die due to choking by aspiration of blood from the site of bleeding, if they remain in an unconscious state unattended. Alcoholic intoxication can also cause death in this fashion; as the cough reflex becomes absent or sluggish.

Asphyxial features will be marked. On autopsy, the foreign body can be detected in the air passage. There will be haemorrhages, interstitial emphysema, severe congestion and edema of the lungs. If blood or vomitus is inhaled, the material will be found even in the terminal bronchioles.

## Agonal Aspiration

Sometimes, at the time of death, stomach contents may regurgitate into the air passage. This is called agonal aspiration. This can also occur due to gas formation in putrefied bodies. Very often, agonal aspiration is mistaken as the death due to choking. If the aspiration was antemortem, the contents will be detected even in the bronchioles and there will be associated changes in the lungs.

## DIRECTIONS TO THE INVESTIGATING OFFICER

Every police officer should be familiar with the first aid measures for choking. The signs of choking are coughing, wheezing, difficulty in breathing, grasping at the throat, bluish discolouration of face, lips and nails. If the obstruction of the airway is partial, the victim will be able to cough and coughing may sometimes expel the foreign body. The method of giving first aid to adults and children are different (Figs 16.9A to C).

### For Adults—Heimlich Maneuver

1. Examine the mouth and carefully remove obstructing articles, if any.
2. Stand behind the victim. Wrap your arms around the victim's abdomen (chest in the case of obese persons and pregnant women)
3. Make your one hand into fist and place it between the lower end of breast bone and umbilicus. This area is known as the 'pit of stomach'.
4. With the other hand grab the hand that was formed into a fist (Fig. 16.9 A).
5. Thrust your hand upwards to expel the object.
6. If the victim is unconscious, check his airway and breathing. Start cardiopulmonary resuscitation (**Refer Chapter 1**) and transfer the person to hospital

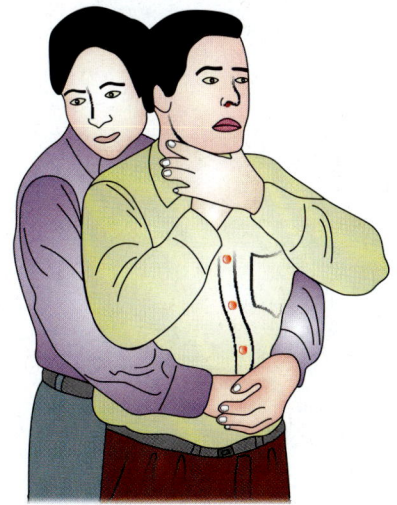

A

**Fig. 16.9A:** Heimlich maneuver for adults

### For Infants

1. Examine baby's mouth and carefully remove obstructing articles, if any.
2. Do not sweep the inside of the mouth (this may push the obstruction further down).
3. Lay the baby face down on your right forearm with your hand beneath the chest and head.
4. Give five quick sharp thumps on his back between the shoulder blades with the heel of your hand (Fig. 16.9B).
5. If the object is not expelled and the baby is still unable to breathe, turn him on his back on your left forearm keeping the baby's head supported.
6. Give five thrusts on the chest with two fingers placed in the center of the chest, a finger width below an imaginary line drawn between the nipples (Fig. 16.9C).

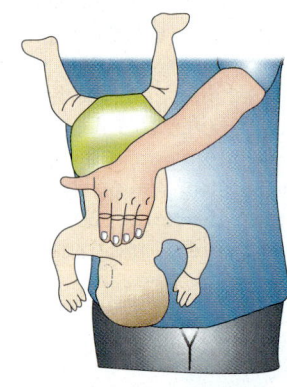

B

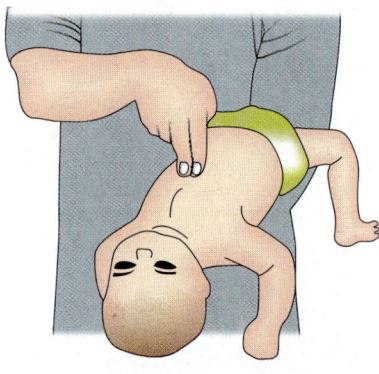

C

**Figs 16.9 B and C:** Heimlich maneuver for infants

7. Repeat the alternate back blows and chest thrusts until the object is expelled.
8. If the baby becomes unconscious, start cardio-pulmonary resuscitation and transfer the baby to a hospital.

### Sexual Asphyxia

This is an autoerotic masochist practice by sexual perverts, mostly males. They tie a ligature around the neck and achieve constriction of neck by partial suspension. Vascular obstruction produces hypoxia which in turn gives erotic sensations and hallucinations. Hypoxia is also obtained by covering the head with a polythene bag. Some of these perverts are transvestites also. During this maneuver, death can occur due to accidental hanging or suffocation.

### DIRECTIONS TO THE INVESTIGATING OFFICER

- Conduct the usual investigations as in a case of hanging.
- Look for pornogrphic material in the scene.
- Look for masochistic injuries on body parts (also healed injuries).
- Presence of semen in the scene (absence does not rule out autoerotic death).

### Death due to Absence of Oxygen and Inhalation of Irrespirable Gases

Asphyxia can be brought about if oxygen is lacking in the atmosphere or due to the inhalation of irrespirable gases like carbon monoxide, carbon dioxide, oxides of nitrogen and sulphur, halogens, etc. In deep wells and in confined spaces, oxygen concentration will be less and carbon dioxide will be more. Inhalation of carbon dioxide of high concentration can produce glottic spasm leading on to suffocation. Carbon dioxide concentration of 25–30% can cause death.

Being heavier than air, carbon dioxide will accumulate at the bottom of wells, mines, cellars, etc. and persons who attempt to rescue the trapped victims may also die if proper precautions are not taken. The best course of action is to pump oxygen through a hose to the area first, before the rescuer descends. Rescuer can also be provided with oxygen masks.

Carbon monoxide is a highly poisonous gas as it combines with hemoglobin to produce carboxy haemoglobin thereby reducing the oxygen carrying capacity of blood. This gas is present in the coal gas, exhaust fumes, and wherever there is incomplete combustion of carbonaceous material. Suicide by inhalation of the exhaust gas of automobiles is not uncommon. Defective exhaust pipes can cause seepage of gases inside the car and the passengers can get poisoned with carbon monoxide. Leaking Geysers working on gas can vitiate the air in a bathroom and cause fatal poisoning to the occupants.

Postmortem findings in these cases will be those of asphyxia. In carbon monoxide poisoning, the blood assumes a cherry red colour. Spectroscopic examination of blood will reveal the presence of carboxyhaemoglobin. Conditions like acute bronchitis, diphtheria, acute pulmonary oedema, acute penumohemothorax, etc. can also cause death due to asphyxia.

## DIRECTIONS TO THE INVESTIGATING OFFICER

Police officers may have to encounter calamities due to inhalation of irrespirable gases. Commonest is death of persons getting into deep wells or confined spaces where oxygen may be sparse or absent. In order to confirm the absence of oxygen, an oil wick lamp can be kept in a suitable container and lowered into the well. If oxygen is absent or less, the light will die out. Take adequate precautions before rescue operations or removal of dead bodies, etc. (vide supra).

Deaths due to inhalation of carbon monoxide are not very infrequent. In suspected cases, request the doctor to preserve samples of blood in air tight containers (vacuette) for the detection of carboxyhemoglobin. The sample may be sent to the forensic scientist who will use modern methods like gas chromatography for the detection of carbon monoxide/carboxyhemoglobin. If the leakage of gas was from a faulty equipment like a geyser or an exhaust pipe or any such device, request an engineer or such other expert to give an opinion after examining it.

## Traumatic (Crush) Asphyxia

When the thoracic wall is compressed as a result of a heavy weight, death can occur due to asphyxia. This is seen in the case of collapse of building and mines, traffic accidents and stampede. A child can die due to overlying by the mother during sleep. The respiratory movements are prevented due to compression of chest and abdomen.

The salient feature is the presence of extreme congestion and petechial haemorrhage above the level of compression and pallor at the site of compression. There may be injuries to the chest wall including fracture of the ribs, sternum, etc. All the internal organs will show signs of asphyxia.

In mass disasters like stampede, earthquakes, collapse of building, etc. victims die due to crush asphyxia. Immediate removal of the compression of chest and administration of oxygen are the first aid measures.

## DROWNING

Drowning is a form of death due to submersion of the body in a fluid medium, whereby the fluid enters into the air passages and prevents entry of air into the lungs. Bodies recovered from water pose the most difficult medicolegal problem, especially when the body is received for autopsy in a putrefied state. The cause of death and manner of death are difficult to be established in most of the cases. The signs of antemortem submersion depend upon the type of drowning.

Drowning occurs when water or any other fluid enters the lungs. This happens when a person is submerged in the fluid medium. But complete submersion is not necessary to cause drowning. An unconscious person can drown in a puddle of water when his face alone is submerged. When water enters the lungs, cough reflex is stimulated and air is driven out of the lungs. There will be more need for air and the person will take deep inspirations which allow more water to enter the lungs. The mechanism of death varies in fresh water drowning and salt water drowning. Death takes place in 3–10 minutes and the drowned body sinks to the bottom. It will raise to the surface of water and float in 12–24 hours when putrefactive gases evolve. The period is highly variable. Bodies of women and children float earlier due to the low specific gravity of their bodies. Fully clothed bodies can float sooner due to trapped air inside the clothes. Higher density of water is also a contributory factor for early floatation. The floating is in a peculiar **floaters attitude,** when the head and limbs will be submerged, back and buttocks will be visible (Fig.16.10). The body will not float, if it is entangled in mud, weeds or rocks.

Persons can die suddenly without water entering into the lungs and this condition is called **dry drowning.** Death is due to spasm of the larynx or reflex vagal inhibition due to the sudden impact of water on the nasopharynx. This type of drowning can occur when the victim falls into the medium vertically from a height. During this act, persons can sustain injuries, which may contribute to death. The postmortem findings depend upon the type of drowning.

### External Signs of Drowning

Lividity of face, cyanosis and petechial haemorrhages may be present in majority of cases. If the body was floating, postmortem staining will be seen on the front aspect of the body, more on the face and limbs.

*Froth at the mouth and nostrils:* Persistent, profuse, fine, white, leathery froth will be present in most cases of drowning (wet). But this is not diagnostic of drowning as it is seen in other conditions also (Fig.16.11). When the drowned body putrefies, the froth becomes pink in colour.

*Washer woman's hands:* Bleaching and soddening of the skin of the hands and soles will be seen, if the body is submerged for about 12–18 hours.

*Goose skin:* The hair on the body stand erect due to the action of cold on the erector pilae

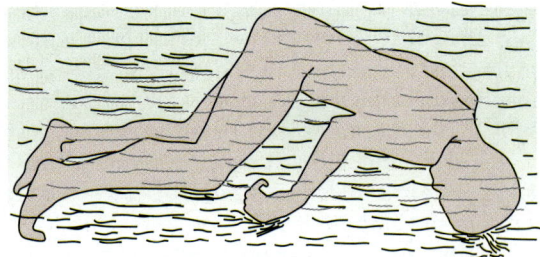

**Fig. 16.10:** Position of a submerged dead body

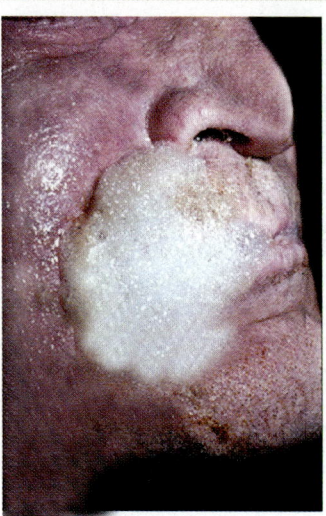

**Fig. 16.11:** Fine froth at mouth and nostrils

muscle fibres attached to the hair follicles. This can occur in a live body in cold climate, fright, etc.

Washerwoman's hands and goose skin are not indicative of death due to drowning. They are only signs of submersion of the body in water.

*Cadaveric spasm:* Sometimes the hands of a drowned body may be found firmly clutching materials like weeds, mud, etc. This is a rare phenomenon, but is conclusive of antemortem submersion.

### Internal Findings

In wet type of drowning, the lungs will be found voluminous, pale and grossly edematous. But these findings are not conclusive of drowning.

*Foreign bodies in the air passages:* During dissection, the trachea and bronchi have to be cut open with clean scissors. Presence of sand, mud, weeds, etc. in the air passages is conclusive of antemortem submersion.

*Water in the stomach:* Water in the stomach has no significance unless it is the same as the medium of drowning. If the water in the stomach contains mud or weeds, it is diagnostic of antemortem submersion. Absence of water in the stomach does not exclude drowning as the drowning person need not necessarily swallow water; swallowing being a voluntary act.

*Water in the middle ear:* Water can be aspirated from the middle ear in the case of drowning. Haemorrhages in the middle ear and mastoid air cells are also diagnostic of drowning.

*Signs of asphyxia:* All the internal organs will be congested. The lungs may be sometimes pale. The signs described above need not be present in all cases of drowning especially in dry type of drowning. The absence of typical signs does not exclude drowning as the mechanism of death varies. To confirm the diagnosis, the following laboratory investigations can be carried out.

## Laboratory Diagnosis of Drowning
### Diatom Test

Diatoms are unicellular algae with a silicaceous coating found in the water of ponds, rivers, sea, etc. (Fig. 16.12). In wet type of drowning, these diatoms also enter the lungs along with water (Fig. 16.13). They are absorbed into the blood and reach the various internal organs. This is an evidence of drowning. To detect diatoms, a sample of bone marrow (minimum 5 gm) can be taken from the sternum or long bones and digested with nitric acid for 1–2 hours. Then the fluid is centrifuged and the deposit is examined microscopically. Through acid digestion, all organic matter will be dissolved except diatoms as they possess a silicaceous covering resistant to acid. There are about 15,000 varieties of diatoms in water and a sample of the drowning medium should also be subjected to microscopic examination. Tincture iodine/Lugol's iodine is added to the water sample and allowed to stand for

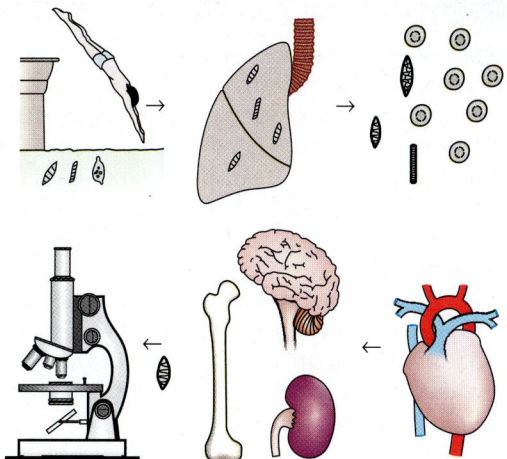

**Fig. 16.13:** Entry of diatoms into the internal organs

24 hours. Then it is centrifuged at 3000 rpm. The supernatant fluid is discarded. The deposit is examined microscopically. If both the medium and the marrow contain the same type of diatoms, it is conclusive of death due to drowning in that medium. Tissues like lungs, kidney, brain, etc. can also be subjected to this test. The sample of the medium and tissues can be sent to the forensic medicine Departments, forensic science laboratory or the chemical examiner's laboratory. Tissues may be collected in double-distilled water and need not be fixed in formalin.

### Chloride Estimation

After opening the chest wall, the pericardium is cut and 10 ml blood is drawn from each ventricle. The sample can be subjected to estimation of chlorides. Normal value of chloride is 600 mg% in both chambers. In salt water drowning, there will 30–40% increase of the chloride level in the blood in left ventricle. In fresh water drowning, the chlorides are reduced to 50%. This change is not seen in dry type of drowning. Samples of blood can be sent to chemical examiner's laboratory or forensic science laboratory for chloride estimation. This test is not valid if the dead body is putrefied as there will be diffusion of blood between the chambers of heart. The test is valid only if it is done within 12–18 hours of death.

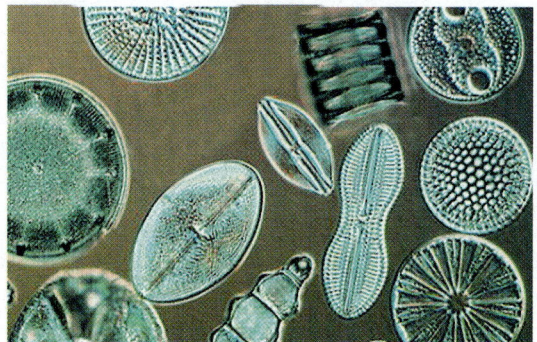

**Fig. 16.12:** Various types of diatoms

## DIRECTIONS TO THE INVESTIGATING OFFICER

Bodies recovered from water will be often found in a putrefied state. Positive findings of drowning will tend to disappear as time elapses. Putrefaction is retarded, if the body remains in water especially if the salinity of the water is more. Once it is taken out, changes of putrefaction occur at a fast rate. Therefore, it is better to protect the dead body from exposure to sun.

Death occurring in shallow waters should be considered as homicide unless otherwise proved. Tying of limbs or attaching a weight to the body may indicate either suicide or homicide. Bodies in water may be attacked by fish and various types of postmortem injuries can occur. Therefore, inquest should be held at the earliest and body should be removed for autopsy. In highly putrefied bodies, identity is to be established by noting the different features. The following tasks may be done:

- Examine the bottom of the well or pond. If possible drain the well by pumping out the water. Examine the material objects if any recovered and note the nature of the floor/bottom of the well.
- Look for the presence of blood/hair on the inner lining of the well/pond.
- Request the doctor to collect viscera and body fluids for chemical analysis.
- Request the doctor to collect vaginal swab and smears, if the victim is a female.
- Collect one litre of water in a clean bottle from the site of drowning and send along with the dead body to the forensic pathologist for conducting a diatom test.
- Arrange for fingerprinting and collection of samples for DNA typing, in the case of unknown dead bodies (especially in homicides).
- Request the doctor to visit the scene of occurrence for correlating the autopsy findings with the findings in the scene.
- Examine the doctor US 161 CrPC to get his opinion as to the cause and manner of death, the nature, mode of causation and age of injuries, if any found on the dead body. The doctor will not be in a position to commit himself as to the manner of death namely accident, suicide or homicide. Accidental drowning can take place

even in shallow waters, if the person falls unconscious due to intoxication or diseases like epilepsy.

## DIVING HAZARDS AND BAROTRAUMA

Diving is becoming popular as a recreation as well as an occupation. There are two types of diving; free diving and diving with the help of breathing equipment. Modern equipment like **SCUBA** (self-contained underwater breathing apparatus) have been developed to facilitate diving especially in deep waters (Fig.16.14). In spite of these new devices and developments, diving is not without danger. Many of the hazards are related to the respiratory physiology and physical laws.

In free diving, breath is held for varying periods. The diver takes a deep breath and descends under water. The length of apnoea depends upon on an individual's lung capacity and the release of carbon dioxide.

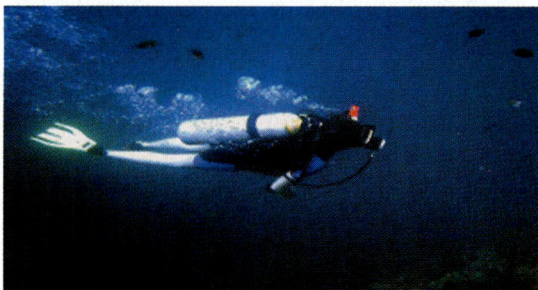

**Fig. 16.14:** Underwater diving with SCUBA equipment

When there is no respiration, carbon dioxide accumulates in the blood and tissues. This will stimulate the respiratory centre and a stage is reached when the person cannot hold the breath any longer. There occurs a long exhalation and release of carbon dioxide. This is called "impulse breathing" which discontinues apnoea. Normally, the period of apnoea is 1–3 minutes.

There are cases when breath was held for 15 minutes after inhalation of pure oxygen and hyperventilation before apnoea. If a person manages somehow to overcome the impulse to breathe, the amount of carbon dioxide can exceed line and can cause unconsciousness or even death due to paralysis of respiratory centre. Physical work under water can precipitate this. Such deaths are common among even trained divers.

At sea level, the atmospheric pressure is about 1 kg per sq.cm. It will be double at a depth of 10 meters in water. As per Boyle's law volume of a gas is inversely proportional to the pressure. Volume will be halved, if the pressure is doubled (temperature remaining constant). In the human body, lungs, middle ear and sinuses are the cavities filled with air. These chambers are unable to cope up with increased pressure. Chest is compressed during descent and the volume of air in the lungs is reduced. During ascent, it expands and the volume is increased. In both these situations, a number of lesions called 'barotrauma' can develop.

## Barotrauma

Because of the increased pressure effect, bleeding in the air sacs of lungs, rupture of air sacs, pneumonia, air in the chest cavities and covering of heart can occur. Rupture of the pulmonary veins may lead to **arterial gas embolism** causing cerebral and myocardial ischemia. The symptoms are chest pain, dyspnoea, cough, cyanosis and shock. In arterial gas embolism, the victim will develop chest pain, dizziness, fatigue, visual disturbances, paralysis, collapse, convulsions, unconsciousness and death. Acute myocardial infarction, arrhythmias, etc. can also develop.

- Take photogrphs of the dead body in the floating posture and after it is taken out of water.
- Take close up photographs of face and injuries.
- Take close up photographs and detailed description of weights and ligatures attached to the body.
- Take photographs of hands, if they contain any foreign articles like weeds, water plants, sand, etc.
- Collect the foreign articles, dry them and preserve.
- Take measurements of the scene of drowning. If it is a well, note the diameter, total depth, depth of water, height of parapet wall, if any. The nature of the side walls is to be examined and recorded in the inquest report.

These symptoms develop minutes after surfacing or after some delay. Arterial gas embolism can also initiate intravascular thrombosis affecting many organs. Barotrauma can tear the tympanic membrane, causing water to enter the middle ear. The vestibular system is affected. The diver becomes dizzy, disoriented and nauseated. This condition is called **labyrinthine crisis**. There will be mucosal bleeding in the air sinuses and severe pain is experienced. During diving, severe pain will be felt in teeth with cavities or fillings, due to increased pressure.

## Decompression Sickness

Air is a mixture of nitrogen (80%) and oxygen (20%). This would mean that 80% of the atmospheric pressure is exerted by nitrogen and 20% by oxygen. During diving, the partial pressure of these gases increases as the depth increases. As a result, more nitrogen will be dissolved into blood and tissues. When a diver surfaces, the dissolved nitrogen bubbles out into blood and tissues similar to opening a bottle of aerated drink. It can occur in dives to depths more than 6 meters.

If the dive is deeper and longer, more nitrogen is taken up by the body. If the assent is slow at a rate of 5 meters per minute, the risk of nitrogen bubbling is minimised. Symptoms occur soon after the dive or after a short period. Generally, symptoms should appear within 24 hours. But climbing mountains or flying soon after diving episode can precipitate symptoms even after 24 hours.

The symptoms of decompression sickness varies because nitrogen bubbles can form in different parts of the body. The bubbles will cause mechanical obstruction producing tissue damage. Respiratory symptoms include dry cough, chest pain, dyspnoea, cyanosis and shock **(chokes)**. The diver may complain of headache, vertigo **(staggers)** fatigue, pain in joints **(bends),** tingling of arms and legs, muscular weakness and paralysis. In serious cases, dyspnoea, shock, unconsciousness and even death can occur.

## Other Diving Hazards

Apart from barotrauma, a diver or swimmer can sustain fatal injuries in water. Diving into shallow waters can cause head injury and cervical spine fractures and dislocations due to a head impact on a hard surface or object. Deaths due to vasovagal attacks are also possible due to panic, agitation and hyperventilation. Use of alcohol, cannabis, cocaine, etc. can also cause problems for swimmer or diver. Antihistamines and tranquilizers can produce drowsiness and fatigue.

The swimmer can be attacked by venomous fishes, ray fish, stone fish, fire fish, coelenterates, octopus, cone shells, snakes, etc. Many of these species can cause fatal poisoning. Ray fish can cause penetrating injuries with its sting. The famous reporter Steve Irwin (National Geographic TV fame) died due to the injury sustained by the sting of a ray fish. The sting had penetrated his heart. Injuries are caused by fishes like barracuda, sharks and eels. Attack by crocodiles is also possible in some waters.

### Diving/Swimming and Pre-existing Diseases

There are several occasions when divers/swimmers die due to drowning. Pre-existing cardiovascular, respiratory, CNS, endocrine disorders contribute to death. Exertion and cold can precipitate coronary spasm. Arrhythmias can be caused by hyperventilation, apnoea and hypothermia. Persons with lung diseases like a critical asthma, emphysema can develop rupture of alveoli, pneumothorax, arterial gas embolism, etc.

Epileptic convulsions are possible in known epileptics due to high partial pressure of oxygen during diving. In diabetics, hypoglycemic episodes are possible due to exertion.

### DIRECTIONS TO THE INVESTIGATING OFFICER

Diving accidents and barotrauma are very rare in our country. However, in such an eventuality, the police officer should be able to take appropriate action.

- If the person is rescued by the police, try to resuscitate him by cardiac massage, artificial respiration and oxygen inhalation if possible. Transport the victim to hospital immediately.
- Preserve the entire diving equipment including the gas cylinders for expert examination. as the faulty diving equipment may be the reason for the fatality.
- X-ray photographs of the dead body to detect air embolism in the brain and lungs prior to autopsy.
- Body should be subjected to autopsy within four hours of death as the air will be reabsorbed into blood and evidence of air embolism will be lost.
- Request the doctor to collect a sample of arterial blood in a vacuette for estimation of blood gases.
- Request the doctor to collect body fluids and viscera for toxicological analysis.

# Death due to Electricity and Lightning

Death due to electric shock and lightning are unnatural deaths. Sometimes the victim's dead body may be found under suspicious circumstances. Proper investigation and autopsy may be necessary to arrive at the exact cause and manner of death. Therefore, a detailed examination of the dead body and the scene have to be conducted during inquest. Assistance of experts from the electrical inspectorate and forensic science laboratory may be obtained.

Electrocution occurs either from the domestic supply or from the open electric lines or due to lightning. The voltage of the domestic supply is around 230 volts alternate current. Industrial voltages may vary up to a few kilovolts. The voltage in lightning stroke may be millions of volts. The effects depend upon the intensity of the electric current, resistance of the body, earthing, and the duration of the passage of current.

Three factors are of importance in electrocution.
1. A charged electrical source
2. A current pathway through the body of the victim
3. Perfect ground contact

For electrocution to occur, all three factors should act simultaneously. A ground has the same electric potential as the earth. A person well insulated from the ground, may contact an electric conductor without sustaining a fatal electric shock. Operating electrical appliances, standing barefoot on a wet floor or in contact with metallic objects can allow the electric current to pass through the body to the ground.

If the ground is perfect, the electrical charge will pass through the body which acts as a conductor. When the current passes through the brain and spinal cord, spasm of the muscles occur. Tetanic spasm of the respiratory muscles will result in respiratory arrest and death. When the current flows through the heart, disturbance of the rhythm of the heart occurs. Current as low as 0.1 ampere can produce ventricular fibrillation. The mechanism of death is due to ventricular fibrillation, respiratory paralysis, spasm and paralysis of the respiratory muscles, cerebral anoxia and neurological damage.

## ELECTRIC BURNS (JOULE BURNS)

If the person is in good contact with the earth, when the electric shock is sustained, the effects will be severe and entrance and exit electric burns will occur. **Entrance burns** will be seen at the site of contact with the electric source (Fig. 17.1). An electric burn may vary from minimal burns to extensive charring and destruction of the tissues. If there is difficulty in identifying the lesion, microscopical examination of a bit of tissue taken from that area will be helpful.

Sometimes a greyish or yellowish mark may be the only sign. If the contact has been for a longer time, the size and shape of the mark will correspond to the size of the source of current. The burnt area will have a characteristic crater like appearance with central charring surrounded by an area of erythema. The areas which are in contact with the earth may show exit burns (Fig. 17.2). They may vary from burns to punched out craters. Usually, they are seen on the soles.

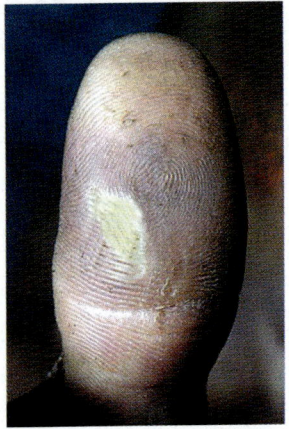

Fig. 17.1: Electric burn—entry (Photo: Dr. V. Prathapan)

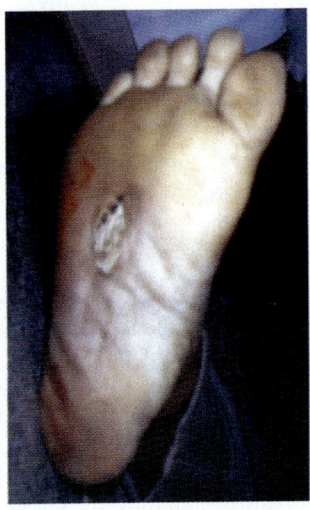

Fig. 17.2: Electric burn-exit (Photo: Dr. V. Prathapan)

The production of electric burns depends upon the voltage, amount of current flow, area of contact and duration of contact. An electrical burn occurs only if the temperature is high and contact is of a longer duration. In majority of the low voltage electrocutions, burns will be absent. But in high voltage electric shock, severe type of high temperature burns will be seen.

## LIGHTNING INJURIES

Lightning is an electrical arc from a negatively charged cloud to the underlying positively charged earth. Motion of water and dust particles during thunderstorms causes the build up of the large negative charge in the clouds. The current flow in a lightning flash is very large and the potential will be millions of volts. The duration of the lightning flash is very short so that the injuries could be sometimes less than those caused by high voltage electricity.

In lightning, apart from the electric charge, there will be considerable amount of heat and explosive expansion of air, producing other types of injuries like contusions, lacerations, fractures, etc. The clothes will be torn and metallic articles on the body will melt. Metallic objects will be magnetised. The electric burns caused in lightning and high voltage contact may sometimes show patterns like **crocodile skin** (Fig. 17.3) or **arborescent villi** (Fig. 17.4) (like the branches of a tree).

Death occurs due to respiratory arrest, ventricular fibrillation and cardiac arrest. It is possible to prevent death by giving immediate resuscitative treatment. Disruption of clothing and blast injuries found on the body of a victim discovered in an isolated place can arouse suspicion of assault. In such cases, a detailed

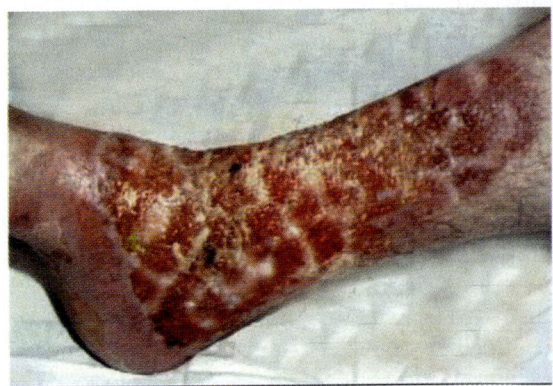

Fig. 17.3: Crocodile skin

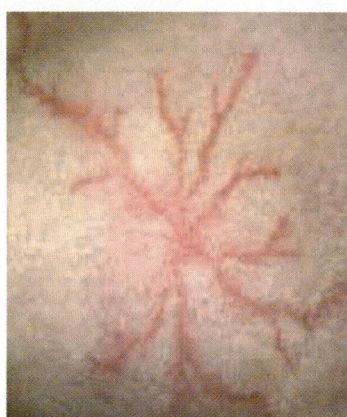

**Fig. 17.4:** Arborescent villi

examination of the dead body will reveal flash burns and other evidences of lightning strike. Examination of the scene may reveal damage sustained to nearby trees or other objects.

In domestic electrocutions, it is necessary to conduct examination of the electric installation and appliances for the presence of faults. Leakage of electricity is possible in domestic appliances, use of which can cause fatal electric shock.

## DIRECTIONS TO THE INVESTIGATING OFFICER

Sometimes the dead body of the victim of electrocution or lightning will be discovered under suspicious circumstances. The victim may be usually found in an open place or under a tall tree. The disruption of the clothes and injuries on the body may create a suspicion of foulplay. Electrocution from domestic or high tension electric circuits will often reveal some evidence. The victim may still be attached to the source of current. The IO

should take all precautions to cut off the electric supply to the scene with the help of persons concerned. Help of the experts from the electricity board or inspectorate may be obtained for collecting evidence. If lightning stroke is suspected, local inhabitants may be questioned to find out whether there was a thunderstorm or rain in the area where the dead body was seen. Examine the trees and buildings near the dead body for damages if any caused by a lightning stroke.

Sometimes electrical appliances and conductors can be the cause of a fire also. Electric sparks can ignite any inflammable substance. Damaged insulation on wires, shortcircuits, excessive load, overheating of electrical equipment, etc. can cause a fire. The victim may be electrocuted and later the body may sustain burns. Fires can also be caused due to lightning. If the lightning hits a dry tree or house directly, it can result in a fire.

Apart from the routine procedures in the inquest, the following steps may also be taken:
- Examine the clothes and personal articles.
- Examine the metal articles on the body like ornaments, spectacles, keys, etc. for signs of melting or magnetisation.
- Look for the presence of electric burns, entrance and exit.
- If the entrance burn is patterned, compare with the conductor by taking exact measurements.
- Examine the soles of feet of the dead body for exit burns due to earthing.
- Examine the footwear if any worn by the deceased for signs of exit of electric current.
- Look for the presence of patterned joule burns—crocodile skin/arborescent villi.

# 18

# Burns

Burns are the localised wounds caused by heat in any form. Exposure to temperatures above 60 °C will produce thermal burns. Tissue damage can occur in 3 minutes. Usually lesions produced by dry heat are called burns and by moist heat are called scalds (Fig.18.3). Lightning, electricity, X-rays and corrosives also produce burns. Burns are classified according to the depth of tissue destruction (Fig. 18.1 and Box 18.1).

First degree burns are superficial. The burnt area is red due to increased blood flow and congestion. It is swollen and painful due to inflammation (Fig. 18.4). In second degree burns, epidermis is destroyed exposing the dermis which is partly affected. Healing may produce scars (Fig. 18.5). In third degree burns (Fig. 18.6), whole thickness of skin, subcutaneous tissues and muscles are involved. Pain is absent due to the destruction of nerve fibres. Scarring will occur after healing. Assessment of the extent of the area involved is of prognostic importance. Wallace's rule of nine' is used to assess the extent of burns involving the body surface of adults and infants (Fig. 18.2 and Box 18.2).

## EFFECT OF BURNS ON THE BODY

Many systems of the body are affected by burns. Skin is the most affected part. Inhalation of smoke and noxious gases cause **respiratory burns**. The air passages and lungs will be affected. Hot air,

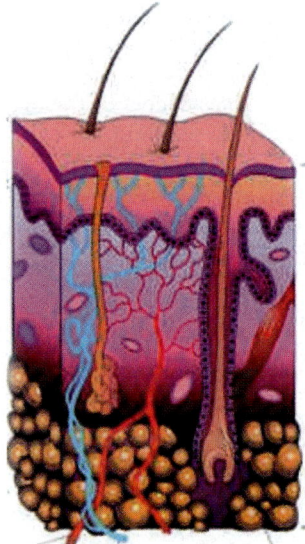

**Fig. 18.1:** Structure of skin and depth of tissue destruction in burns

| Box 18.1: Wilson's classification of burns | | |
|---|---|---|
| *Degree* | *Tissues involved* | *Features* |
| First degree | Epidermis | Erythema, and blistering. Peeling of skin seldom develops. Lesions heal without scarring |
| Second degree | Epidermis and dermis | Whole thickness of skin is involved. The epidermis is destroyed. Scarring is inevitable. |
| Third degree | Skin and deeper tissues | Extensive destruction of subcutaneous tissues and muscles, exposing bones |

**Box 18.2:** Wallace's rule of nine

| Adult | | Infant | |
|---|---|---|---|
| Head and neck | 9% | Head and neck | 18% |
| Upper limbs | 9% each | Upper limbs | 9% each |
| Trunk | 18% each | Trunk | 18% each |
| (front and back) | | (front and back) | |
| Lower limbs | 18% each | Lower limbs | 13.5% each |
| Perineum | 1% | Perineum | 1% |

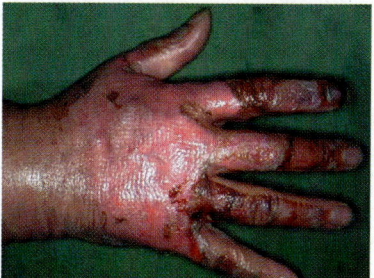

Fig. 18.4: First degree burns

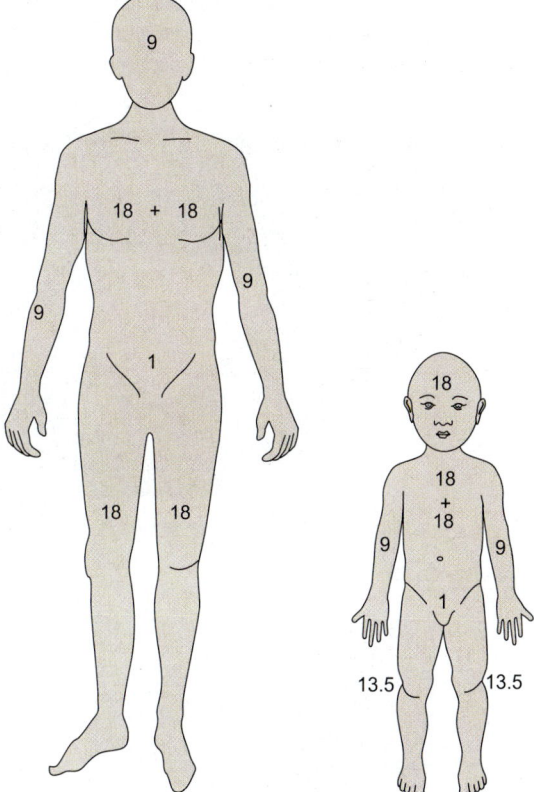

Fig. 18.2: Wallace's rule of nine — A Adult, B. Infant

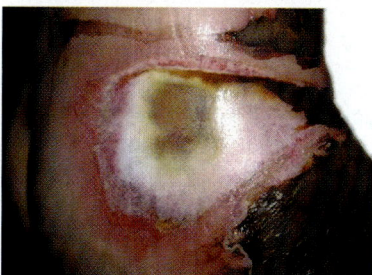

Fig. 18.5: Second degree burns

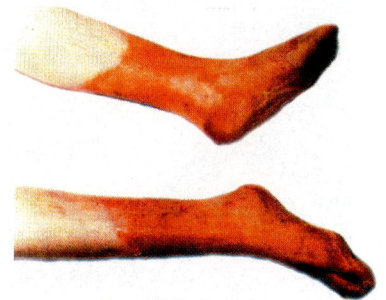

Fig. 18.3: Scalds

Fig. 18.6: Third degree burns

smoke and fumes inhaled by the victim will cause burns of the mucosa of the air passages. Mucosa will become swollen. Laryngeal swelling and shedding of the epithelium of the lower air passages and alveoli are also possible in burns due to inhalation of hot vapours. This can also block the air passages and cause death due to asphyxia.

A fire will generate irrespirable gases like carbon dioxide, carbon monoxide, methane, hydrogen cyanide, etc. The affinity of carbon monoxide to combine with haemoglobin is 240 times greater than oxygen.

More than 10% concentration of carboxy-hemoglobin in the blood can be dangerous. Death occurs with concentrations around 40–60%. House fires can produce highly toxic hydrogen cyanide gas due to the burning of wool, nylon, plastic, etc. Death will be due to the interference with mitochondrial respiration. Inhaled smoke and soot particles will stick to the alveoli and produce an intense reaction. Pulmonary edema and pneumonitis will decrease the exchange of gases and can lead to death.

A burn is like an open bleeding wound. The permeability of the blood vessels will increase and large quantity of fluid escapes into the extra-vascular space. The passage of large quantity of water, solutes and proteins from the blood vessels will produce circulatory shock. If the total surface area is more than 25%, the inflammatory reaction will cause fluid loss from blood vessels, remote from the site of burns. Ulcers **(Curling's ulcer)** will also develop in the gastroduodenum as early as 5 hours after burns. Fatal bleeding can occur from these ulcers.

Burns cause increased capillary permeability and fluid loss which may lead to reduction of blood volume and fall of blood pressure and circulatory failure. Intravenous fluid replacement is necessary in persons who have sustained burns involving more than 10–15% of body surface area. Burns involving more than 20% of the body surface area is serious and more than 30% may be fatal. Cause of death could be due to primary or secondary shock. Delayed deaths are due to toxaemia and septicaemia. Asphyxia, fat embolism and hypo-proteinemia can also cause death.

### Burns—Are they Antemortem or Postmortem?

The main medicolegal problem is to find out whether the burns are antemortem or not. In first and second degree burns, an external examination of the burns will reveal the nature. An antemortem burn will show a line of redness in the periphery of the burnt area. Vesicles may be formed which will contain a serous exudate. The floor of the vesicle will be red in colour. Histological examination will reveal inflammatory/reparative processes. In a body showing third degree burns or extensive charring (Fig. 18.7), the antemortem

features of burns will not be evident. Extensive heat will coagulate muscle proteins and the limbs will show stiffening simulating rigor mortis. This appearance is called **pugilistic (boxer) attitude** (Fig.18.9).

In such cases, presence of soot particles in the air passages, especially below the larynx will prove that the person was alive at the time of the fire (Fig.18.8). Presence of soot in the small air passages (bronchioles) and alveoli (air sacs) is a sure indication that the deceased was alive at the time of sustainig

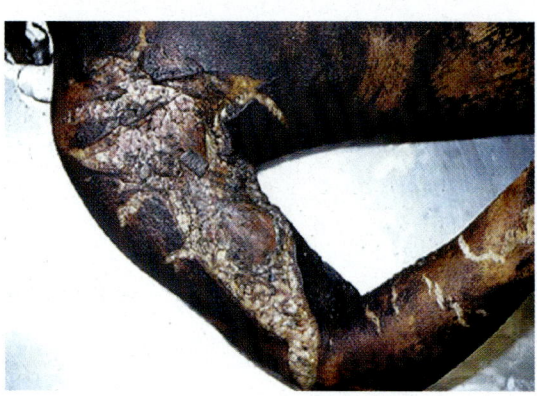

**Fig. 18.7:** Charring of tissues

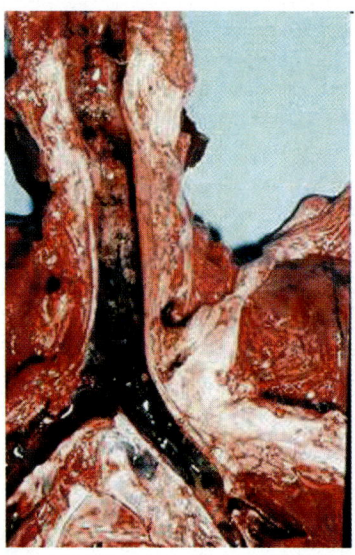

**Fig. 18.8** Soot in the air passages

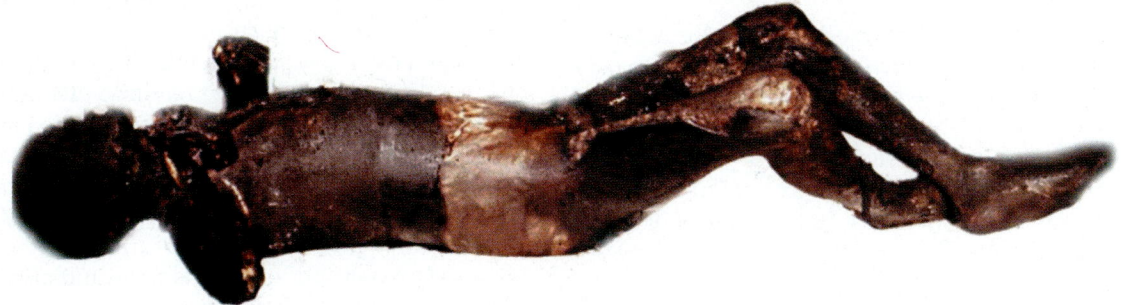

**Fig. 18.9:** Charred body—pugilistic attitude—third degree burns

the burns. A sample of blood taken from the dead body can be subjected to spectroscopic examination and may reveal high carboxyhemoglobin content. Absence of carboxyhemoglobin will not rule out antemortem burning because carbon monoxide may not be formed in open fires. It may also not be present, if the victim dies quickly in flash burns or explosive burns.

Extreme heat can produce postmortem injuries like splitting of skin and fractures of skull (**heat fracture**) which will simulate antemortem violence. Blood in the dural sinuses and meningeal vessels may extravasate and be cooked showing an appearance of extradural hematoma. Analysis of blood from these **heat hematomas** will also yield carboxyhemoglobin. To find out the manner of death, an examination of the scene is also necessary. The majority of the cases are either suicidal or accidental. A person wearing synthetic clothes can sustain severe and extensive burns when the clothes catch fire. Those who attempt to commit suicide will pour some adjuvant like kerosene or petrol over their body and set fire. Homicidal burning is rare, but not uncommon. The victims are rendered unconscious or killed when the bodies are burnt. In all cases of burns, careful examination is necessary for excluding ante-mortem violence.

## CHEMICAL BURNS

Injuries caused by acids, alkalies or corrosive chemicals when they come into contact with skin, are called chemical burns. These lesions are produced by destruction of tissues by the corrosive action of the chemicals (Fig.18.10). Severity of the lesions depends upon the type of chemical, its concentration and length of exposure to the skin or tissues. Acids and alkalies penetrate the deeper tissues and the burns will be more serious in nature. The action of the corrosives will continue till they are washed off or neutralised.

Acids precipitate proteins and the tissues will be necrosed. On the other hand, alkalies dissolve proteins and liquefy tissues. In acid burns, tissues are charred. Alkalies produce mucilaginous/slough. Chemical burns can also be produced by phosphorus, petrol and other hydrocarbons. Treatment consists of immediate removal of the victim from the site of accident and irrigate the affected area with plenty of water. If eyes are affected irrigate with plenty of water. Treat the chemical burns by giving routine treatment of a thermal burn.

Throwing or spraying acids or alkalies on the face of a person due to rivalry is not uncommon. Corrosive acid is filled in a damaged electric bulb (acid bulb) or bottle and thrown at the victim. Injury to the eyes and loss of vision are possible. Permanent scarring of face and disfiguration are the results of these chemical burns. This is legally classified as grievous hurt. Consumption of corrosives to commit suicide is commonly seen. Chemical burns of hands, face, lips, oral cavity and oesophagus with perforation of stomach and intestine are caused.

## DIRECTIONS TO THE INVESTIGATING OFFICER

A good majority of dowry deaths are due to burns. First information given in many of the cases may not be correct. The history given may be that the victim had sustained burns from a stove while cooking or that the stove had burst accidentally. Whatever be the information received, it is the duty of the IO to find out the cause and manner of death.

The following task may be performed:

- Examine the scene thoroughly and meticulously. Locate the source of arson. Look for containers of inflammable substance if any. Examine the containers for fingerprints and preserve them for chemical analysis. Look for disturbance in the scene.
- Take photographs of the body and scene using wide angle and close up lenses.
- Examine the burnt areas for signs of redness and bleb formation (antemortem burns).
- Examine the extent of burns. Find out areas which are burnt more severely and areas spared.
- Identify smell of inflammable substances like kerosene oil, etc.
- Preserve stove or any such device for forensic examination.
- Look for weapons especially blunt ones in the scene.
- Collect trace evidences like burnt hair, clothes, debris and all foreign materials.
- Question the witnesses to find out: (i) The alleged time of the incident, (ii) movements of the inmates of the house including the deceased, (iii) time of consumption of last meal by the deceased, (iv) motive for committing suicide/homicide, etc. and (v) letters/documents received or written by the deceased.
- Examine other inmates of the house for signs of burns or injuries on their person.

- Request the autopsy surgeon to look for the presence of soot in the air passages.
- Request the autopsy surgeon to collect a sample of blood for the estimation of carboxyhemoglobin. The blood sample should be collected in a vacuote or in an airtight container. The sample should be sent to forensic science Laboratory for conducting special analysis like spectroscopy/gas chromatography.
- Request for collection of viscera, blood and urine for routine chemical analysis.
- Request the doctor to collect vaginal swabs and make vaginal smears in the case of female victims.

### Examining the Autopsy Surgeon U/S 161 of Criminal Procedure Code

The medical officer may be questioned on the following aspects.

- What is the probable time of death?
- Whether the burns were antemortem?
- What is the extent and nature of burns?
- Were injuries or signs of violence present?
- Was there any evidence of sexual assault/pregnancy?
- What was the nature of last meal?
- Were there any signs of poisoning/alcohol/drugs?
- Was there any smell of kerosene or other inflammable substances on the body?
- Were trickle marks of any inflammable substance present on the body?
- What were the areas severely burnt and what were spared?
- What could be the probable position of the victim at the time of conflagration?
- What are the features of identification, such as sex, age, stature, dental/bony peculiarities and other features to establish identity (in unidentified and unknown dead bodies).

# 19

# Virginity

Ascertaining the virginity of a woman is required in certain criminal and civil cases like assault, rape, nullity of marriage, divorce, allegations of sexual abuse, etc. Recent signs of defloration or loss of virginity is a positive sign of sexual intercourse or an attempt of sexual act in a case of rape or sexual assault.

Consummation of a marriage happens only if a successful sexual intercourse has taken place. If not, the marriage can be declared as null and void by a court of law. If the marriage is not consummated, the bride can file a petition before the civil court for dissolution of marriage. To verify the allegation, the bride is subjected to examination for signs of virginity.

Virgin is a woman who has never had sexual intercourse. Defloration is the loss of virginity. Signs of virginity are seen in the genitalia. Female external genitalia has four lip like folds of skin. Labia majora are two elongated folds of skin beginning from the mons veneris and covering vaginal orifice. Their lower portions fuse in the midline to form posterior commissure. Labia minora are two soft, thin, pink folds of skin within the labia majora. Their lower portions fuse to form a fold called 'fourchette' (Fig.19.1).

In a virgin, labia majora will be thick, firm, rounded, closely opposed and covering the vaginal orifice completely. Labia minora of a virgin will be within the labia majora and will not be visible outside. The space between the labia minora (vestibule) will be narrow. The posterior

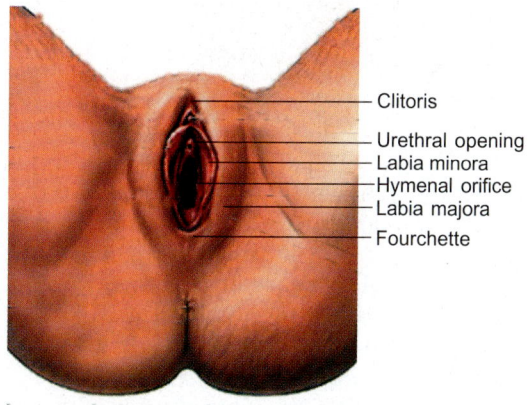

**Fig. 19.1:** Female external genitalia

- Clitoris
- Urethral opening
- Labia minora
- Hymenal orifice
- Labia majora
- Fourchette

commissure and fourchette will be intact. Clitoris will be small. Breasts will be firm and rounded.

## HYMEN

Hymen is named after the Greek god of marriage Hymenaeus, son of goddess Venus. It is a thin fold of mucus membrane at the vaginal orifice, partially concealing it. There is an orifice in the hymen, the shape of which varies considerably (Fig. 19.2). It may be annular, crescentic, fimbriate or septate. Menstrual blood and vaginal secretions flow out through the hymenal opening. In some women, the hymen will not have an opening (imperforate hymen). It will be detected during puberty, when menstrual blood will stagnate in the vagina resulting in pain and infection.

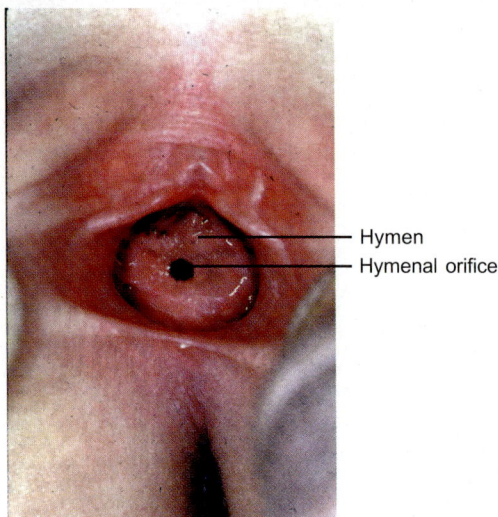

Hymen

Hymenal orifice

**Fig. 19.2:** Intact hymen with a circular orifice

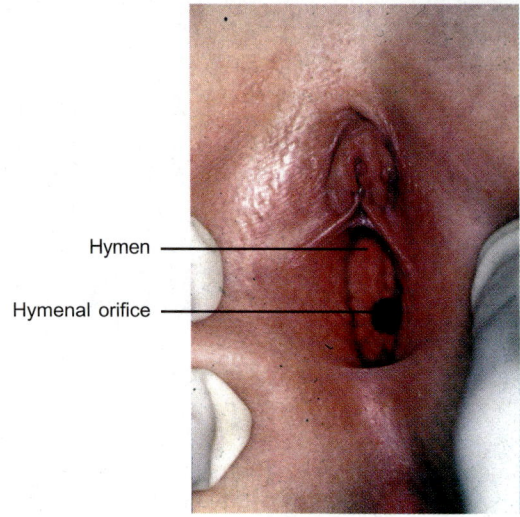

Hymen

Hymenal orifice

**Fig. 19.3:** False virgin—thick, fleshy, elastic hymen

Normally, the hymen will admit only tip of a small finger (diameter 20–25 mm). Diameter of an erect adult penis is 30–40 mm (two fingers). Penile penetration will rupture and dilate an intact hymen. A torn and stretched hymen will never assume its original size. Rupture of the hymen may cause slight bleeding. Hymen ruptures due to sexual act, masturbation by introduction of fingers or a foreign body, violent exercises, introduction of tampons, etc. The structure and consistency of the hymen also varies. It may be thin, fleshy, thick or elastic. In elastic hymen, the hymenal orifice can be stretched without a tear. Sexual act will not cause tears in such an elastic hymen. A woman with an intact hymen which admits only the little finger can be considered as a **virgo intacta,** a virgin. Prior vaginal intercourse can be absolutely ruled out. Women with an elastic hymen can allow a penis to enter without tearing. But it does not mean that such a woman is not a virgin. Woman having an elastic hymen, and who had sexual act is called a **false virgin** (Fig.19.3).

Hymen will be ruptured and dilated in a woman used to sexual act. There will be multiple tears which will extend up to the vaginal wall. In women used to sexual act, the margins of the hymen will have rounded tags of torn hymen

known as **carenculae hymenalis** (Fig. 19.4). Natural clefts in the hymenal margin may be mistaken as tears. Nowadays hymen repair surgery is done in prospective brides!! Hymenorrhaphy is by suturing the remnants of the ruptured hymen together with a gelatin capsule containing a blood-like substance. The husband will be convinced of his bride's virginity when the capsule bursts and stains the bedsheet during first intercourse!!

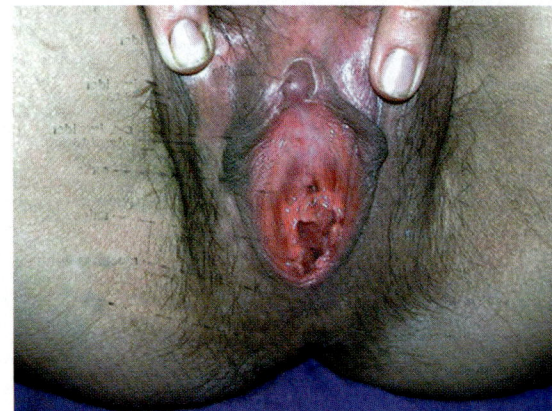

**Fig. 19.4:** Genitalia of a woman used to sexual act. Carenculae hymenalis (tags of hymen) present

## VAGINA

Vagina is a funnel-shaped distensible passage 6–9 cm deep and 4–6 cm wide. Vagina will be narrow and tight in virgins. The mucosa will be rugose. In a woman used to sexual act, the vagina will become lax and elongated. The rugosity will be lost. Unusually in some virgins, mucosa will not be rugose. Frequent sexual act can also cause rupture of fourchette. Labia majora will not be opposed. Labia minora will be exposed and separated from the labia majora. Presence or absence of hymen in no way indicates whether a woman is virgin or not. **Virginity can be proved; but cannot be disproved.** A woman is a virgin until she has sexual intercourse. In women used to sexual act, the hymenal orifice will admit two fingers easily.

## DIRECTIONS TO THE INVESTIGATING OFFICER

When it is necessary to ascertain the virginity of a woman involved in a criminal case, she may be sent to a government medical expert, preferably a doctor specialised in obstetrics and gynaecology. Examination of the victim should be conducted only with the written informed consent of the woman. If the victim is a minor, permission of the lawful guardian should be obtained. The victim should be accompanied by a woman police constable. The IO may write a request to the medical officer giving a gist of the case and the nature of examination to be conducted. In sexual offences like rape, apart form the general and genital examination, material evidences have to be collected from the person of the victim. The details are given in Chapter 20.

# 20

# Sexual Offences

## RAPE

Rape is defined as unlawful sexual intercourse by a man with a woman against her will, without her consent or with her consent when it is obtained by fraud, or putting her in fear of death or hurt or by impersonation or by drugging.

The female should be aged above 16 years, for consensual sexual intercourse. Sexual intercourse with a girl aged below 16 years is statutory rape, even if the intercourse was performed with her consent. Mere penetration (without ejaculation) will constitute an offence of rape.

Rape is always not a surprise attack by a stranger. When a man rapes a woman he knows, it is called **acquaintance rape.** Some times, the woman is given a drink containing a drug like robypnol/GHB/ketamine in a party and she is violated in a drugged state. This is called **date rape**.

Marriage is a contract and consent to sexual intercourse is implicit. Therefore, a husband cannot be held for raping his wife. But now English, US and Canadian laws recognise rape within a marriage as a crime. It is considered as a part of domestic violence. Sexual intercourse with a wife against her will and consent is termed **marital rape.**

**Custodial rape** is the rape of a woman by authorities, like police officers, jail authorities, hospital authorities, etc. who, by virtue of their authority exploits the woman under their custody and commits the offence. **Gang rape** is a rape of a woman by a group of persons acting in furtherance of common intention.

## Legal Aspects

Sections 375 and 376 of Indian Penal Code deal with rape. These sections have been substantially amended in 1983 by incorporating several new sub-sections.

Section 375 of IPC defines rape as follows:

A man is said to commit "rape" who except in the case hereinafter excepted, has sexual intercourse with a woman under circumstances falling under any of the following six descriptions:-

*First:* Against her will

*Secondly:* Without her consent

*Thirdly:* With her consent, when her consent has been obtained by putting her or any person in whom she is interested in fear of death or of hurt.

*Fourthly:* With her consent, when the man knows that he is not her husband, and that her consent is given because she believes that he is another man to whom she is or believes herself to be lawfully married.

*Fifthly:* With her consent, when, at the time of giving such consent, by reason of unsoundness of mind or intoxication or the administration by him personally or through another of any stupefying or unwholesome substance, she is unable to understand the nature and consequences of that to which she gives consent.

*Sixthly:* With or without consent, when she is under sixteen years of age.

*Explanation:* Penetration is sufficient to constitute the sexual intercourse necessary to the offence of rape.

*Exception:* Sexual intercourse by a man with his own wife, the wife not being under fifteen years of age, is not rape.

The above section has two ingredients:

a. Sexual intercourse by a man with a woman.
b. The sexual intercourse must be under circumstances falling under any of the six clauses of the section.

**Section 376 IPC** prescribes the punishment for rape.

(1) "Whoever, except in the cases provided for by subsection (2), commits rape shall be punished with imprisonment of either description for a term which shall not be less than 7 years but which may be for life or for a term which may extend to 10 years and shall also be liable to fine unless the woman raped is his own wife and is not under 12 years of age, in which case, he shall be punished with imprisonment of either description for a term which may extend to 2 years or with fine or with both:

Provided that the court may, for adequate and special reasons to be mentioned in the judgement, impose a sentence of imprisonment for a term of less than 7 years."

(2) Whoever,

a. Being a police officer commits rape: (i) within the limits of his police station to which he is appointed; or (ii) in the premises of any station house whether or not situated in the police station to which he is appointed; or (iii) on a woman in his custody or in the custody of a police officer subordinate to him; or
b. Being a public servant, takes advantage of his official position and commits rape on a woman in his custody as such public servant or in the custody of a public servant subordinate to him; or
c. Being on the management or on the staff of a jail, remand home or other place of custody established by or under any law for the time being in force or of a women's or children's institution takes advantage of his official position and commits rape on any inmate of such jail, remand home, place or institution; or
d. Being on the management or on the staff of a hospital, takes advantage of his official position

and commits rape on a woman in that hospital; or

e. Commits rape on a woman knowing her to be pregnant; or
f. Commits rape on a woman when she is under 12 years of age; or
g. Commits gang rape.

Shall be punished with rigorous imprisonment for a term which shall not be less than 10 years but which may be for life and shall also be liable to fine:

Provided that the court may, for adequate and special reasons to be mentioned in the judgement, impose a sentence of imprisonment of either description for a term of less than 10 years.

*Explanation 1:* Where a woman is raped by one or more in a group of persons acting in furtherance of their common intention, each of the persons shall be deemed to have committed gang rape within the meaning of this subsection.

*Explanation 2:* "Women's or children's institution" means an institution, whether called an orphanage or a home for neglected women or children or a widow's home or by any other name, which is established and maintained for the reception and care of women or children.

*Explanation 3:* "Hospital" means the precincts of the hospital and includes the precincts of any institution for the reception and treatment of persons during convalescence or of persons requiring medical attention or rehabilitation.

### Section 376 A

Whoever, has sexual intercourse with his own wife, who is living separately from him under a decree of separation or under any custom or usage without her consent, shall be punished with imprisonment of either description for a term which may extend to 2 years and shall also be liable to fine.

### Section 376 B

Whoever, being a public servant, takes advantage of his official position and induces or seduces, any woman, who is in his custody as such public servant or in the custody of a public servant subordinate to him, to have sexual intercourse with him, such sexual intercourse not amounting to the offence of rape, shall be punished with imprisonment of either description for a term which may extend to 5 years and shall also be liable to fine.

## Section 376 C

Whoever, being the superintendent or manager of a jail, remand home or other place of custody established by or under any law for the time being in force or of a women's or children's institution takes advantage of his official position and induces or seduces any female inmate of such jail, remand home, place or institution to have sexual intercourse with him, such sexual intercourse not amounting to the offence of rape, shall be punished with imprisonment of either description for a term which may extend to 5 years and shall also be liable to fine.

*Explanation 1:* "Superintendent" in relation to a jail, remand home or other place of custody or a women's/children's institution includes a person holding any other office in such jail, remand home, place or institution by virtue of which he can exercise any authority or control over its inmates.

*Explanation 2:* The expression "women's or children's institution" shall have the same meaning as in explanation 2 to subsection 2 of Section 376.

## Section 376 D

Whoever, being on the management of a hospital or being on the staff of a hospital takes advantages of his position and has sexual intercourse with any woman in that hospital, such sexual intercourse not amounting to the offence of rape, shall be punished with imprisonment of either description for a term which may extend to 5 years and shall also be liable to fine.

*Explanation:* The expression 'hospital' shall have the same meaning as in explanation 3 to subsection (2) of Section 376.

These new sections were introduced with a view to stop sexual abuses of women in custody, care and control by various categories of persons, which though not amounting to rape, were nevertheless considered highly reprehensible. The amended Section 376 IPC now prescribes a minimum punishment of 7 years imprisonment for the offence of rape. For custodial rape, rape on pregnant women, rape on girls under 12 years of age, and gang rape, a minimum punishment of 10 years imprisonment has been made obligatory.

**Section 114 (a) of Indian Evidence Act** states that: "In a prosecution for rape under clause (a) or clause (b) or clause (c) or clause (d) or clause (e) or clause (g) of subsection (2) of Section 376 of the Indian Penal Code (45 of 1860) where sexual intercourse by the accused is proved and the question is whether it was without the consent of the woman alleged to have been raped and she states in her evidence before the court that she did not consent, the court shall presume that she did not consent." Addition of this section has made the prosecution of a case of rape easier. The statement of the victim of rape that she had not consented for the act is accepted by the court.

**Section 327 (2)(3) of Criminal Procedure Code**

As per the provisions of this Section, trial of rape cases shall be conducted **in camera** and forbids the disclosure of the identity of the victim. These provisions of law protect the honour of the victim and make it possible for her to depose in the court fearlessly.

## Examination of the Victim

As per the new **Section 164 A** of Cr. P. C:
1. Where, during the stage when an offence of committing rape or attempt to commit rape is under investigation, it is proposed to get the person of the woman with whom rape is alleged or attempt to have been committed or attempted, examined by a medical expert, such examination shall be conducted by a registered medical practitioner employed in a hospital run by the government or a local authority and in the absence of such a practitioner, by any other registered medical practitioner, with the consent of such woman or of a person competent to give such consent on her behalf and such woman shall be sent to such registered medical practitioner within 24 hours from the time of receiving the information relating to the commission of such offence.

2. The registered medical practitioner, to whom such woman is sent shall, without delay, examine her person and prepare a report of his examination giving the following particulars, namely:

   i. The name and address of the woman and of the person by whom she was brought;

  ii. The age of the woman;

 iii. The description of material taken from the person of the woman for DNA profiling;

 iv. Marks of injury, if any, on the person of the woman;

  v. General mental condition of the woman; and

 vi. Other material particulars in reasonable detail.

3. The report shall state precisely the reasons for each conclusion arrived at.

4. The report shall specifically record that the consent of the woman or of the person competent to give such consent on her behalf to such examination had been obtained.

5. The exact time of commencement and completion of the examination shall also be noted in the report.

6. The registered medical practitioner shall, without delay forward the report to the investigation officer who shall forward it to the magistrate concerned (Sec 173 Cr. P. C).

7. Nothing in this section shall be construed as rendering lawful any examination without the consent of the woman or of any person competent to give such consent on her behalf.

## Investigation of a Case of Alleged Rape—General Directions

Most often the first information as to the commission of the offence is received from:

1. The medical officer who attended the sexually assaulted victim brought to the hospital with general and genital injuries. Intimationed only with the consent of the victim.

2. The victim of sexual assault who directly lodges a complaint before the station house officer.

In all these cases, the most important aspect is the collection of physical evidence without delay. The evidence is collected from the victim, accused and the scene. Therefore after recording the first information statement, the victim should be sent to a doctor of the nearest government hospital for physical examination after obtaining her written informed consent. If she is a minor, the consent should be obtained from her lawful guardian. If such a medical officer is not available the victim can be got examined by any other registered medical practitioner. The woman shall be sent for medical examination within 24 hours from the time of receiving the first information. In my opinion, it is better to get the victim examined by a gynaecologist who is an expert in conducting genital examination.

The medical officer should be requested to conduct a physical examination and collect of samples for laboratory analysis. A detailed history should also be obtained prior to the examination. The doctor may be requested to collect clothes of the victim worn at the time of the assault. The clothes should be examined and preserved for forensic examination.

In cases of rape or attempted rape, medical examination of the victim and the accused soon after the incident will yield a lot of corroborative evidences. Delay in the examination will result in the loss of valuable evidences. At the same time, absence of medical findings does not rule out the offence of rape. For example, mere penetration need not produce any tell tale physical evidence. Sexual intercourse with a married woman need not produce any injuries to the genitalia.

Marks of violence on the body of a victim indicate that she had offered resistance. But if the act was done under threat or in an intoxicated state, there will not be any general injuries on the body of a victim. Presence of bodily injuries like bite marks, nail marks, etc. on the body of the accused also prove that the victim had offered resistance. Genital injuries can be serious if the act is done on a virgin or a young girl (Fig. 20.1). Genital injuries will be minimal in a woman used to sexual act. Trivial general injuries can be seen on the victim as well as the accused in violent sexual act. Generally speaking, if there are signs of general and genital violence, it can be assumed that the sexual act was

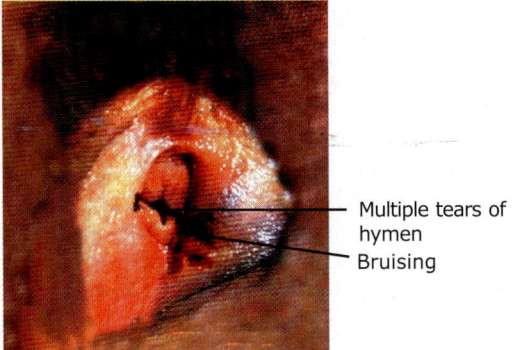

Multiple tears of hymen

Bruising

**Fig. 20.1:** Injuries to the genitalia of a victim of rape

done against the will and without the consent of the victim.

Request the doctor to collect the following materials from the victim for examination:

- Blood —for grouping, DNA typing and toxico-logical analysis (in drug-facilitated rape).
- Hair —scalp and pubic (to be cut and combed)
- Loose hair on the body — for DNA typing.
- Swabs from stained areas — prepare smears.
- Vaginal and cervical swabs and smears.
- Rectal swab (if anal penetration is alleged).
- Oral swabs and smear (if oral penetration is alleged).
- Swabs from bite marks (if bite marks are present).
- Clothes (worn at the time of assault) dried in shade and each item packed separately.

If bite marks are present, the same may be photographed with a scale. Help of forensic odontologist should be sought for further necessary examination. If the age is disputed, the victim should be sent to a medical expert* for determination of age.

## Medicolegal Aspects

Rape is a legal term and it is not proper or correct to form an opinion that rape has/has not taken place based on physical findings. However, the following points may provide corroborative evidence:

- Clothes torn and stained with blood, semen, mud, etc.
- Presence of foreign hairs on the body.

- General injuries may suggest a struggle.
- Genital injuries like abrasions and contusions involving the vulva, thigh, pubic region may indicate an attempt of penetration.
- Recent injuries of the hymen or fourchette may indicate penetration.
- Presence of semen. Spermatozoa may remain motile for 6–8 hours. Non-motile forms are detected up to 48 hours and rarely up to 72–96 hours (spermatozoa need not be present, e.g. vasectomy, azoospermia). Semen in the vagina is an indication of recent sexual act.
- Venereal diseases—if the accused is suffering from venereal disease and the time of onset is within the incubation period in the victim who was previously free from such disease.

(Detection of DNA materials of the accused from the samples collected from the person of the victim will be a positive evidence to prove the guilt of the accused.)

## Molestation

Assault or criminal force to a woman with intend to outrage her modesty is punishable u/s 354 of IPC. Generally, this is termed as an indecent assault. This is an offence of lesser gravity than rape. Touching the body parts of a woman with a malicious intention will amount to outrage of her modesty. There may not be any physical evidence in this type of offence. However, if necessary, with the consent of the victim, a medical examination may be conducted.

## False Accusation

A woman, with ulterior motive may falsely accuse a man of raping her. She may give a falsified history and even fabricate evidence such as torn clothes with stains of blood and semen. One should remember the saying: **Rape is an allegation, easily made; difficult to prove and hard to disprove.** As per the provisions of Section 214 of Evidence Act, if the victim states that it was not a consensual intercourse, the act is considered as rape.

*Police surgeon, Superintendents of Govt Hospitals, Radiologists

A detailed history, thorough physical examination and laboratory examinations including DNA typing of the semen collected from vagina and other trace evidences will help the investigators to arrive at accurate conclusions.

## Drug-facilitated Sexual Assaults

Certain drugs like robypnol, GHB, ketamine are added to a drink and given to the victim in deceit. When the drug is dissolved in the drink, they will be colourless and odourless. Some drugs are tasteless also. The drug makes the victim confused, weak and unconscious. These drugs are called rape/club drugs. The incapacitated victim is sexually assaulted. The victim will be unable to resist the rapist or even call out for help.

## Treatment

The victim might have sustained injuries during the sexual assault. Minor injuries can be treated in the outpatient department. Severe injuries can occur and may require surgical repair, especially in children. The victim may contract venereal diseases like gonorrhoea, chlamydia, syphilis, hepatitis, and even HIV from the accused. This will be an evidence to substantiate the offence of rape. Therefore, the doctor may be asked to conduct tests initially and after 6 weeks and thereafter at 3 and 6 months as the incubation period of the venereal infections vary. Pregnancy after rape is possible. Pregnancy tests can be conducted 4–6 weeks after the incident. Pregnancy can be prevented by giving contraceptive (morning after) pills within 48 hours after rape. If pregnancy occurs after rape, it can be terminated as per the provisions of Medical Termination of Pregnancy Act.

Rape is a psychological trauma to the victim. The victim may develop acute stress reactions which may last for weeks. The victim will have uncontrollable crying and trembling. She will be frightened, embarrassed and feel degraded **(rape trauma syndrome—RTS).** Most of the women may adjust quickly and return to normal. But in some, long-term effects like flash backs, aversion to sex, anxiety, phobia, depression, nightmares, etc. may develop. They need psychological counselling and psychiatric help.

## Rape and Murder

Sometimes a sexual assault ends in death of the victim. The woman sustains fatal injuries or she is choked or strangled to death, when the accused attempts to overcome her resistance. Some psychopathic offenders murder the victim and mutilate the dead body after rape. Young children and old women succumb to violence easily. Sometimes, the raped woman is murdered to prevent detection of the offence. The usual modes of killing are by strangulation, smothering or blunt violence. Sadistic murderers use sharp weapons and inflict a number of mutilating injuries.

While holding inquest on the dead body of a female, if sexual assault is suspected care must be taken to identify injuries caused by the sexual act and collect material evidence from the scene and dead body. Help of a forensic surgeon and forensic scientist may be obtained. All the steps taken in the examination of a living victim of rape should be taken in the case of a dead victim also. Sometimes, the penetration was effected after death.

A careful search should be made on the dead body and the scene for trace evidences. Loose hair, salivary stains, seminal stains, blood stains, etc. may be present on the body and clothes. If bite marks are present, forensic odontologist may be called to conduct necessary investigations. Photographs of all the injuries and marks of violence should be taken. In all cases, the anus and oral cavity should be examined. Many of the offenders may be sexual perverts. There could be evidence of anal or oral coitus. Swabs should be taken from the rectum and oral cavity. Some perverts may use instruments or fingers to penetrate the vagina or anus. In such case, severe injuries may be present and semen may be absent in the orifices.

## Examination of an Accused in a Case of Rape

According to the new Section 53 A in the Criminal Procedure Code (25/2005):

1. When a person is arrested on a charge of committing an offence of rape, or an attempt to commit rape and there are reasonable grounds for believing that an examination of this person will afford evidence as to the commission of

such offence, it shall be lawful for registered medical practitioner employed in a hospital run by the government or by a local authority and in the absence of such a practitioner within the radius of 16 kilometers from the place where the offence has been committed by any other registered medical practitioner, acting at the request of a police officer not below the rank of a subinspector, and for any person acting in good faith in his aid and under his direction, to make such an examination of the arrested person and to use such force as is reasonably necessary for that purpose.

2. The registered medical practitioner conducting such examination shall, without delay, examine such person and prepare a report of his examination giving the following particulars, namely:

   i. The name and address of the accused and of the person by whom he was brought,

   ii. The age of the accused,

   iii. Marks of injury, if any, on the person of the accused,

   iv. The description of the material taken from the person of the accused for DNA profiling

   v. Other material particulars in reasonable detail.

3. The report shall state precisely the reasons for each conclusion arrived at.

4. The exact time of commencement and completion of the examination shall also be noted in the report.

5. The registered medical practitioner shall, without delay, forward the report to the investigating officer, who shall forward it to the magistrate concerned (vide Sec. 173 CrPC).

The following points, if present, may offer corroborative evidence:

- Tearing of the clothes with detection of stains such as blood, semen, mud, etc.
- Detection of scalp hair and pubic hairs of the female on the body of the accused.
- Injuries like bite marks and nail marks.
- Absence of smegma in the uncircumcised male
- Presence of vaginal epithelial cells in the glans penis.
- Venereal diseases — if the victim is suffering from venereal diseases and the time of onset is within the incubation period in an accused who was previously free from such disease.

Genital injuries such as rupture of frenulum (attachment of the foreskin of penis) or subsequent paraphimosis (slipping of the foreskin). This may not occur, if the victim is used to sexual act.

Smegma is an yellowish secretion seen as a coating under the foreskin of the penis. During intercourse, the smegma coating will be removed from the penis. It is also removed due to bathing or washing. It takes 24 hours for smegma to accumulate again. Therefore, if smegma is absent when the accused is examined immediately after the sexual act, the presumption is that he had a recent sexual act. In circumcised males, as the foreskin is removed, there will not be any smegma.

Vagina is lined by cells called squamous epithelial cells. These cells contain a substance called glycogen. During penile penetration, the vaginal epithelial cells will be transferred to the penis. A cotton swab, wet with saline or distilled water is applied around the glans and smears are prepared on glass slides. Another method is to wash the penis in normal saline or distilled water and collect washings. The washings are centrifuged and smear is prepared from the dposit. The smear is stained with iodine or per iodic acid Schiff reagent. The glycogen content in the vaginal epithelial cells will take up the stain and will appear brown. If vaginal epithelial cells are detected in a smear, the dried swab and a few unstained smears can be used for DNA typing.

Clothes of the accused should be sent as a whole for examination. Stained areas should not be cut or marked. Clothes have to be dried in the shade before packing. Detection of the DNA material of the prosecutrix/deceased in the trace evidence collected from the person of the accused will prove the guilt of the accused.

If the accused is pleading impotence, an examination and certification regarding his potency should also be conducted. Any government doctor is competent to conduct potency examination and issue a certificate.

## Discussion

*"A murderer destroys the physical frame of the victim, a rapist degrades and defiles the soul of a helpless woman."*

Justice Arjit Pasayat, Hon.Judge,<br>Supreme Court of India.

In the present circumstances, sexual assaults and harassments are on the rise. For a successful prosecution, medical and scientific evidences play a vital role. Delay in reporting cases will cause valuable trace evidence from the body of the victim to disappear. Medical examination of the victim soon after the assault will yield evidences to prove that sexual intercourse has taken place. DNA analysis of the semen or its stains found on the body of the victim will be the best evidence to connect the accused with the crime, even if he is apprehended after years.

Marks of violence on the body of the victim (as well as the accused) are indicative of resistance offered by the victim. This would support the allegation of rape. But a victim may not resist, if the accused threatens to kill or maim her. Therefore, absence of general injuries on the body does not prove that the victim was a consenting party. But Sec. 114(A) of Evidence Act states that court shall presume that the victim did not consent to the act, if she states so. Genital injuries may also be absent or minimal in the case of women accustomed to sexual act. Partial penetration also may not produce any genital injuries. Absence of genital injuries does not rule out rape.

The investigating officer and the medical officer should also be aware of false allegations and accusations. Therefore, care and attention should be exercised in the physical examination and collection of scientific evidence without delay from the victim, accused and the scene.

## UNNATURAL SEXUAL OFFENCES

**Section 377 of IPC** deals with unnatural sexual offences. "Whoever voluntarily has carnal intercourse against the order of nature with any man, woman or animal, shall be punished with imprisonment for life, or with imprisonment of either description for a term which may extend to 10 years, and shall also be liable to fine."

*Explanation:* Penetration is sufficient to constitute the carnal intercourse necessary to constitute the offence described in this section.

## Sodomy

Sodomy is an unnatural sexual offence punishable under this section. It is anal intercourse by a man with another man or a woman. Sometimes, the victim may be a habitual passive agent. Even if the act is done with the consent of the victim, both the accused and the victim are liable to punishment. If the act is done without the consent of the passive agent, the active agent alone is punished. It is very difficult to accomplish the act against the will and without the consent of the victim unless the victim is weak, intoxicated or unconscious. Sometimes the sodomite is murdered after accomplishing the act.

## Discussion

If there are general injuries on the body, inference is that the act was done against the will and without the consent of the victim. Anal injuries indicate stretching and are consistent with penetration. Normally, the anal opening will admit one finger. If two fingers can be passed without difficulty, the anal opening being patulous with loss of tone of sphincter, the inference is that victim could be a habitual passive agent. If recent dilatation has taken place, semen might be detected in the rectum or anal canal. The doctor may be requested to take swabs from the anal canal, prepare smears, dry the swabs and smears and send them for chemical/forensic examination. Intercourse in between the thighs of a passive agent is another unnatural sexual offence. Moist swabs are to be appliezd on the thighs of the victim, dried and sent for chemical examination. Clothes of the accused and victim are also to be examined for seminal stains. If the accused is pleading impotence, he should be sent for examination and certification for signs of impotence. Habitual passive agents will show recent and old injuries in the anus which is dilated, lax, funnel-shpaed and fissured with keratinised margins. The tone of anal sphinctre is lost. Fresh injuries are due to recent violence (Fig. 20. 2).

## Bestiality

Rectal or vaginal intercourse with an animal is termed bestiality. The accused is examined by a medical officer. The animal is to be examined by a veterinary surgeon. Swabs should be collected from the rectum/vagina of the animal.

## Buccal Coitus

Buccal coitus or fellatio is also an unnatural sexual offence under Section 377 of IPC. In this case, apart from the routine physical examination, swabs from the oral cavity of the victim are to be taken for detection of sperms/semen. Swabs from the penis of the accused have to be taken and examined for the presence of saliva and buccal epithelium.

## Lesbians and Gays

Homosexuality is sexual orientation towards people of the same sex. Female homosexuals are called lesbians. Male homosexuals are 'gays'. Nowadays both are called gays. Lesbianism (tribadism) is the practice of a woman obtaining sexual gratification from another woman. Lesbians practice mutual masturbation and use artificial phallus. Gay men practice sodomy and oral coitus.

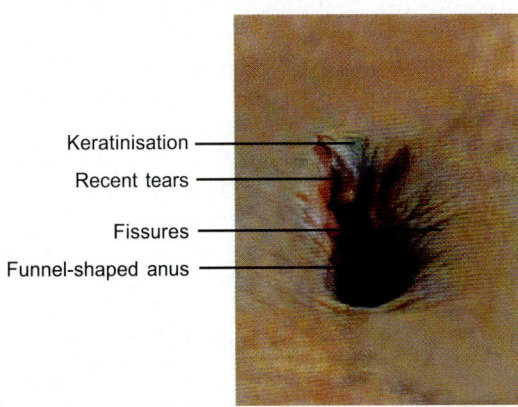

Keratinisation
Recent tears
Fissures
Funnel-shaped anus

**Fig. 20.2:** Anus of habitual passive agent (Recent and old injuries in the anus which is dilated, lax, funnel-shaped and fissured with keratinised margins. The tone of the anal sphinctre is lost. Fresh injuries are due to recent violence)

This is considered as a mental deviation and not as an unnatural sexual offence. Many gays and lesbians marry each other or cohabit.

## Incest

Incest is sexual intercourse between people who are legally prohibited from marrying because of their close blood relationship. Degree of relationship within which marriage is forbidden varies in different cultures and societies. However, relation between the parents and children and between brother and sister are forbidden. Incest is not a cognisable offence in India. When a complaint is lodged, the case is charged U/S 376 of IPC. Incest is considered as a personality disorder.

## SEXUAL PERVERSIONS (PARAPHILIA)

According to Sigmund Freud, perversions are sexual activities which either extend, in an anatomical sense, beyond the regions of the body that are designed for sexual union. These are habitual acts to obtain sexual gratification without sexual intercourse.

### Sadism

This is a sexual disorder, in which erotic excitement or gratification is derived from inflicting physical or mental pain on others. This is seen commonly in males. Biting, whipping, inflicting sharp force injuries, cigarette burns, etc. are the usual methods. Sometimes a sadist may murder the victim by inflicting serious injuries on the body of the victim **(lust murder)**. In this type of murder, the genital organs may be mutilated. A sadist may sometimes indulge in intercourse with the dead body **(necrophilia)**. Some may even drink the blood of the victim or eat the flesh **(necrophagia)**. Many serial killers are sadists.

### Masochism

Sexual pleasure is derived from pain that is either self-inflicted or inflicted by another person usually a female. The disorder occurs rarely alone; instead, it is usually combined with sadism. The combination is called sadomasochism. Masochists engage in autoerotic practices like applying nooses around the neck and inducing asphyxia (sexual asphyxia).

Accidental death is common during the masochistic practices.

## Fetishism

In psychology, the term applies to a sexual disorder in which sexual urges and fantasies persistently involve the use of non-living objects by themselves or, at times, with a sexual partner. Common fetish objects are feet, shoes, brassiere, undergarments and articles of female apparel. Sometimes, the pervert may masturbate on these articles. These articles are often stolen by the fetish. In general, psychologists believe that fetishism serves to alleviate feelings of sexual inadequacy, usually among males.

## Transvestism

This is the practice of wearing the clothing of the opposite sex for emotional or sexual expression. Transvestism does not include all instances of wearing such clothing. Transvestites have a desire to be identified with the opposite sex. The transvestite gains emotional satisfaction from dressing in the clothing of the opposite sex. Transvestism occurs among both sexes, but is more common among men than among women and more common among heterosexuals than among homosexuals. Persons who practice autoerotic practices often dress up in female attire. In one of the temples in Kerala, transvestism is practised by males of all ages as a ritual during the temple festival. Transvestism is considered as a deviant behaviour.

## Exhibitionism

This is a psychological disorder seen in males who exhibit their genitals in the presence of women. Occasionally, this is seen in women also. Some males may masturbate in public. All these are obscene acts and are punishable U/S 294 IPC.

## Voyeurism (Scoptophilia)

It is a practice of obtaining sexual excitement and pleasure by looking, especially secretly, at other people's naked bodies or watching the sexual activity of other people (peeping tom). Voyeurs enter hostels and houses at night and peep into bedrooms and bathrooms.

## Frotteurism

It is a practice of rubbing the genitalia against another person. This is commonly practised by a pervert male in crowded public transports and other places. It is associated with fondling the breasts and body parts of the females. Some may even ejaculate on the clothing or body of the women.

## Uranism

According to Sigmund Freud (1856–1939), this is a psychological disorder due to fixation of the libido at earlier levels of anal phase or sucking phase. The person gets sexual gratification by sucking or licking the genitals of another person. They practice fellatio (sucking the penis) or cunnilingus (licking the clitoris). These persons are interested in drinking the semen after oral intercourse. In a survey conducted in Kerala (Project SASI - Trivandrum), this perversion is seen in many persons of varying ages. The pervert may even pay the active agent for allowing him to do oral sex.

## Troilism

This is a practice of getting sexual pleasure by a male by watching his wife or another female engaged in sexual intercourse with another man. He may engage in masturbation while observing the act. The pervert will entice another male to his home and induce his wife to have intercourse with him. This is a deviant behaviour.

## SEXUAL HARASSMENT OF WORKING WOMEN: DIRECTIONS OF SUPREME COURT

Sexual harassment of working women at work places is not uncommon. The present penal laws do not adequately provide for specific protection of women from this social evil. A lady social worker was brutally raped at her work place in a village in Rajasthan. That incident revealed the hazards to which a working woman is exposed and the necessity for urgent measures for safeguards.

Following this incident, a group of social activists and Non-governmental organisations filed writ petitions before the Hon: Supreme Court. A three judges bench chaired by the Hon: Chief Justice Sri J S Verma, laid down the following guidelines and norms applicable to both public and private sectors. This was done in exercise of the powers of the court under article 32 of the Indian Constitution for enforcement of the fundamental rights. These are to be treated as law declared under Article 141 of the Constitution.

1. *Duty of the employer or other responsible persons in work places and other institutions:* It shall be the duty of the employer or other responsible persons in work places or other institutions to prevent or deter the commission of acts of sexual harassment and to provide the procedures for the resolution, settlement or prosecution of acts of sexual harassment by taking all steps required.

2. *Definition:* For this purpose, sexual harassment includes such unwelcome sexually determined behaviour (whether directly or by implication) as:
   a. Physical contact and advance,
   b. A demand or request for sexual favours
   c. Sexually coloured remarks
   d. Showing pornography
   e. Any other unwelcome physical, verbal or non verbal conduct of sexual nature.

Where any of these acts is committed in circumstances whereunder the victim of such conduct has a reasonable apprehension that in relation to the victim's employment or work whether she is drawing salary, or honorarium or voluntary, whether in government, public or private enterprise, such conduct can be humiliating and may constitute a health and safety problem. It is discriminatory for instance when the women has reasonable grounds to believe that her objections would disadvantage her in connection with her employment or work including recruiting or promotion or when it creates a hostile work environment. Adverse consequences might be visited if the victim does not consent to the conduct in question or raises any objection whereto.

3. *Preventive steps:* All employers or persons in charge of work place whether in the public or private sector should take appropriate steps to prevent the sexual harassment. Without prejudice to the generality of this obligation, they should take the following steps:
   a. Express prohibition of sexual harassment as defined above at the work place should be notified, published and circulated in appropriate ways.
   b. The rules/regulations of government and public sector bodies relating to conduct and discipline should include rules or regulations prohibiting sexual harassment and provide for appropriate penalties in such rules against the offender.
   c. As regards private employers, steps should be taken to include aforesaid prohibitions of the standing orders under the Industrial Employment (or standing orders) Act 1946.
   d. Appropriate work conditions should be provided in respect of work, leisure, health, hygiene and to further ensure that there is no hostile environment towards women at work places and no employee woman should have reasonable grounds to believe that she is disadvantaged in connection with her employment.

4. *Criminal proceedings:* Where such conduct amounts to a specific offence under the Indian Penal Code or under any other law, the employer shall initiate appropriate action in accordance with law by making a complaint with the appropriate authority. In particular, it should be ensured that victim or witnesses are not victimised or discriminated against while dealing with complaints of sexual harassment. The victims of sexual harassment should have the option to seek transfer of the perpetrator or their own transfer.

5. *Disciplinary action:* Where such conduct amounts to misconduct in employment as defined by the relevant rules, appropriate disciplinary action should be initiated by the employer in accordance with the rules.

6. *Complaint mechanism:* Whether or no such conduct constitute an offence under law or a breach of the service rules, an appropriate complaint mechanism should be created in the employer's organisation for redressal of the complaint made by the victim. Such complaint mechanism should ensure time-based treatment of complaints.

7. *Complaints committee:* The complaint mechanism, referred to (in 6) above should be adequate to provide where necessary, a complaints committee, a special counsellor or other support service including the main-tenance of confidentiality. The complaints committee should be headed by a woman and not less than half of its members could be women. Further to prevent the probability of any undue pressure or influence at senior levels, such complaints committee should involve a third party, either NGO or other party who is familiar with the issue of sexual harassment. The complaints committee must make annual report to the government department concerned of the complaints and action taken by them. The employers and person in charge will also report on the complaint with the aforesaid guidelines including on the reports of the complaints committee to the government departments.

8. *Worker's initiative:* Employees should be allowed to raise issues of sexual harassment at worker's meeting and in other appropri-ate forum and it should be affirmatively discussed in the employer-employee meetings.

9. *Awareness:* Awareness of the rights of female employees at this regard should be created in particular by prominently notifying the guidelines (and appropriate legislation when enacted on the subject) in a suitable manner.

10. *Third party harassment:* Where sexual harassment occurs as a result of an act or omission by any third party or outsider, the employer and person in charge will take all steps necessary and reasonable to assist the affected person in terms of support and pre-ventive action.

11. **The Central/State Governments** are req-uested to consider adopting suitable measures including legislation to ensure that the guidelines laid down by this order are also observed by the employers in private sector.

12. **These guidelines** will not prejudice any rights available under the protection of Human Rights Act, 1993. Accordingly, we direct that the above guidelines and norms would be strictly observed in all work places for the preservation and enforcement of the right to gender equality of the working women. These directions would be binding and enforceable in law until suitable legislation is enacted to occupy the field.

## Trial of Child Sex Abuse or Rape—Directions of The Supreme Court

A writ petition was filed by way of public interest litigation by 'Sakshi' an organisation to provide legal, medical, residential, psychological or any other help or assistance or charitable support for women who are victims of sexual abuse or harassment, violence or any kind of atrocity. The main reliefs sought were as follows:

1. Issue a writ in the nature of declaration/direction that sexual intercourse as contai-ned in Section 375 of IPC shall include all forms of penetration such as penile/vaginal, penile/anal, penile/oral, finger/vaginal, finger/anal or object/vaginal penetration.

2. To register all such cases found to be true on investigation, offences falling within the broadened interpretation of sexual inter-course set out in the prayer aforesaid as offences under Sections 375 and 376 A to D.

The writ petition was disposed of with the following directions:

1. The provisions of **Section 327(2) of Cr.P.C** shall also apply to inquiry or trial of offences under **Section 354 and 377 IPC.**

2. In holding trial of child sex abuse or rape:
   i. A screen or some such arrangements may be made where the victim or witness (who may be equally vulnerable like the victim) do not see the body of the accused.
   ii. The questions put in cross-examination on behalf of the accused, in so far as they relate directly to the incident, should be given in writing to the presiding officer of the court who may put them to the victim or witness in a language which is clear and not embarrassing.
   iii. The victim of child abuse or rape, while giving testimony in court, should be allowed sufficient breaks when required.

These directions are in addition to those given in Gurmit Singh Vs State of Punjab given below:
   a. Should not ignore the mandate of the provisions of **Sections 327(2) and (3) of CrPC.** and the trial of rape cases should be conducted in camera.
   b. As far as possible trial of such cases should be conducted by lady judges wherever available so that the prosecutrix can make statements with greater ease and assist the court to properly discharge their duties.

## DIRECTIONS TO THE INVESTIGATING OFFICER

### Rape Victim

- Treat the victim gently with kindness and compassion.
- After recording the first information, the victim should be sent to the nearest government doctor for examination and collection of material evidence without delay.
- Request the doctor to collect the following:
  Blood — for grouping, DNA typing
  Blood for chemical analysis (if drugging is alleged)
  - Hair — scalp and pubic (to be cut and combed)
  - Loose hairs on the body- for DNA typing
  - Finger nail scrapings/clippings
  - Swabs from stained areas like breasts, thighs— prepare smears
  - Vaginal and cervical swabs and smears
  - Rectal swab (if anal penetration is alleged)
  - Oral swabs and smear (if oral coitus is alleged)
  -- Swabs from bite marks (if bite marks are present)
  - Clothes (worn at the time of assault) dried in shade and each item packed separately
- If bite marks are present on the body, same may be photographed with a scale.
  Obtain the help of a forensic odontologist for further necessary examination.
- If there is no definite proof of the age of the victim, she should be sent for determination of age.
- Obtain a detailed statement from the victim taking into account the following facts:
  i. Name, age, address, marital status
  ii. Emotional demeanour of the victim (crying/agitated/angry/frightened/shocked)
  iii. Description of victims appearance (torn and disheveled clothes/bruised face/nail marks
  iv. Date and time of alleged assault
  v. Accused/s known details, if unknown describe features which will help to identify him
  vi. Offering resistance—details
  vii. Coercion used–threats/weapons—details
  viii. Victims description of the alleged assault-vaginal/anal/oral penetration-? ejaculation
  ix. Injuries on the victim (her statement only— no examination!!)
  x. Injuries on the assailant caused by the victim
  xi. Any concensual coitus in the last 3–4 days
  xii. Victims menstrual history
- Request the doctor to test the victim periodically for venereal diseases.
- If the victim is emotionally upset, help her undergo psychiatric/psychologic counselling
- Give her moral support throughout the investigation and trial of the case.

### Accused

- After the preliminary procedures, the accused should be sent to the nearest government doctor for medical examination.

- Request the doctor to collect the following material evidence.
    - i. Clothes worn at the time of committing the offence.
    - ii. Blood for grouping and DNA typing.
    - iii. Scalp and pubic hair samples.
    - iv. Loose hairs found on the body especially pubic area.
    - v. Finger nail scrapings/clippings.
    - vi. Penile swabs/washings for the detection of vaginal epithelial cells.
    - vii. Tests for venereal diseases.
    - vii. Odontological examination, if bite marks are present on the victim.
- The accused may be sent to the nearest government doctor for examination and certification of potency as impotence may be one of the defences.

## Crime Scene

Examination of the scene of occurrence of sexual assault may yield trace evidences which may help in detecting the crime. Apart from taking photographs, preparing sketches, developing latent fingerprints and footprints, detailed search of the scene to collect trace evidences should be made. The following trace evidences may be present in the scene:

- Loose hair and fibres.
- Blood-stained and seminal-stained bed spreads, illows, briefs, etc.
- Weapons, ligatures, gags, etc.
- If the scene is in the open, collect soil/vegetation/debris for comparison.

# 21

# Pregnancy

Medical examination of a woman for signs of pregnancy is required in the following situations:

1. For exemption from appearing as a witness on the grounds of pregnancy.
2. Woman convicted for rigorous imprisonment or execution (pregnancy has to be excluded as per Section 416 of Criminal Procedure Code).
3. Women accused of criminal abortion, neonaticide or concealment of birth.
4. Woman claim pregnancy in maintenance cases, breach of promise of marriage, allegation of seduction or for blackmailing.

Pregnancy due to illicit sexual intimacy may be the reason for a woman to commit suicide. In such cases, signs of pregnancy have to be looked for while doing an autopsy. Before terminating the pregnancy of a woman under the Medical Termination of Pregnancy Act, pregnancy has to be confirmed beofre termination.

Pregnancy is the development of an embryo in the female when an ovum is fertilised by a spermatozoa (Fig. 21.1). Fertilisation takes place in the fallopian tube. The fertilised ovum moves to the uterine cavity, gets implanted in the endometrium and grows into a foetus. Fertile period in the life of a woman is from puberty to menopause. Signs of pregnancy in the living are presumptive signs, probable signs and conclusive signs.

## PRESUMPTIVE SIGNS

### Cessation of Menstruation (Amenorrhoea)

Menstruation ceases (amenorrhoea) with the implantation of a fertilised ovum in the uterus (Fig. 21.1). Amenorrhoea can occur in anemia, hormonal imbalance, psychological conditions, etc. On the contrary, slight menstrual bleeding can occur during the first 2 or 3 months of pregnancy. Pregnancy can develop during lactational amenorrhoea.

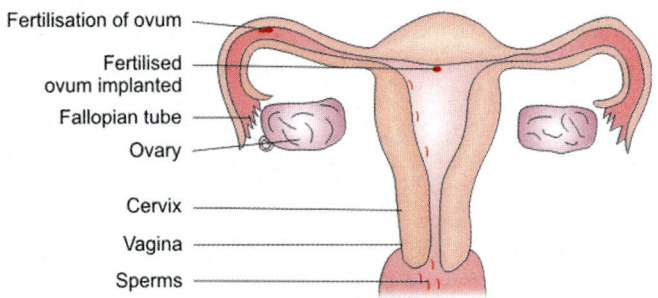

Fertilisation of ovum
Fertilised ovum implanted
Fallopian tube
Ovary
Cervix
Vagina
Sperms

**Fig. 21.1:** Uterus with appendages—implantation of the fertilised ovum

## Morning Sickness

Symptoms such as excessive salivation, nausea, vomiting, dizziness, perverted appetite, etc. appear during the first month of pregnancy. These symptoms usually disappear by 2–3 months. In some women, these symptoms will be absent; but in some other, these will be severe. The symptoms are due to increased levels of hormones (human chorionic gonadotropin—(hCG and oestrogen) and sympathetic disturbance.

## Changes in the Breasts

Breasts will become swollen and tender in the early weeks. Breasts will enlarge from the second month. During that period, areolae become pigmented and small round tubercles (**Montgomery's tubercles**) appear around the areolae due to the enlargement of sebaceous glands. Breasts will start secreting colostrum, a thin yellowish fluid consisting of fat globules and phagocytic cells by the third month of pregnancy. Colostrum will be present until a week after delivery and it is replaced by milk.

## Changes in the Vagina

By the end of second month, mucosa of the vagina changes its colour from pink to blue. The vaginal tissues will become soft and mucus secretion increases.

## Pigmentation of Skin

Vulva, abdomen and armpits become dark and a dark line extends from pubis to umbilicus (**linea nigra**). After 6 months, silver coloured lines called 'striae gravidarum' appear on the abdomen due to stretching of skin and rupture of its deeper layers.

## Quickening

The pregnant woman starts feeling the movement of the foetus from the beginning of 18th week. As pregnancy advances, the movements will increase in intensity.

## Urinary Disturbances

Pressure of the gravid uterus on the bladder will cause frequency of micturition in the early months of pregnancy, when the uterus remains in the pelvis. When the uterus enlarges and rises up in the abdominal cavity, the urinary symptoms will disappear. When the head of the foetus descends to the pelvis near full term, the urinary symptoms will reappear.

## PROBABLE SIGNS

### Enlargement of Abdomen

As the uterus enlarges in size, the abdomen gradually enlarges. Up to third month, uterus will be in the pelvic cavity. By fourth month, it will be above the symphysis pubis. At fifth month, it will be between the pubis and umbilicus. At sixth month, the fundus of uterus will be at the level of umbilicus and at seventh month, it will be 5 cm above umbilicus. At 8th month, it will be 5 cm below xiphisternum. At ninth month, it will be at the level of xiphisternum. At full term, uterus will sink downwards and reach to a level, 5 cm below xiphisternum (Fig. 21.2).

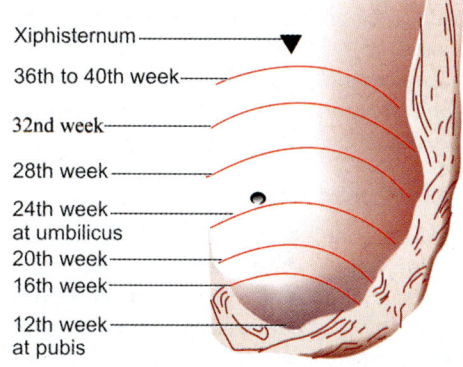

Xiphisternum

36th to 40th week

32nd week

28th week

24th week
at umbilicus

20th week

16th week

12th week
at pubis

**Fig. 21.2:** Level of fundus of uterus at various stages of pregnancy

## CONCLUSIVE SIGNS

Conclusive signs of pregnancy can be appreciated from fourth month of gestation. They are the following.

### Foetal Heart Sounds

By 18–20 weeks of gestation, foetal heart sounds can be heard on auscultation of the abdomen of the pregnant woman. The foetal heart rate is 120–160 per minute. It is not synchronous with the mother's heart beat.

The heart sounds can be now monitored and recorded accurately by an electronic foetal monitor.

### Foetal Parts and Foetal Movements

Palpation of foetal parts per abdomen is a positive sign of pregnancy from fourth month of gestation. Foetal movements can be appreciated from 18–20 weeks of gestation. Foetal skeleton can be visible by radiological examination from 20 weeks of pregnancy. But this is contraindicated as radiation may adversely affect the growth of the foetus.

### Prenatal Diagnostic Imaging Ultrasonography

Ultrasonography (Figs 21.3A and B) is a safe, non-invasive, accurate and costeffective method of diagnosing pregnancy and foetal abnormalities. Pregnancy can be diagnosed as early as 4–5 weeks. The embryo can be observed and measured by 5–6 weeks. Heart beat is detectable by Doppler ultrasound by about 6 weeks. The foetal age can be assessed by measuring the embryo's crown-rump length, biparietal diameter of the head, length of femur, etc. Foetal malformations, abnormal localization of the placenta, multiple pregnancies, hydramnios or oligamnios can be detected by ultrasonography.

### Immunological Tests

At present, with the help of hormonal assays, pregnancy can be diagnosed accurately before the development of physical signs and symptoms. Urine of the pregnant woman contains chorionic gonadotrophin, a hormone secreted by the chorionic villi of the embryo. The presence of this hormone can be identified by testing the urine. Chromatographic rapid pregnancy diagnostic test kits are available in the market. One drop of urine is placed in the well of the test device. Positive reaction appears as a band in the test window of the device. This test will be positive 4 weeks after the implantation of the ovum.

### PRECONCEPTION AND PRENATAL DIAGNOSTIC TECHNIQUES (Prohibition of Sex Selection Act 1994)

As per this Act, sex selection is prohibited before or after conception and prenatal diagnostic techniques

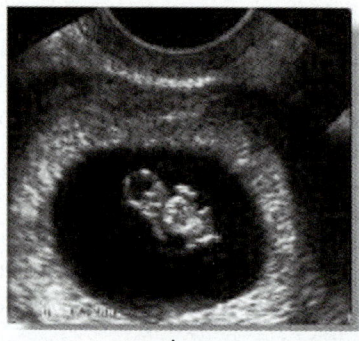

A

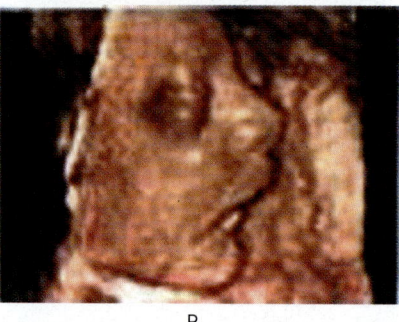

B

**Figs 21.3A and B:** Ultrasonographic diagnosis of pregnancy: A. Foetus 9 weeks, B. 3 D scan of face of foetus

for the purposes of detecting genetic abnormalities or metabolic disorders or chromosomal abnormalities or certain congenital malformations or sex-linked disorders are regulated. This is to prevent misuse of sex determination leading to female foeticide.

### Salient Aspects of the Act

- Genetic counselling centres, genetic laboratories and genetic clinics should be registered and only qualified geneticist, gynaecologist or paediatricians should be employed in these centres.
- No person shall conduct sex selection on a man or woman or on any tissue, embryo, conceptus or gametes.
- No person shall sell any ultrasound machine or imaging machines or any equipment capable of determining the sex of a foetus to any clinic or centre not registered under this Act.

- No place or clinic or centre shall conduct prenatal diagnostic techniques except for the purpose of detecting chromosomal abnormalities, genetic metabolic disorders, sex-linked genetic disorders, hemoglobinopathies or congenital anomalies.
- Prenatal diagnostic techniques shall be conducted only on pregnant women aged above 35 years, or on women who have undergone two or more spontaneous abortions or foetal loss or on pregnant woman exposed to teratogenic drugs, radiation or chemicals, or on women or her spouse has a family history of mental retardation or physical abnormalities.
- Person conducting ultrasonography on a woman shall keep complete records thereof in the clinic.
- No person including a relative or husband of a pregnant woman shall seek any prenatal diagnostic techniques or sex selection techniques except for the purposes mentioned supra.
- Written consent of the woman is required for conducting prenatal diagnostic procedures and sex of the foetus should not be communicated to the pregnant woman or her relatives or any other person by words or signs or in any other manner.

## Central Advisory Board

A Central Advisory Board under the chairmanship of the Union Minister for Health is constituted to advise the central government on policy matters relating to the use of prenatal diagnostic and sex selection techniques and against their misuse. The board reviews and monitors the implementation of the Act and rules and recommend to the government changes in the said Act and rules. Public awareness is created against the practice of preconception sex.

## State Advisory Board

A State Advisory Board under the chairmanship of the State Minister for Health is constituted in every state and union territory. The main function is to monitor the implementation of the provisions of the Act and rules. State board also creates public awareness against the practice of sex selection and prenatal diagnosis of sex of foetus leading to female foeticide. State board has to send consolidated reports to the Central Advisory Board.

## Appropriate Authority and Advisory Committee

Central government shall appoint appropriate authorities in the union territories and state government shall appoint appropriate authorities in each state. Advisory committee are also constituted to aid and advise the appropriate authority in the discharge of its functions. Appropriate authority consists of an officer above the rank of a joint director of health services as chairman, an eminent woman representing women's organisation and an officer of the law department of the government.

Advisory committee consist of three medical experts: gynaecologist-obstetrician/paediatrician/medical geneticist/one legal expert/one officer to represent the department of information and publicity and three eminent social workers.

Appropriate authority has powers to summon any person possessing any information regarding to the violation of the provisions of the Act or rules, or to order for the production of any document or material object relating to the case or to issue search warrant for any place suspected to be indulging in sex selection techniques or prenatal sex determination. Appropriate authority issues certificate of registration to the genetic laboratories, centres or clinics after holding proper enquiries. The authority can cancel the registration, if the centre contravenes the provisions of the Act or rules. Any person who contravenes the provisions of the Act shall be punishable with imprisonment for a term which may extend to 3 years and with fine which may extend to Rs 10,000/-. The court (metropolitan magistrate/judicial I class magistrate) will take cognizance of the offence on a complaint made by the appropriate authority.

Prenatal Diagnostic Techniques (Regulation and Prevention of Misuse) Rules, 1996 contains various proformas for use in a genetic laboratory/ clinic/centre.

## DIRECTIONS TO THE INVESTIGATING OFFICER

- When medical examination of a woman is required to find out whether she is pregnant or not, she should be sent to a medical expert, preferably a gynaecologist with a requisition and escort of a woman police constable.

- In early pregnancy, immunological tests may be necessary.

- If the woman is an accused and under arrest, no consent is needed for examination of her person and collection of body fluids like blood or urine (Sec 53 of CrPC).

- If the woman is not an accused, written, informed consent is necessary for physical examination and collection of body fluids.

# 22

# Delivery

## MEDICOLEGAL ASPECTS

Examination of woman for signs of delivery may be required in several medicolegal situations like neonaticide (murdering newborn baby), criminal abortion, concealment of birth, feigned delivery, legitimacy, maintenance case, divorce, nullity of marriage, etc.

Delivery is the process by which the foetus is expelled from the uterus. Normal duration of the pregnancy is 40 weeks (280 days) from the first day of the last menstrual period. Maximum duration of pregnancy has been a moot point in cases of legitimacy. Medically, pregnancy is unlikely to extend for more than 42–43 weeks. At present, to solve issues of legitimacy, DNA typing is resorted to. Normally, a woman will deliver near full term. She undergoes a process called labour, in which rhythmic contractions of the uterus expel the baby through the vagina.

The onset of labour is triggered by the hormone oxytocin. Symptoms of labour are backache, abdominal cramps, blood-stained discharge (show), leaking of amniotic fluid due to rupture of membranes and uterine contractions. Labour is divided into 3 stages; dilatation of cervix, delivery of the baby and then the expulsion of placenta.

In the first stage, uterine contractions grow progressively stronger. Each contraction will shorten the muscle fibres of the uterine wall, pulling the cervix wider (Fig. 22.1A). Cervix will dilate gradually. As the labour progresses, the cervix reaches the maximum dilatation of 10 cm in diameter. The second stage begins after full dilatation of the cervix. Uterine contractions grow stronger and the baby descends down through the birth canal (Fig. 22.1 B). In the third stage, uterus continues to contract, placenta is detached from the uterus and expelled (Fig. 22.1C). The duration of each stage is highly variable. Usually in primiparae, the first stage lasts for 8–12 hours; second stage 45 minutes to 2 hours and the third stage lasts for 5–15 minutes.

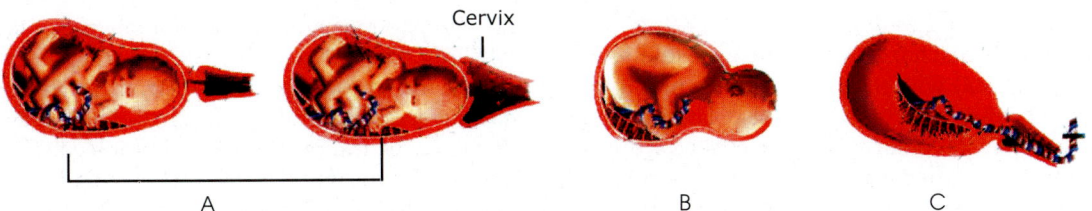

Cervix

A B C

**Figs 22.1A to C:** Stages of labour— A. I stage, B. II stage, C. III stage

## SIGNS OF DELIVERY

### General Findings

The woman will be pale and have a languid appearance. She may have slight rise of temperature with increased pulse rate. Intermittent contractions of uterus known as after pains will be present for 5 to 6 days after delivery.

### Breasts

Breasts will be enlarged and the nipples and areolae will be dark. Montgomery's tubercles will be seen. Colostrum may be present for about a week after delivery and is replaced by milk. Colostrum corpuscles will be seen in the milk for some more days.

### Abdomen

Abdomen will be lax, pendulous and will show striae gravidarum or linea albicantes. Fundus of uterus can be felt at the level of umbilicus just after delivery. It involutes at the rate of 2 cm a day and in 10 days it will reach the level of symphysis pubis.

### Vagina and Cervix

Perineum may show tears. The labia will be swollen. Vaginal walls will be congested and tears or excoriations may be seen. The cervix will be soft and dilated. The edges of the external os will be torn. The external os will remain patulous for 10–14 days. Internal os will close within 24 hours; but external os will close only by 2 weeks. Vagina will be dilated and mucosa will be congested. Blood-stained discharge may be seen. In dead bodies, uterus can be preserved for histological examination.

### Lochia

A reddish discharge with disagreeable smell (lochia rubra) will be present for the first 3 to 4 days. It will contain blood clots also. The discharge will change its colour and becomes serous during the next 4 days (lochia serosa). After the ninth day, the colour becomes turbid or yellowish white (lochia alba).

### Pregnancy Tests

Blood or urine can be tested for human chorionic gonadotropins. A positive test indicates that there was a recent delivery or abortion. HCG will disappear within 10 days after delivery.

### Microscopic Examination of the Lining Membrane (endometrium) of Uterine Cavity

A uterine curettage can be done and curettings can be sent for histology. On histological examination, a decidual reaction, presence of chorionic villi or trophoblastic cells, hypertrophied endometrium with or without signs of inflammation, etc. indicate the presence of products of conception.

## SIGNS OF RECENT DELIVERY IN THE DEAD

In the dead body, all genital and breast changes described in the living will be seen. Immediately after the delivery, the weight of the uterus will be about 1000 gm. Uterus will be enlarged and will contain placental remnants and blood clots. The placental site will be irregular and granular. After a full term delivery, the site will be 15 cm in diameter, covered with blood, lymph and portions of decidua. The area will become normal in 8 weeks after delivery. In abortion, sometimes foetal parts may also be seen. The uterus with appendages can be preserved for histology, and also for chemical analysis to exclude the application of abortifacients. If abortion was induced by mechanical means, uterus may show injuries or perforation. From the size of the perforation, the nature of the instrument used can be inferred sometimes.

## SIGNS OF PARITY IN A WOMAN

It is possible to find out whether a woman had delivered vaginally in the past or not. Pregnancy will cause permanent changes in the woman, if it had attained full term. But it is not possible to detect signs of a previous termination of a pregnancy of short-term. Abdomen will be lax and show linea nigra in the midline extending from pubis to umbilicus and striae gravidarum on the flanks. The breasts may be lax, pendulous and wrinkled. The nipples will be large with dark areolae and Montgomery's tubercles. The labia majora may not completely cover the vaginal opening. Labia minora will be visible externally. Hymen will show hymenalis carenculae. Vagina will be lax. Rugosity of the vagina will be absent. The perineum will show scars of healed lacerations. Previous caesarean section will show evidence of healed incisions on the abdomen and uterus.

Apart from the changes mentioned above, examination of the uterus in a dead woman will provide clues to the status of parity. Uterus of a parous woman will be larger with thicker walls when compared to that of a nulliparous woman. In old women, it is not possible to differentiate, because the uterus will be atrophic. Cavity of a nulliparous uterus will be triangular while a parous uterus will have a rounded cavity. The fundus of uterus will be convex in a parous woman and it will be above the level of broad ligaments. The nulliparous uterus will be at the level of broad ligament. In a parous woman, the body of the uterus will have twice the length of the cervix. They are of the same length in the nulliparous. In the nulliparous woman, there will be several mucosal folds in the cervical canal (**arbor vitae**). These will be lost during delivery. The external os will show a transverse opening with irregular edges in a parous woman; while in a nulliparous woman, it will be circular with rounded edges.

Histology of the placental site will show presence of blood pigments up to 6 months after delivery. Endarteritis obliterans of the blood vessels can be noted. This change can be seen for many years after the delivery.

## Duties of Doctors in Criminal Abortion

When criminal abortion is suspected, another doctor should be consulted. If the person is about to die, recording of a dying declaration should be arranged. If death occurs, the matter should be reported to the police.

## DIRECTIONS TO THE INVESTIGATING OFFICER

Investigating officers should direct the mother who is alleged to have delivered/terminated the pregnancy in cases like neonaticide, criminal abortion delivery, etc. for examination and certification to a medical expert in nearest government hospital. It will be better, if the woman is examined by a forensic specialist or a doctor specialised in obstetrics and gynaecology.

The requisition to the doctor should contain the following queries:

- Whether the woman was pregnant?
- If so, what was the duration of pregnancy?
- Was the pregnancy terminated before confinement?
- If so, what was the method used?
- When was it carried out ?

# 23

# Abortion

Abortion is the expulsion of the products of conception at any period of pregnancy before full term. Abortion could be natural or induced. Natural abortion could be spontaneous or accidental. Induced abortion could be criminal or therapeutic. Criminal abortion is punishable and punishment varies according to the term of pregnancy. Abortion induced in a woman who is "quick with child" invites enhanced punishment. Quickening is the feeling of the movement of the child in utero and occurs at about 4 to 6 months of pregnancy. Up to that period, the product of conception is called an **embryo** and thereafter it is called a **foetus**.

Indian Penal Code (1860) contains penal provisions regarding termination of pregnancy. Abortion is a crime for which the pregnant woman and the abortionist are punished except when it was induced to save the life of the mother. In spite of stringent laws, women seek the help of quacks and unqualified persons for terminating unwanted pregnancy. Most often death or serious complications are the result of these abortions induced secretly by using crude and unhygienic methods.

*Section 312 of Indian Penal Code:* Whoever voluntarily causes a woman with child to miscarry shall, if such miscarriage be not caused in good faith for the purpose of saving the life of the woman, be punished with imprisonment of either description for a term which may extend to 3 years, with fine, or with both, and if the woman be quick with child shall be punished with imprisonment of either description for a term which may extend to 7 years and shall also be liable to fine.

*Section 313 of Indian Penal Code:* Whoever commits the offences defined in the last preceding section without the consent of the woman, whether the woman is quick with child or not, shall be punished with imprisonment for life or with imprisonment of either description for a term which may extend to 10 years and shall also be liable for fine.

*Section 314 IPC:* If death of the woman is the result of such miscarriage, punishment will be for a term of 10 years, if the act is done with consent and life imprisonment for an act done without consent.

## TYPES OF ABORTION

### Natural Abortion

Clinically expulsion of the foetus before term due to natural causes is called natural abortion. Diseases of the mother, diseases of the uterus, faulty development of the embryo, diseases of the decidua or placenta, etc. can cause spontaneous abortion. Strenuous exercise, travel, fall, blunt impacts on the abdomen, etc. can cause abortion. Bleeding can occur between the uterus and membranes. Detachment of the membranes will cause contraction of the uterus and the foetus will be expelled.

## Therapeutic Abortion

It is the intentional termination of pregnancy done in good faith to save the life of the mother, if her life is endangered by the continuance of pregnancy. Pregnancy can also be terminated, if the prenatal testing shows that the foetus has severe congenital abnormalities (Medical Termination of Pregnancy Act provides for other reasons). Therapeutic abortions can be safely performed within the first 6–10 weeks. There are several methods for therapeutic abortion. Menstrual extraction is done between 5 and 7 weeks. Contents of uterus are suctioned out through a thin tube, 3–4 mm diameter, inserted through the undilated cervix. Suction is applied by a small pump or a syringe. As the foetus is small, the abortion may become an incomplete one. Medical abortion is brought about by taking medicines. The procedure is simple and non-invasive. The procedure resembles a natural abortion. But the method is not very effective after 7 weeks. Bleeding after expulsion of the products will be more.

Abortions after 3 months of pregnancy are performed by dilatation of the mouth of the uterus (cervix) and scraping (curettage) of the uterus. An alternative is to induce labour by dilatation of cervix and injection of saline into the uterine cavity. Contractions begin by 8–24 hours and the foetus is expelled. After 14 weeks of pregnancy, foetus is removed by opening the uterus (histerotomy).

## Criminal Abortion

Incidence of criminal abortion has considerably reduced with the liberalisation of abortion under the Medical Termination of Pregnancy Act of 1973. Criminal abortion is resorted to by unmarried women, widows, etc. Most of the abortions are conducted during the second or third month of pregnancy. Abortion is induced by the administration of drugs or by mechanical means. Drugs are usually tried during the first and second months of pregnancy. Mechanical interference is done during the third and fourth months of pregnancy. Mechanical methods are used by abortionists who are mostly quacks. Very often the woman develops serious or fatal complications due to the toxic effects of the drug or injuries sustained to genitalia and uterus.

## Abortifacients

Vegetable irritants, drugs and toxins which are used to induce abortion are called abortifacients. But most of them are ineffective; but in higher doses they will produce toxic effects. Vegetable compounds like juniper, savin, pennyroyal, aloes, colocynth, croton oil, calotropis, plumbago rosea, castor oil, etc. are popular. In south India, unripe fruits of papaya and pineapple are sometimes used. These can produce purgation, congestion and haemorrhage in the uterine mucosa leading to uterine contractions.

Some substances like ergot, quinine and pituitary extracts (ecbolics) have a contractile effect on the uterus. But these drugs do not act well on the uterus in early pregnancy. Chemicals like potassium permanganate are applied to the cervix or vaginal vault. This can produce severe local reaction and haemorrhage. Calotropis juice is also used locally to induce abortion.

## Mechanical Methods

Direct violence like hitting or kicking on the abdomen is applied to induce abortion. Syringing is a common method used to induce abortion. Soap water or saline is injected into the uterus using an enema can or a large syringe. The fluid under pressure will detach the membranes and placenta leading to haemorrhage and contraction of uterus. When fluid is injected under pressure, air will enter the uterine sinuses and can cause air embolism. The irritant substances added to the fluid will be absorbed and can produce toxic effects.

Instrumentation is widely practiced. Foreign bodies like laminaria tent (dried sea weed), elm bark, etc. are placed in the cervix. These will absorb moisture and swell causing dilatation of cervix. Subsequently, uterus will contract and expel the products. Abortion sticks are introduced into the uterus through the cervix to rupture the membranes. Metal rods, wooden sticks, surgical probes, bougies, etc. are used as abortion sticks. When the amniotic fluid escapes, uterus will contract and expel the foetus. Instrumentation can cause perforation of the uterus and intestines. Bleeding, infection and inflammation of the lining membrane of the abdomen (peritonitis) are the usual complications.

## DEATH DUE TO ABORTION

Sudden death due to neurogenic shock can occur in criminal abortion. Sudden dilatation of cervix, perforation of uterus, syringing, etc. can cause sudden stoppage of heart (reflex vagal inhibition). Perforation of vagina, uterus and incomplete separation of the membranes are the usual causes of bleeding and secondary shock. In death due to bleeding, all internal organs including uterus will be pale. Death can occur as a result of syringing to induce abortion. Syringing will detach the fetal membranes and air will enter the uterine venous sinuses. Air will reach the right side of the heart through the pelvic veins and inferior vena cava. Death will occur within minutes.

Along with air, amniotic fluid may also enter the maternal circulation. The amniotic fluid contains foetal epithelial cells, lanugo hair, lipoid from vernix, meconium and cells from chorion/amnion. These elements will occlude the pulmonary capillaries. These are rarely seen in systemic circulation. Amniotic fluid will produce severe anaphylactoid reaction and sudden death. Amniotic fluid embolism can also cause disseminated intravascular coagulation (DIC) leading to generalized bleeding, thrombus formation, infarction and end organ damage.

Infection is almost certain in all types of criminal abortion. Unsterile instruments will introduce infection into the uterine cavity. Placental remnants act as a substrate for infection. Infection can spread to the peritoneal cavity through the fallopian tubes. Infection can lead to septicaemia and death.

Death due to suspected criminal abortion leads to medicolegal investigation. History, circumstances of death, findings of uterus, histological findings and report of toxicological analysis will help the medicolegal expert to come to definite conclusions. Spontaneous abortion should be differentiated from criminal abortion. Autopsy and histological examination of the expelled products of conception will be helpful to differentiate spontaneous abortion from criminal abortion. During autopsy, the signs of pregnancy can be identified by noting the changes in the breasts and abdomen. Skin may show bronze discolouration in clostridial septicemia. Injuries present in the vulva, vagina, cervix and uterus are indicative of instrumentation. Absence of mucus plug in the external os, patent cervical opening with bleeding are signs of recent abortion. The following investigations are to be conducted:

1. Collection of vaginal fluid for chemical analysis.
2. Swabs taken from vagina and uterus for microbiological examination.
3. X-rays or CT scans must be taken if air embolism is suspected
4. Examination of abdomen for evidence of peritonitis.
5. Examination of intestines for the presence of injuries if uterus is found perforated.
6. Examination of uterus with appendages.
7. Measurements and weight of the uterus.
8. State of dilatation of the cervical canal
9. Ascertain the age and development of the foetus if present.
10. Bits of tissues to be taken from appropriate sites for microscopy.
11. Chemical analysis of uterus and ovaries to detect abortifacients.

## ASSAULT AND ABORTION

Women who are victims of assault may allege that they aborted after the assault. It could be a real allegation or a fabricated one. It is very difficult to establish a cause and effect relation with trauma and abortion. The woman must be subjected to a thorough general and genital examination for evidence of recent abortion. An ultrasound scan should be taken to study the uterus and appendages. Blood or urine should be tested for hCG. Aborted material if any available should be subjected to visual and histological examination.

## DIRECTIONS TO THE INVESTIGATING OFFICER

When a woman who is accused of criminal abortion, she has to be subjected for a physical examination by a medical expert. If death has occurred due to alleged criminal abortion, it has to be ascertained whether it was spontaneous or due to any criminal interference. The following facts have to be ascertained:

- Was the woman pregnant?
- What was the term of pregnancy?
- Is there evidence of abortion?
- Was it spontaneous or induced?
- If it was induced,what was the method used?
- Who induced it? Self or assisted?
- What were the complications?
- What was the cause of death?
- What is the result of chemical analysis?
- What are the microscopical findings?

If the medical expert/forensic surgeon is of opinion that the abortion was induced by illegal means, further investigation can be started. The investigation should be directed to find out whether the abortion is criminal or not. Any abortion which does not come under the purview of Medical Termination of Pregnancy Act of 1973 is to be considered as criminal.

If the abortion is induced by drugs or by mechanical intereference, the IO should find out the source of abortifacients and recover the implements used for the same. Examination of the scene of occurrence may be helpful in collecting incriminating evidence.

When the aborted material or foetus is recovered the same has to be sent for examination by a medical expert. The details are given in chapter "infanticide". The nature of offence and section of law are decided after ascertaining the age of the foetus by the medical expert.

# 24

# Medical Termination of Pregnancy

## MEDICAL TERMINATION OF PREGNANCY (MTP) ACT

The Act was passed by the Parliament in the year 1971 to liberalise and legalise abortion. As per this law, pregnancy can be terminated as a health measure or on humanitarian or eugenic grounds. Some of the provisions of this Act were amended in 2002. MTP rules were laid down in 1975 and 2003 and regulations were laid down in 2003.

According to the provisions of this Act, pregnancy can be terminated on the following grounds:

1. Continuation of the pregnancy would involve a risk to the life of the pregnant woman or of grave injury to her physical or mental health.
2. There is a substantial risk that if the child were born, it would suffer from such physical or mental abnormalities as to be seriously handicapped.
3. The pregnancy is alleged by the pregnant woman to have been caused by rape; the anguish caused by such unwanted pregnancy may be presumed to constitute a grave injury to the mental health of the pregnant woman.
4. Pregnancy occurs as a result of failure of any device or method used by any married woman or her husband for the purpose of limiting the number of children; the anguish caused by such pregnancy may be presumed to constitute a grave injury to the mental health of the pregnant woman.

In determining whether the continuation of a pregnancy would involve such risk of injury to the health, account may be taken to the pregnant woman's actual or reasonable foreseeable environment. Pregnancy can be terminated only with the written informed consent of the woman in Form C (Proforma 24.1). If the woman is under 18 years of age or is mentally ill, consent of the guardian is necessary.

The Act does not specify the conditions which can endanger the life of the pregnant woman. It is left to the decision of the doctor. With regard to ground no.3, the statement of the woman alone is enough. It is not necessary that a case of rape has been registered by the police. The ground no.4 is applicable only in the case of a married woman.

## Who can Terminate Pregnancy?

Pregnancy can be terminated by a registered medical practitioner;

1. Who has registered in a State Medical Council before 1971 and who possesses experience in the practice of obstetrics and gynaecology for a period not less than 3 years; or
2. Who is registered in a State Medical Council and if he has completed 6 months housemanship in obstetrics and gynaecology or who has experience in any hospital in the practice of obstetrics and gynaecology for a period of not less than one year; or
3. Who has assisted another doctor in the performance of 25 cases of medical termination

**Proforma 24.1:** Form C (MTP Rule 9) Consent Letter of the Pregnant Woman

I.................................................daughter/wife of............................................................ aged about...................years at present residing at ........................................... (permanent address) do hereby give my consent to termination of my pregnancy at.......................................................
(State the name of place where the pregnancy is to be terminated).

Place.........................                                     Signature.............................................
Date.........................

**(To be filled in by guardian where the woman is a mentally ill person or a minor)**

I ...............................son/daughter/wife of ........................aged about...........years at present residing at (permanent address)...................................................do hereby give my consent to the termination of the pregnancy of my ward...............................who is a minor/mentally ill person at ............................................. .......
(place of termination of my pregnancy)

Place......................                                     Signature.......................................

---

of pregnancy of which at least five have been performed independently in a hospital or training institute approved by the government. But this training would enable the RMP to do only terminations up to 12 weeks of pregnancy.
4. Who possesses postgraduate degree or diploma in obstetrics and gynaecology. Termination of pregnancy up to 20 weeks duration can be conducted only by the doctor who possesses the qualifications specified in 1, 2 and 4.

## Place Where Pregnancy can be Terminated

1. A hospital established or maintained by the government.
2. A place approved for the purpose of the Act by the government or a committee constituted by the government, or a district level committee constituted by the government with the district medical officer as chairperson.
3. The place should have all facilities for conducting termination of pregnancies safely under hygienic conditions. A gynaecology examination table, sterilization and resuscitation equipment, drugs including IV fluids, facilities for treatment of shock, transportation facilities are needed for termination up to 12 weeks of pregnancy.

4. For termination of pregnancies up to 20 weeks, an operation theatre with facilities for performing gynaecological surgery, anaesthetic and sterilisation equipment, drugs including IV fluids, etc. are necessary.
5. Termination of pregnancy conducted in a place other than an approved one is also punishable. Owner of that place will also be prosecuted.

*Duration of pregnancy:* As per the provision of the Act, pregnancy up to 20 weeks can be terminated. But if the pregnancy is between 12 and 20 weeks, another doctor should be consulted. Both doctors shall issue a certificate in Form I (Proforma 24.2).

In the case of termination of pregnancy up to 7 weeks using **RU486 (mifipristone)** with **misoprostol**, the same may be prescribed by a registered medical practitioner with postgraduate degree or diploma in obstetrics and gynaecology at his clinic provided that such practitioner has access to a place approved by the government for conducting termination of pregnancy under the Act. The practitioner should obtain a certificate to this effect from the owner of that approved place.

*Immediate termination of pregnancy (Section 5 of MTP Act):* If a registered medical practitioner forms an opinion in good faith that the termination of a pregnancy is immediately necessary to save the life of the pregnant woman, conditions like duration of the pregnancy and necessity of opinion of two doctors shall not apply to the termination of that pregnancy. In this context, the hospital where the termination was conducted need not be an institution approved by the government for the purpose of medical termination of pregnancy under MTP Act. Medical practitioners who terminate pregnancy shall also certify the termination in the same form within 3 hours of the procedure. However, termination of pregnancy conducted by a person who is not an RMP amounts to a criminal offence.

*Hospital registers:* The name of the pregnant woman admitted for MTP shall not be entered in any case sheet, operation theater register or any records other than the MTP admission register **(Form III—Proforma 24.4)**. In all other documents,

the number assigned to each patient in the MTP register shall be used as a reference number.

*Custody of forms:* The consent given by the pregnant woman for MTP, certified opinion of the doctors and the intimation of MTP shall be placed in an envelope and sealed. On every envelope, the serial number allotted to the pregnant woman in the MTP admission register shall be written and marked secret. The doctor who performed the termination of pregnancy shall send the envelope to the head/owner of the hospital. The name of doctor and the date of termination are also to be written on the envelope. The head/owner of the hospital shall keep all the envelopes under safe custody. He shall send a monthly statement in **Form II** (Proforma 24.3) to the director of health services. When pregnancy is terminated in an unapproved place or hospital,

---

**Proforma 24.2:** Form I (Regulation 3) Certificate of Termination of Pregnancy

I...................................................................................................................
(Name and qualifications of the registered medical practitioner in block letters)
...................................................................................................................
(Full address of the registered medical practitioner)
I...................................................................................................................
(Name and qualifications of the registered medical practitioner in block letters)
...................................................................................................................
(full address of the registered medical practitioner) hereby certify that *I/We/am /are/of opinion, formed in good faith, that it is necessary to terminate the pregnancy of
.......................................................................................... (full name of pregnant woman in block letters) resident of...................................................................................................................
(Full address of pregnant woman in block letters) for the reasons given below**.
          *I /We hereby give intimation that *I/We terminated the pregnancy of the woman referred to above who bears the serial no. ..................................... in the admission register of the hospital/approved place.

Place..................Signature of the Registered Medical Practitioner........................Regn. No........
Date..................Signature of the Registered Medical Practitioner........................Regn. No........

Strike out whichever is not applicable,

** Of the reasons specified in items (i) to (v) write the one which is appropriate:
  i.  In order to save the life of the pregnant woman,
  ii. In order to prevent grave injury to the physical and mental health of the pregnant woman,
  iii. In view of the substantial risk that if the child was born it would suffer from such physical or mental abnormalities as to be seriously handicapped,
  iv. As the pregnancy is alleged by pregnant woman to have been caused by rape,
  v.  As the pregnancy has occurred as result of failure of any contraceptive device or methods used by the married woman or her husband for the purpose of limiting the number of children

**Note:** Account may be taken of the pregnant woman's actual or reasonably foreseeable environment in determining whether the continuance of her pregnancy would involve a grave injury to her physical or mental health.

**Proforma 24.3:** Form II ((As per Regulation 4 (5) Monthly Statement)

1. Name of the state
2. Name of the hospital/approved place
3. Duration of pregnancy (Total No )................ a) Up to 12 weeks.................. b) Between 12–20 weeks.......................
4. Religion of woman—Hindu/Muslim/Christian/others............... total No----.........
5. Termination with acceptance of contraception: a. Sterilisation - total No........... b. IUCD..........total no...............
6. Reasons for termination (give total number under each subhead)
   a. Danger to life of pregnant woman
   b. Grave injury to the physical health of the pregnant woman
   c. Grave injury to the mental health of the pregnant woman
   d. Pregnancy caused by rape
   e. Substantial risk that if the child was born, it would suffer from such physical or mental abnormalities as to be seriously handicapped
   f. Failure of any contraceptive device or method

Signature of the Officer in charge with date:

**Proforma 24.4:** Form III (Regulation 5) Admission Register

(To be destroyed on the expiry of five years from the date of the last entry in the register)
1. S. no.
2. Date of admission
3. Name of the patient
4. Wife/daughter of
5. Age
6. Religion
7. Address
8. Duration of pregnancy
9. Reasons on which pregnancy is terminated
10. Date of termination of pregnancy
11. Date of discharge of patient
12. Result and remarks
13. Name of registered medical practitioner (s) by whom the opinion is formed
14. Name of registered medical practitioner (s) by whom pregnancy is terminated

the owner of that place shall send all the relevant documents in a sealed envelope to the DHS by registered post on the same day or not later than the next working day.

## MAINTENANCE OF RECORDS

### Admission Register (Form III—Proforma 24.4)

The owner or the head of the hospital shall maintain an admission register for recording the details of admission of women for termination of their pregnancy. The register should be kept for a period of 5 years from the end of calendar year it relates to. The entries in the registers shall be made serially and a fresh number shall be started at the commencement of each calendar year, e.g. '5/05', '26/06', etc. Admission register is a secret document and the information regarding the particulars of the pregnant women should not be disclosed to any person. The register shall be kept under safe custody. It shall not be open for inspection by any person except under the authority of law. A certificate can be issued to an employed woman who had undergone termination of pregnancy; if she applies for the same for official purpose

### Approval of Hospitals

Applications in **Form A** (Proforma 24.5) has to be submitted to the DMO of the district for getting approval of an institution. DMO after necessary enquiries and verification of the facilities, will recommend to the district level committee for approval of the institution. The committee will consider the application and issue a certificate of approval in Form B (Proforma 24.6). The certificate has to be exhibited in a conspicuous place in the institution. DMO has the authority to inspect the place periodically and recommend to the committee to cancel or suspend the approval if the facilities are not properly maintained. Appeal against the order of cancellation of approval has to be preferred within 60 days to the government.

## DIRECTIONS TO THE INVESTIGATING OFFICER

As per the provisions of the MTP Act, abortion has been liberalised. A qualified registered doctor shall not be guilty if any pregnancy is terminated by him in accordance with the provisions of the MTP Act 1971 (amended in 2004). However, any abortion induced in defiance to any one of the provisions of the MTP Act will amount to criminal abortion. The doctor and the person in charge of the hospital are liable. When a case of abortion is investigated the investigating officer should be able to find out whether the pregnancy terminated was lawful.

The IO should find out whether the:
- Doctor has the requisite qualifications?
- Hospital is a recognised centre?
- Centre is equipped with facilities for conducting MTP?
- Termination of pregnancy was indicated as per the Act?

---

**Proforma 24.5:** Form A (Sub-Rule 2 of Rule 4) Application Form for the Approval of a Place

1. Name
2. Address in full
3. Non-government/private/nursing home/other institution
4. State if the following facilities are available at the place
   i. An operation table and instruments for performing abdominal or gynaecological surgery
   ii. Drugs and parenteral fluid in sufficient supply for emergency cases.
   iii. Anaesthetic equipment, resuscitation equipment and sterilisation equipment

Place........................

Date........................                    Signature of the owner of the place...........................................

---

**Proforma 24.6:** Form B (Sub-Rule 6 of Rule 4) Certificate of Approval

The place described below is hereby approved for the purpose of Medical Termination of Pregnancy Act 1971(34 of 1971)

Name of the place

Address and other descriptions

Name of the owner

Place............................                    For the Govt of ..............................

- Duration of pregnancy was below 20 weeks?
- Doctors have issued proper certificates?
- Consent of the pregnant woman has been obtained?
- Registers are maintained properly?

Above 20 weeks of pregnancy can be terminated only on therapeutic consideration for the mother, when continuation of pregnancy will involve a risk to the life of the mother. In such cases, decision can be taken by a single doctor and termination can be performed even in an unrecognised centre.

Consent of the woman will be invalid, if she is a minor or mentally challenged. In such cases, consent of the lawful guardian should be obtained. Consent of the husband is not needed in the case of a married woman.

If death or damage occurs to the woman during the termination of pregnancy due to inadvertent action of the doctor or other paramedical personnel, a separate case can be registered and investigated as per the Sections of law concerned.

# 25

# Neonaticide and Infanticide

Neonate is a child within 24 hours of life. Killing a newborn child is called neonaticide. Beyond that period, till one year of age, it is termed infanticide. Most of the neonaticides and infanticides are committed by the mother, who may be an unmarried woman, widow, or divorcee. Female newborns are also killed sometimes.

## LEGAL ASPECTS

*Section 315 IPC:* Act done with intent to prevent a child from being born alive or to cause it to die after birth is also punishable under ths Section.

*Section 316 IPC:* Causing the death of quick unborn child by an act amounting to culpable homicide is punishable as per this Section.

*Section 317 IPC:* Exposure and abandoning infants are punishable under this Section.

*Section 318 IPC:* Concealment of birth by secret disposal is punishable as per this Section.

In all the instances, the foetus and the mother are to be examined. Mother is examined for noting the recent signs of delivery or abortion. If death of the woman has occurred, it has to be ascertained whether the death was due to the act of miscarriage or not.

## GENERAL DIRECTIONS FOR INVESTIGATION OF NEONATICIDE AND INFANTICIDE

Examination of the foetus is required in neonaticide, criminal miscarriage, concealment of birth, etc. Neonaticide and infanticide are considered as murder. Causing the death of a child in the mother's uterus is criminal miscarriage. To constitute the offence of neonaticide, the foetus should be viable and the child should be born partly or completely and shown signs of live birth. A foetus is said to be viable when it can lead an independent existence when born out of the mother's womb. Viability will be attained after the completion of 7 months of intrauterine age.

Infanticide can be considered as a secret homicide!. Usually, the newborn child is murdered and the body is buried or discarded. Sometimes, the foetus is abandoned and death may be due to causes other than homicide. In all these cases, it is necessary to find out the accused and connect her with the crime. A detailed inquest and investigation are to be conducted. The following facts have to be ascertained:

- Intrauterine age of the foetus
- Signs of live birth
- Signs of survival
- Cause of death
- Time of death.

### Examination of the Foetus (Columns 7 and 8 of Inquest Report)

#### Postmortem Changes

Cooling, rigor mortis, postmortem lividity, signs of putrefaction, etc. are to be noted. These changes will help to estimate the time since death.

#### Signs of Maceration

A dead born child is one which had died inside the uterus. Because of the absence of microorganisms in the amniotic fluid, instead of decomposition, the dead foetus will undergo a series of changes known as maceration. Body becomes soft, flaccid and will emit a disagreeable odour. Body flattens out when placed on a flat surface (Fig. 25. 1). Skin will be purple in colour and will peel off easily. Skull sutures separate and the skull bones slide over one another (Spaulding's sign). Sometimes the body will be mummified or calcified. If signs of maceration or mummification are present, live birth can be ruled out.

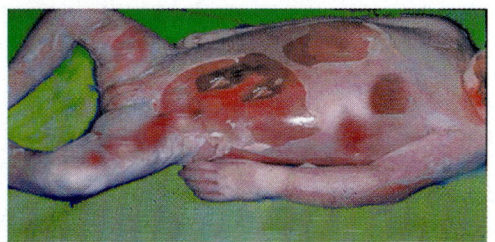

**Fig. 25.1:** Intrauterine death of the foetus—signs of maceration

### Umbilical Cord and Placenta

If umbilical cord is present, it should be examined carefully. Note whether it is tied or torn. Blood in the cut end clots within 24 hours. The cord shrinks and dries up in a day. The cord will be mummified in 2–3 days. It will fall off in 5–6 days leaving a raw ulcer which will heal and a scar is formed in 10–12 days. Sometimes the cord may be attached to the placenta. The placenta should be examined for the presence of diseases, infarcts, etc.

### Length

Using a flexible tape (better by a thread), length of the foetus is taken from the crown to heel. From the length, the age can be calculated **(Haase rule)**. Up to 25 cm, take the square root (square root of 25 = 5 months). The intrauterine age of a 25 cm long foetus is 5 months. Beyond 25 cm, the length in cm is divided by five (30 cm ./. 5 = IU age is 6 months).

### Scalp Hair

Hair appears on the scalp at 4th month and will be more than 0.5 cm in length at 7th month. At full term, it will be 2 to 2.5 cm long.

### Eyebrows and Eyelashes

These appear at the age of 6th month and will become distinct at 7th month.

### Finger and Toe Nails

These appear at 4th month and will be just below the tip of finger at 7th month. At full term, the nails will project beyond the fingertips.

By observing these, the minimum age of the foetus can be ascertained. The doctor who performs the autopsy will be able to estimate the age more accurately by examining the growth of bones (ossification centres in the bones). The doctor will also be looking for signs of live birth by examining the lungs, stomach and other internal organs. Live birth can be confirmed by performing a **hydrostatic test** and microscopy of lungs.

### External Signs of Live Birth

Changes in the umbilical cord are helpful in determining live birth and also the time of survival. Apart from it, there are other signs to indicate live birth. The superficial layers of skin will show desquamation from the 2nd day onwards. There will be physiological jaundice as evidenced by yellow colouration of the sclera from the 2nd day. The shape of the chest will be arched. When the thorax is opened, the level of the dome of diaphragm will be at the level of 6th or 7th ribs. The size of the lungs will increase. Weight of an unrespired lung is 30 gm; while after respiration it will weigh 60 gm **(Ploucquet's test)**. This is due to the establishment of pulmonary circulation. The respired lungs will be crepitant and the margins will be rounded. The margins of an unrespired lung will be sharply defined.

### Hydrostatic Test

This test is performed during the autopsy of the foetus. The principle of this test is that an aerated lung will float in water. The lungs, heart and thymus are removed en masse. The organ en masse is placed in a trough filled with water. If the lungs are respired fully, it will float. Then lungs are separated and put in water independently. If one lung is not aerated, it will sink. Then the lungs are cut into small pieces and put in water to find out whether there is any partial respiration. The floatation is either due to trapped respired air in the alveoli or due to the presence of putrefactive gases. To exclude putrefaction, the floating pieces are taken out, squeezed between wooden planks to expel gases of putrefaction from the interstitial spaces and then put in water again. If the lung bit which was floating previously, sinks after squeezing, the floatation was due to putrefaction. A respired lung will sink due to diseases. Hence the confirmatory test to prove live birth is a microscopical examination of lungs.

Similarly, the stomach is ligated at cardiac and duodenal ends, severed and put in water **(Breslau's second life test).** Floatation is indicative of live birth. But this test can be fallacious and is not much significant.

### Presence of Milk/Food

Presence of food/milk in the digestive tract is a good evidence of live birth. Milk in the stomach can be identified by taking a drop and staining it with fat stains like sudan III and examining for fat globules under the microscope.

### Survival

Changes in the cardiovascular system of the infant after birth will help to determine the time of survival. The umbilical arteries are obliterated on the 3rd day. The umbilical vein and ductus venosus are obliterated in 4–5 days. The ductus arteriosus closes in 10–12 days and foramen ovale by 1 to 3 months.

If the head is the presenting part, there will be bleeding under the scalp. This is a good evidence to rule out sudden delivery (precipitate delivery). Meconium is completely excreted from large intestine in 24–28 hours after birth except in breech presentations. Blood can be examined for nucleated red cells and foetal hemoglobin. Nucleated red cells disappear in 24 hours. The percentage of foetal hemoglobin is 80% and will be reduced after birth. Kidneys will show orange coloured deposits of uric acid in the pyramids of the medulla from the second day of life.

### Cause of Death

If the foetus is neither live born nor dead born, it could be still born. There are many factors which may cause a stillbirth. Natural causes include congenital abnormalities of heart and other organs, prolonged labour, intrauterine asphyxia, prematurity and birth trauma. Assisted delivery can result in head injury. Sometimes, the child will be delivered precipitously. This usually occurs in multiparous women. If the delivery is in the standing posture, the foetus will fall on the floor and sustain injuries to the head. If delivery occurs when the woman is straining while sitting in a water closet, the child can fall into water and drown. In a case of neonaticide by inflicting injury on the head of the child, the accused mother may put forward a defence of **precipitate delivery**. If the delivery was a normal one with the usual first and second stages of labour, the presenting part will be compressed. There will be extravasation and diffusion of blood in the subcutaneous tissues. The condition is called **caput succedaneum** (Fig. 25.2). Its presence proves that the labour was a slow process and not precipitous. It also shows that the foetus was alive during delivery. **Cephalhematoma** is the extravasation of blood in the head due to instrumental delivery. Its presence indicates that the child was alive at the time of delivery.

Aim of the medicolegal foetal autopsy is to find out whether the death was due to a criminal act of commission or omission. Common methods of commission include drowning, throttling, strangulation, suffocation, injuries, poisoning, etc. Acts of omission are exposure, not tying the cut umbilical cord, etc. Smothering or strangulation are the common methods of neonaticide. Injuries

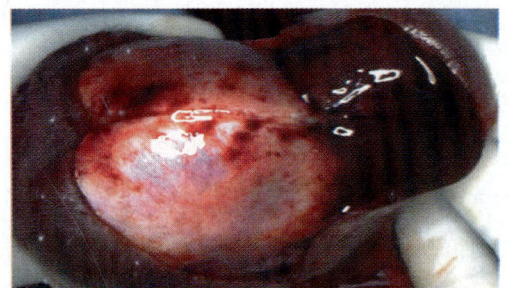

**Fig. 25.2:** Caput succedaneum. Effusion of blood beneath the scalp and galea aponeurotica

like nail marks and contusions will be seen around the mouth and inside the oral cavity. Ligature strangulation will show evidence of a ligature mark and signs of violence in the region of neck. Sometimes umbilical cord is used to strangle the child. A nuchal cord found at the time of delivery should not be mistaken for a sign of violence. If the cord is used for strangulation, the Wharton's jelly may be displaced.

The law presumes that a woman who is about to deliver should take all precautions to save her child. Failure to do so amounts to criminal negligence. Mother has to make necessary preparations for delivery, remove the child from the discharges, tie and separate the umbilical cord, protect the child from cold and heat and give proper food. Exposure and abandonment of a child under 12 years is punishable under Section 317 of IPC. Under this section, exposing or leaving a child in any place with the intention of abandoning is an offence.

In cases where neonaticide cannot be proved due to putrefaction or other reasons, the mother will be charged with a lesser offence of concealment of birth. As per Section 318 IPC, whoever by secretly burying or otherwise disposing of the dead body of a child, whether such child dies before or after or during its birth intentionally conceals or endeavours to conceal the birth of such child, is punishable. For the purpose of this Section, the foetus should have attained viability. Another common method of neonaticide is the administration of poison. In ancient times, opium was the poison of choice. Calotropis juice, datura, insulin, tranquilizers and hypnotics are also used to kill the child. Signs of poisoning can be easily detected in the autopsy. Viscera should be preserved for chemical analysis in all cases of neonatal deaths.

## Time of Death

This can be inferred from the postmortem changes like lividity, rigor mortis, putrefactive changes, etc. Usually, the dead body of the child is buried or thrown in water and will be detected in a putrefied state. In such instances, it will be difficult to find out the time of death. Assessment of the time of death of the child is to correlate with the time of delivery. The signs of recent delivery in the mother can be detected by a physical examination and can be correlated with the time since death of the child.

## Cot Deaths

Sudden, unexpected, unexplained death of a child, who was otherwise well and normal is known as cot (crib) death. Very often, autopsy may not reveal the cause of death. Most of the babies die during sleep in the crib or cot and hence the name. It is usually seen in children aged 6 weeks to 6 months. There are many theories regarding the cause of death. Viral infection, milk allergy, parathyroid malfunctioning, adrenal insufficiency, laryngospasm and cardiac arrhythmia are believed to be the reasons. Nasal obstruction in mild respiratory infection can cause apnoea which will lead to cerebral anoxia and death. Suffocation by bed clothes can also result in death due to asphyxiation.

## Battered Baby

Various forms of domestic violence are seen in our society. Violence against the elderly, wife and children are common in many families. The perpetrator of violence against children is not always the male, females are also involved in the crime. Alcoholism, drug addiction, personality problems, stressful situations, poverty, etc. are the basic causes for domestic violence. Usually the baby will be an illegitimate one or born out of an unwanted pregnancy.

As the babies are defenceless, they are battered most. Battering is not the only method of violence inflicted. All sorts of injuries are seen on children. The common feature of non-accidental violence are multiple injuries of varying nature and in different stages of healing. Physical assault, deprivation of food, intentional drugging, sexual abuse and lack of medical care are the common methods of child abuse.

Acts of omission include abandoning the child and exposing it to intemperate climate. Wild animals and rodents may attack the child, if it is left in the open. Child can develop pneumonia due to exposure. If the cut umbilical cord is not ligated the child may bleed to death. But the cord may contract and get occluded with clot after it is cut. Depriving the child of milk or fluids is also an act of omission (Fig. 25.3).

Head and visceral injuries are inflicted through beating and kicking as a result of sudden loss of temper. Apart from the recent fatal injuries, many old injuries may be present. Bruises, burns and healing fractures will be present. Usually there will be delay in providing medical attention. The history given by the parents will not be consistent with the nature of injuries. Children employed as servants are also subjected to ill treatment and violence. They are beaten up, branded with hot irons, scalded and deprived of food.

### Shaken-Baby Syndrome

Vigorous shaking of the baby or a young child by the arms, legs or shoulders will result in brain damage leading to mental retardation, speech and hearing disabilities, paralysis, seizures and death. This condition is known as shaken-baby syndrome. A baby's head and neck are vulnerable to trauma as the head is large and neck muscles are weak. They can be damaged by whiplash injuries easily.

In shaken-baby syndrome, retinal haemorrhages, subdural hematoma, damage to spinal cord and

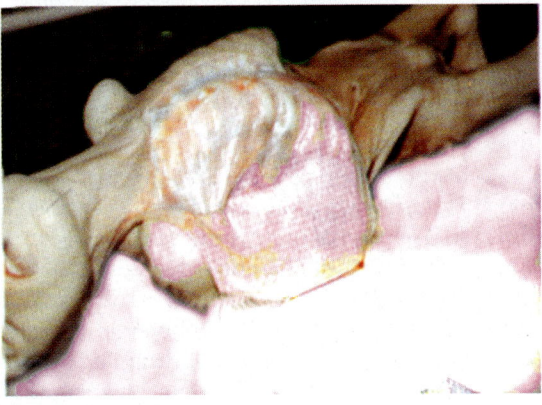

**Fig. 25.3:** Child deprived of nutrition-absence of fat under the skin

broken ribs are seen. CT scan or MRI scan will reveal the lesions. The child will show symptoms of vomiting, seizures, difficulty in breathing and altered consciousness. Sometimes the child will be unconscious and present signs of a closed head injury.

Usually the perpetrator of shaken-baby abuse is the mother, father or the baby sitter. Many babies survive the shaking, but later they may show a variety of disabilities such as visual and hearing disabilities, cerebral palsy, autism, cognitive impairments, developmental disorders and behavioural abnormalities.

### DIRECTIONS TO THE INVESTIGATING OFFICER

- Take photographs of the dead foetus and scene.
- Recod detailed description of the scene.
- Record the description of the pit if the foetus was found buried.
- Examine the clothes/wrappings and record detailed description.
- Look for evidences which will help in establishing the identity of the child. (In hospital deliveries, identification tag may be seen.)
- Collect samples for DNA typing to establishing identity in future.

After the inquest, send the foetus to the medical officer preferably a forensic specialist for conducting the autopsy. After ascertaining the age, live birth, cause of death and time since death further investigation can be started. If it is proved to be a case of infanticide, the next step is to find the woman who delivered the foetus. It may be possible to find out who has recently delivered near the area where the dead foetus was discovered. Sometimes there may be some identifiable articles like clothes or wrappings on the dead body. Once the woman is identified, the next step is to find out whether she has signs of recent delivery. The suspect may be subjected to a medical examination, preferably by an obstetrician or by a forensic specialist. DNA typing of the foetal blood/tissue and the suspect will provide concrete evidence.

# 26

# Impotence

## MEDICOLEGAL ASPECTS

In various civil and criminal cases, a male person may be subjected to medical examination and certification regarding his potency. The civil cases include nullity of marriage, disputed paternity, litigations for compensations, maintenance, etc. Criminal cases include rape, sodomy and other sexual offences.

Potency is defined as the ability of a male to perform the sexual act. The sexual act comprises erection, intromission and ejaculation as far as the male is concerned. The main defect is erectile dysfunction. The female being a passive agent, is considered as normal if she has no sexual dysfunction to partake in the sexual act. The commonest civil case where the question of potency arises is nullity of marriage. A marriage is said to be consummated only when a successful sexual act has taken place. If not, one of the parties can approach the court for dissolution of marriage on the grounds of impotence. In civil litigations, persons may sustain injuries and claim for damages complaining of impotence developing after the trauma. In criminal cases like rape, the accused persons will plead 'not guilty' on the grounds of impotence, and request for a medical examination as per the provisions of **Section 54 (1) of Criminal Procedure Code** which states as follows:

"When a person, who is arrested, whether on a charge or otherwise, alleges, at the time when he is produced before a magistrate or at any time during the period of his detention in custody that the examination of his body will afford evidence which will disprove the commission by him of any offence or which will establish the commission by any other person of any offence against his body, the magistrate shall, if requested by the arrested person so to do, direct the examination of the body of such person by a registered medical practitioner unless the magistrate considers that the request is made for the purpose of vexation or delay or for defeating the ends of justice."

The new subsection 2 states that "where an examination is made under subsection 1, a copy of the report of such examination shall be furnished by the registered medical practitioner to the arrested person or the person nominated by such arrested person."

## PHYSIOLOGY OF ERECTION

Male sexual organs are penis, testes, epididymis, vas deferens, seminal vesicle, prostate, bulbourethral (Cowper's gland) and periurethral glands (glands of Littre). The male sexual arousal is characterised by excitation, erection, and ejaculation with orgasm. Erection is not essential for ejaculation. Ejaculation can be induced in paraplegics by vibratory stimulation of the glans penis. Similarly, orgasm can occur without ejaculation. Each of these has a separate mechanism.

The shaft of the penis consists of erectile tissue in the form of three longitudinal chambers, two corpora cavernosa, placed side by side and one corpus spongiosum underneath them. The erectile tissue consists of sinusoids, lined with trabecular smooth muscles and endothelium. Spongiosum covers the urethra (Figs 26.1A and B).

Sexual excitation causes increased heart rate, blood pressure and more blood flow to the genital organs. Even though all the chambers are filled with blood, pressure in the spongiosum will be half of that in the cavernosa. This mechanism will keep the urethra patent for the emission of semen. The venous outflow is blocked due to the compression of the veins.

Ejaculation is due to stimulation of the sympathetic nerves. Emission of semen occurs at the highest level of sexual arousal and starts with the movement of genital secretions in seminal vesicles and prostate. Thirty percent of the secretions come from prostate and sixty percent from the seminal vesicles. When the fluid reaches and distends the prostatic urethra, ejaculatory reflex is initiated. The sphincter of the bladder closes to prevent the reflux of semen into the bladder during ejaculation. When the ejaculatory reflex starts, clonic contractions of the muscles in the cavernosa and spongiosum occur and semen is ejected along the urethra with force.

The volume of the human ejaculate varies from 2–6 ml. Immediately after voiding, it will be gel like, but liquefies within 15 minutes. Orgasm is an extremely pleasurable sensation just before ejaculation. Following ejaculation, penis becomes flaccid again. There will be a refractory period after the ejaculation during which erection will not occur. This period increases with age.

## Causes of Impotence

Andrological research over the past years has proved that in 80–90% of cases of impotence, there will be some organic cause. Impotence since birth is called primary impotence. Impotence which sets in after years of normal sex is called secondary impotence. Causes of secondary impotence are diabetes mellitus, hypertension, atherosclerosis, renal failure, heart disease, neurological disorders, hormonal deficiency, injuries, pelvic surgeries, penile diseases, use of tobacco, drugs, etc.

Arteriosclerotic narrowing of the arteries supplying penis can result in diminished supply of blood to the erectile tissues. Diabetes, hypertension, pelvic and genital injuries, etc. can cause reduction of blood flow. Low grade gradual injuries sustained to bicycle riders can result in clot formation in the arteries causing blockade. Ultrasonogram and penis angiogram can make accurate study of penile blood supply. Nowadays, microvascular surgery, epigastric-dorsal artery bypass grafting, etc. are available to cure the vascular problems.

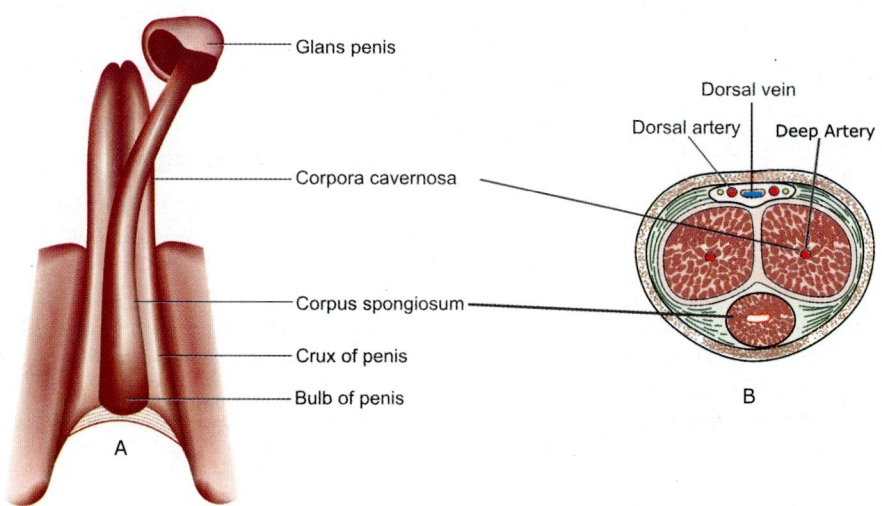

**Figs 26.1A and B:** A. Gross anatomy of penis, B. Transverse section of penis

During erection, the corpora cavernosa are filled with blood and the veins close down almost completely. Practically no blood flows out of the erectile tissues and erection is maintained. Leakage of blood from penile veins can occur in adult life after years of normal sexual life. Surgical correction is possible by tying and removing the deep dorsal vein of penis.

Injuries to the spine, pelvic or perirenal injuries and pelvic surgeries can cause injuries to the nerves of the penis. Operation of the rectum, prostate, urinary bladder, retroperitoneum, etc. can injure the nerves and cause impotence. Disorders of the nervous system such as multiple sclerosis, myelitis, Alzheimer's disease, Parkinson's disease, spinal cord injuries and pelvic irradiation, etc. can cause erectile dysfunction. Diabetitence. It is estimated that as many as 50% of all diabetics are impotent!!

Deficiency of sex hormones can cause impotence. Testicular androgen secretion decreases progressively with age. Low levels of testosterone, luteinising hormone and prolactin can cause impotence. Usually, hormone deficiency affects the libido or sexual desire. Hormone replacement therapy can enhance potency and improve libido. Hypothyroidism and Cushing's syndrome are some of the other endocrinological causes for impotence.

Substance abuses such as alcoholism, anabolic steroids, heroin and marijuana can cause erectile dysfunction. Tobacco use is one of the major causes of impotence. Thrombosis (blood clots) can develop in the penile arteries of heavy smokers. Many drugs affect the neurotransmitters at the nerve endings resulting in impotence. Notable among these drugs are antihypertensives, opiates, psychotropics and tranquilizers. Congenital and acquired malformations and diseases of the penis can cause impotence. Penis may be congenitally absent or infantile.

## PSYCHOGENIC IMPOTENCE

Twenty per cent of erectile dysfunction is due to psychogenic causes. When there is no organic cause for impotence, the cause could be psychological. Before diagnosing psychogenic impotence, organic causes should be excluded. Depression, anxiety, fear, anger and other mental conditions can cause impotence. **Honeymoon impotence** is a typical example of impotence caused by anxiety and fear. Sexual counselling and sex therapy are effective in such patients. **Quoad hanc** is the condition when a person is impotent towards his wife, but potent towards other women.

Organic causes can be ruled out by a physical examination, but psychological impotence cannot be excluded. A psychosocial examination can be conducted to rule out psychogenic conditions. Monitoring erections that occur during sleep (nocturnal penile tumescence) can rule out certain organic causes. Healthy men have involuntary erections during sleep. If nocturnal erections occur, the erectile dysfunction is considered as due to psychological causes and not due to physical causes. But tests for nocturnal erections are not reliable completely. Such tests have not been standardised yet.

As defined earlier, potency actually means the ability to have and sustain an erection, sufficient for intromission and ejaculation. However, ejaculation can occur without an erection. Some medical officers test for erection by asking the subject for self-stimulation. This procedure is irregular and not at all conclusive. The reaction is that due to psychological reasons the person may not have an erection.

In medicolegal cases, the medical officer will conduct a thorough examination of all the systems with special attention to central nervous system and endocrine glands. A detailed examination of the genitalia is also conducted to rule out organic causes. If a male is free from congenital or acquired malformations or diseases of the genital organs and has no abnormality in the systemic examination or baseline laboratory investigations, he can be declared as potent. But a certificate to that effect is not given by the doctors, as psychological impotence cannot be ruled out. Hence a certificate in double negative form is given: **"there are no findings to suggest that the person is impotent."**

### Medicolegal Points

A person can be declared as impotent, if he suffers from absence or abnormalities of penis, infantile penis, diseases of the hypopituitarism or Addison's disease will also produce impotence. Nervous system disorders such as paraplegia, neurosyphilis, disseminated sclerosis, etc. can render a person impotent. Injuries involving the lumbar vertebrae affecting the sacral segments, operations like bilateral lumbar sympathectomy, administration of parasympatholytic and ganglion blocking drugs can also produce impotence.

Regarding potency, extremes of age is of no significance. Persons in the prepubertal age as well as old age are also found to be potent. But normally, a person becomes potent when he attains puberty. Potency may diminish as age advances, but it is difficult to fix an upper age limit.

## FEMALE SEXUAL DYSFUNCTION

Examination of a woman for sexual dysfunction is necessary in cases of dissolution of marriage on the grounds of non-consummation. A marriage can be declared null and void, if a successful sexual act has not taken place. The husband can file a case for nullity, if the wife is not capable of partaking in the sexual act due to genital reasons. The causes for female sexual dysfunction could be due to functional causes or organic causes.

### Functional Causes

Anxiety, stress, fear of pain, guilt complex, etc. can cause strong contractions of the para vaginal muscles at the time of intercourse. Even an attempt of penile penetration can cause this change called **vaginismus.** Intercourse is impossible in severe vaginismus. This condition may have deep rooted psychological reasons. Psychotherapy and counseling can cure this condition which is only temporary in nature.

Some women may not have sexual desire. This condition is called **frigidity.** The reason is usually psychological. Frigidity can develop in a woman who does not experience an orgasm in sexual intercourse. She gradually loses interest in intercourse. Repulsion towards the partner can develop lack of libido and frigidity. Vaginismus can lead to sexual aversion and frigidity. Some women will be selectively frigid. Lesbians are usually selectively frigid to male partner.

Other causes for frigidity are usage of sedatives or depressants, diseases like hypothyroidism, neurological disorders, menopause, etc.

### Organic Causes

Agenesis of vagina, atresia of vagina, septate vagina, imperforate or tough hymen, etc. can make intercourse impossible. Vaginal infection with ulceration is a common cause for painful intercourse **(dyspareunia)**. Bartholin's cyst, ulceration of vulva, prolapsed uterus, large cystocoel, etc. can be impediments for intercourse. After menopause, changes in the vaginal mucosa can also cause pain during coitus.

### Medicolegal Aspects of Female Sexual Dysfunction

In the case of a female, if she has no abnormality in the genitalia, she can be considered as a **vera copula**. If the woman is having congenital malformations like absence or atresia of vagina, thick imperforate hymen, diseases like tumours or elephantiasis of vulva, she can be declared as sexually dysfunctional. But vaginismus, dyspareunia and thick imperforate hymen are the conditions which will produce only temporary incapacity. Sexual intercourse could not have taken place in patients with vaginismus. But some of the congenital abnormalities and vaginismus can be treated and corrected.

Wife can file a petition to declare the marriage as null and void on the grounds of non-consummation due to the impotency of the husband. In that case, the allegation is proved by the examination of the wife rather than the husband.

If the hymenal orifice does admit only a finger with difficulty, the inference is that sexual intercourse has not taken place and marriage could not have been consummated. Admission of two or more fingers indicates that intercourse could have taken place even though some virgins possess a large hymenal orifice due to the use of sanitary tampons or regular masturbation using foreign bodies. If the hymenal orifice is wide enough to admit a penis, the laxity and rugosity of the vagina has to be noted. A woman who had regular intercourse will possess a lax vagina with less rugosity of the vaginal mucosa. A woman may possess an elastic hymen which will admit two fingers, at the same time she will be a virgin.

A doctor can declare a woman a virgin, if her hymen is intact and the hymenal orifice admits only a little finger. But it is not proper to state that a woman is not a virgin based on the findings that her hymen has ruptured or is absent. A virgin is defined as a woman who has not experienced sexual intercourse.

## DIRECTIONS TO THE INVESTIGATING OFFICER

The accused in a case of sexual offence should be subjected to potency examination as he is likely to plead impotence. If the accused is apprehended immediately after committing the offence of sexual assault, he should be sent to a registered medical practitioner, (preferably an expert) for physical examination U/S 53 A of CrPC. The same doctor may be asked to conduct a potency examination also. When the accused is arrested after a considerable lapse of time, a physical examination may not yield incriminating physical evidence. However, there is a possibility of detecting old injuries. Collection of blood samples for DNA typing, laboratory tests for venereal diseases and potency examination should be conducted.

# 27

# Drunkenness

## ALCOHOL

Alcohol produced by fermentation of substances containing sugar is commonly used as a beverage. The chemical name is ethyl alcohol. It is a transparent, colourless, volatile liquid having a spirituous smell and burning taste. It has medical and industrial applications also. Toddy, wine, beer, etc. are fermented beverages containing varying concentrations of alcohol ranging from 5 to 15%. Fermented materials are distilled to produce various types of liquors such as whisky, brandy, rum. Universally, it is the most commonly consumed substance.

**Proof** is the standard strength of distilled alcoholic liquors. Proof spirit is a mixture of alcohol and water having proof strength. It is the minimum concentration of alcohol in a solution of alcohol and water, which will retain the ignitability of gun powder soaked in such a mixture. Hundred degree proof spirit contains 57.1% of ethyl alcohol by volume. According to Indian Abkari Act, distilled liquors having a strength of 75% proof (25° under proof) alone can be sold for public consumption. Approximately, the concentration of alcohol in all those liquors will be 42.83%. Absolute alcohol contains 99.95% of alcohol, while rectified spirit contains 90% of alcohol. Methylated spirit or denatured alcohol is a mixture of 95% ethyl alcohol and 5% methyl alcohol.

**Illicit liquor** or country arrack is produced by distilling fermented toddy, rice or a mixture of fruits and jaggery. The distillation is by using various ingenious contraptions. The distilled liquor contains 20 to 30% ethyl alcohol. Toddy and country arrack are mixed with datura, chloral hydrate and even organic phosphate insecticides to make it more strong!! Sometimes, methyl alcohol is added to it. This has resulted in mass fatalities. The liquor tragedies which frequently occur in Kerala and other southern states of India have a heavy toll on human lives.

When alcohol is consumed, 20% of it is absorbed from the stomach and 80% from the small intestine. Factors like food in the stomach, concentration of alcohol, etc. modify the rate of absorption. Alcohol in low concentration (15%) is absorbed fast. Food, especially fatty foods in the stomach retard the rate of absorption. Absorption starts within five minutes of consumption and will be completed in one and a half to two hours and maximum concentration of alcohol in blood is reached. About 60% of alcohol is absorbed within one hour. Blood alcohol concentration **(BAC)** cannot be accurately determined from the quantity of alcohol consumed. Approximate estimations are only possible. BAC depends upon many factors like rate of absorption, concentration of the liquor consumed, weight of the person, time elapsed after consumption, etc.

Alcohol is mainly metabolised in the liver (90%). The rest is excreted through the kidneys and lungs. Ethyl alcohol is oxidised to acetaldehyde by the enzyme alcohol dehydrogenase in the liver.

Acetaldehyde is converted into acetic acid by an enzyme aldehyde dehydrogenase. It is finally converted to carbon dioxide and water. The rate of elimination of alcohol is approximately 10 gm (equivalent to 30 ml whisky or one pint beer or one glass of wine) per hour. Elimination will be reduced in persons with liver damage. Relative concentration of alcohol in blood and urine is in the ratio of 1:1.3.

## Effect of Alcohol

Alcohol acts on the nerve cells of brain. This is the reason for the behavioural changes seen in alcohol consumption. The toxic properties of the meta-bolites are also injurious. Alcohol is a depressant of the central nervous system. First of all the depression of the higher centres releases their inhibitory tone on the lower centres. The loss of inhibition results in the more primitive and unrestrained behaviour. As the concentration increases; other parts of the brain are affected leading to depression of the vital centres. The stages of alcohol intoxication are graphically shown in Fig. 27.1.

### Stage of Sobriety (Decent)

Up to a blood concentration of 30–50 mg%, the person may remain apparently sober. But recent studies indicate that concentrations varying from 30–50 mg% of alcohol in blood may cause impair-ment of visual acuity, coordination and reflex activity, which are essential for safe driving. There will be deterioration of driving ability.

### Stage of Euphoria (Delighted)

At blood concentrations between 50 and 100 mg%, the person may have a feeling of well-being. He will be excited and talkative. Face will be flushed. Conjunctivae will be congested. Pupils will be dilated. Pulse will be rapid. He may lose the inhibi-tions. Concentration and judgement may be affected.

### Stage of Excitement (Delirious)

At a BAC of 100–150 mg%, the person may show signs of intoxication as evidenced by slight ataxia. In such situations, reflexes will be sluggish.

Reaction time will be slow. Alcohol gaze nystagmus may also appear at this stage. This is jerking movement of the eye in the direction of the gaze and independent of the position of the head. But this is not constantly seen. Concentration and judgement are affected.

### Stage of Confusion (Dazed)

At concentrations between 150 and 200 mg%, the person will be definitely under the influence of alcohol and show marked signs of intoxication. He will be disoriented and confused. Ataxia will be marked. Speech will be slurred and incoherent. Skilled movements are affected. Reaction time is very much increased. Vision will be blurred. Diplopia and vertigo will be seen.

### Stage of Stupor (Dejected)

The person will reach this stage at a BAC of 200–250 mg%. There will be loss of facial muscle tone resulting in an 'owlish' facial appearance. He will not be able to walk. There will be hiccup, nausea and vomiting. Response to external stimuli will be diminished.

### Stage of Coma (Dead Drunk)

The person will become unconscious when the concentration reaches 300–400 mg%. Reflexes will be abolished. There will be incontinence of faeces and urine. Alcoholic coma is characterised by symptoms like rapid pulse, subnormal tempera-ture, constricted pupils, etc.

### Death

Death due to acute alcoholism can occur due to respiratory paralysis when the BAC is above 400 mg%. Respiratory paralysis is caused by prolonged hypoxia of brain affecting the higher centres. There is considerable variation in the individual reaction towards alcohol.

## Treatment of Acute Alcoholism

An excessively drunken person may require hospitalisation and treatment. Normally, an intoxicated person recovers within a few hours even without any treatment. An excited person will require sedation. Stomach wash is indicated in a

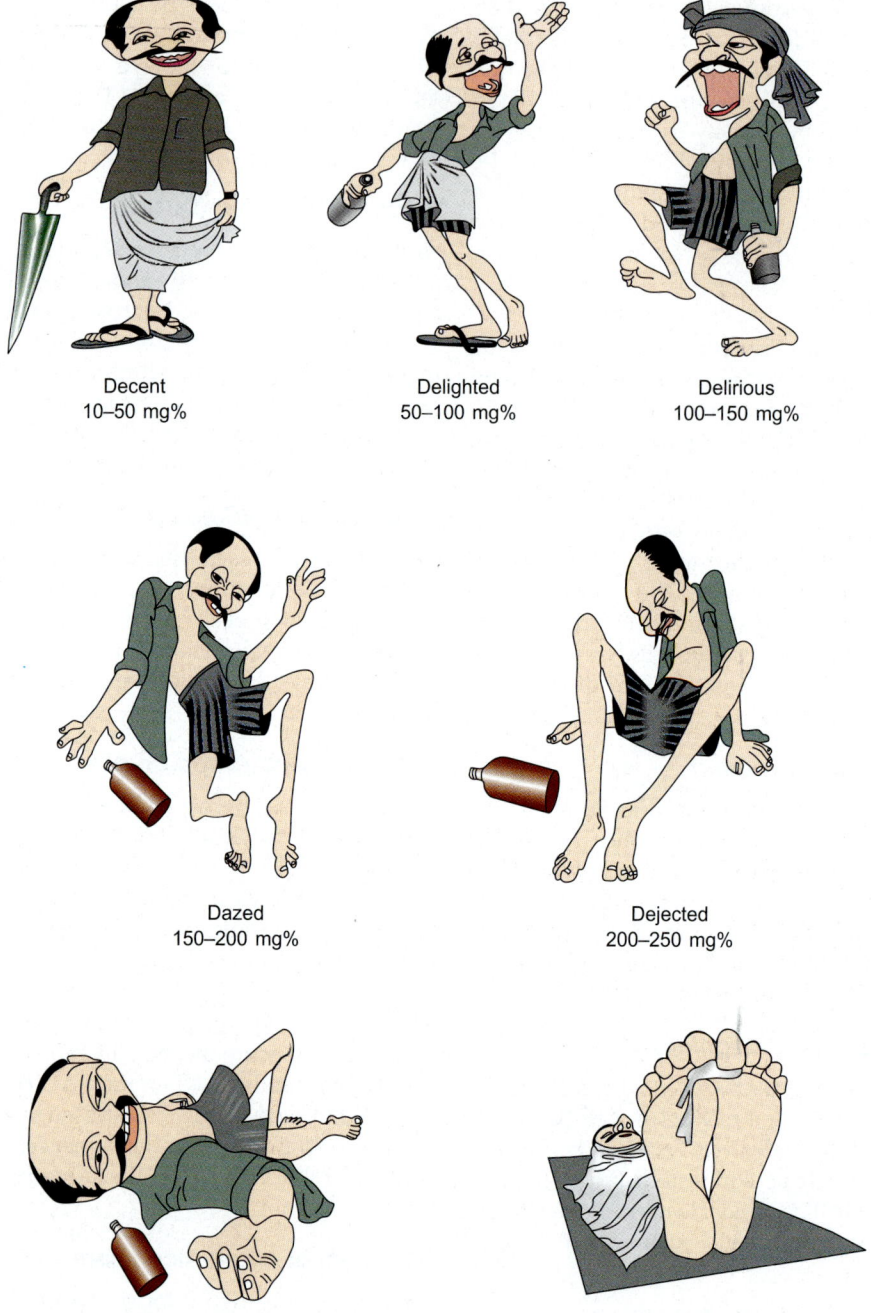

Decent
10–50 mg%

Delighted
50–100 mg%

Delirious
100–150 mg%

Dazed
150–200 mg%

Dejected
200–250 mg%

Dead drunk
300–400 mg%

Dead
400–500 mg%

**Fig. 27.1:** Blood alcohol concentration in different stages of alcoholic intoxication '7 Ds' (Drawing by Br. Vimal, M.A.Math)

highly intoxicated person who is likely to become unconscious. An unconscious person needs prompt treatment according to the standard regimen.

## Drunkenness and Crime

Legally, drunkenness means a state of intoxication due to the consumption of alcoholic drinks. It is the condition produced in a person who has taken alcohol in a quantity sufficient to make him loose control of his faculties to such an extent that he is unable to execute safely the occupation in which he is engaged in at the material time. Drunkenness is an offence under the following circumstances:
1. Drunken driving
2. Drunken and disorderly behaviour in a public place
3. Drinking in a prohibited area.

Moreover, drunkenness has relation to crimes, contracts, consent and medical practice.

## Drunkenness and Driving

The Motor Vehicles Act of 1939 was amended in the year 1988. It was further amended in the year 1993, 1994, 2000 and 2001. According to Section 185 of the 1988 Act, driving or attempting to drive a motor vehicle, after consuming even a small quantity of alcohol was punishable. It was amended in 1994. Section 185 of motor vehicle Act of 1988 (amended in 1994) states that "Whoever, while driving or attempting to drive a motor vehicle, has, in his blood, alcohol exceeding **30 mg per 100 ml** of blood detected in a test by a breath analyser or is under the influence of a drug to such an extent as to be incapable of exercising proper control over the vehicle shall be punishable for the first offence with imprisonment for a term which may extend to 6 months or with fine which may extend to Rs. 2000/- or with both; and for a second or subsequent offence if committed within 3 years of the commission of the previous similar offence, with imprisonment for a term which may extend to 2 years or with fine which may extend to Rs. 3000/- or with both (legal aspects of the breath test, collection of samples, etc. are given in Chapter 17.

According to the **MV Act 1988 (amended), Sections 185-203-204 and 205,** driving or attempting to drive a motor vehicle with a blood alcohol level exceeding 30 mg% or under the influence of an inebriating drug is an offence. A police officer in uniform can conduct breath test on the driver of any motor vehicle. If breath test yields a positive result, the driver can be arrested without warrant. The arrested person is brought before a registered medical practitioner for collecting sample of blood or urine. As per Section 205, if such a person refuses, omits or fails to consent to the taking of a specimen of breath or blood, his refusal, omission or failure will go as evidence against him unless reasonable cause is shown.

But according to **Sec. 53 of Cr. PC** consent is not necessary for physical examination of an accused, if he is arrested and brought before a medical officer by a police officer not below the rank of a subinspector. Even reasonable force can be used for this purpose. As per the amendment of the Criminal Procedure Code in 2005, an explanatory clause has been added to Section 53. Examination under Section 53 shall include the examination of blood, blood stains, semen, swabs in case of sexual offences, sputum and sweat, hair samples and finger nail clippings by the use of modern and scientific techniques including DNA profiling and such other tests which the registered medical practitioner thinks necessary in a particular case. Therefore, it is lawful for the doctor acting at the request of the police officer to collect blood and other body fluids as is reasonably necessary for the purpose of laboratory examination.

The doctor has to collect 10 ml of venous blood using a sterile syringe and needle in a clean glass bottle. Hundred milligrams of sodium fluoride should be added as the preservative. The area from which blood is drawn should not be cleaned with spirit. The bottle should be made airtight by sealing it with molten paraffin poured over the stopper and the mouth of the bottle. The bottle should be labelled, packed, sealed and despatched to the chemical examiner with a requisition and a sample seal.

## Drunkenness and Disorderly Behaviour in a Public Place

Under the **Police Act (51)**, whoever in any street or public place or in any court, police station or other public office or in any place of public amusement or resort or on board any passenger boat or vessel or in any public passenger vehicle, is found drunk and incapable of taking care of himself or behaves in a disorderly manner under the influence of drink shall, on conviction be punished:

a. For a first offence, with imprisonment for a term which may extend to one month and with fine which may extend to 200 rupees. Provided that in the absence of special and adequate reasons to the contrary to be mentioned in the judgement of the court, such imprisonment shall not be less than 15 days and fine shall not be less than 50 rupees; and

b. For a subsequent offence, with imprisonment for a term which may extend to 6 months and with fine which may extend to 500 rupees. Provided that in the absence of special and adequate reasons to the contrary to be mentioned in the judgement of the court, such imprisonment shall not be less than one month and fine shall not be less than 50 rupees; and for a subsequent offence, with imprisonment for a term which may extend to 6 months and with fine which may extend to 500 rupees; provided that in the absence of special and adequate reason to the contrary to be mentioned in the judgment of the court, such imprisonment shall not be less than one month and fine shall not be less than 100 rupees. For the purposes of this Section "Public Passenger Vehicle" means a vehicle used for carrying passengers for hire or reward other than a vehicle which carries passengers for hire or reward under a contract expressed or implied for the use of the vehicle as a whole or for a fixed or agreed rate or sum.

To support a conviction under this section, it is necessary to prove that the accused was drunk and incapable of taking care of himself or behaved in a disorderly manner under the influence of drink. The court will be guided by medical opinion and also direct evidence rendered by the witnesses.

Single bench of the High Court of Kerala in the case Varghese Vs State of Kerala (1990 (2) KLT 416) had held that it cannot be conclusively proved that a person has consumed alcohol unless urine or blood test was carried out and mere smelling of alcohol, unsteady gait, dilatation of pupils,

incoherence of speech are not enough to come to any such conclusion. Accordingly, examination of blood was mandatory when an accused is examined for signs of drunkenness in a case of drunken and disorderly behaviour in public place.

Division bench of the Hon'ble High Court of Kerala set aside the decision of the single bench on the grounds that it does not lay down the law correctly *(Georgekutty Vs State of Kerala- 1991(2) KLT 570)*. Based on this decision, the medical officer is expected to conduct a physical examination and arrive at a conclusion as to whether the person has consumed alcohol or not and if consumed whether he is under its influence or not.

The law only states that it is not mandatory to collect blood or urine in cases of offence under the police Act. But the law does not prevent a doctor from collecting blood or urine, if the accused has given consent. On examination, if a person is found to be under the influence of alcohol, analysis of blood/urine will prove that the intoxication was due to consumption of alcohol. It is true that clinical examination is more valid in giving an opinion as to the intoxication, rather than the level of alcohol in the blood or urine. Analysis of blood or urine will be helpful for the physician to support his finding that the intoxication was due to the consumption of alcohol and not due to other disease conditions simulating intoxication.

Mental disease, shock, head injury, hypoglycemia, uremia, brain and spinal cord tumours, Parkinsonism, cerebellar ataxia, multiple sclerosis, Meniere's syndrome, etc. can cause muscular incoordination and other signs mimicking alcoholism. Consent for collection of blood is not necessary under the newly amended (2005) **Section 53 of CrPC.** But the doctor should confirm whether the accused is under arrest and brought by a police officer of and above the rank of a sub-inspector of police.

## Drunkenness and Criminal Responsibility

In olden days, a drunken person committing an offence would get more severe punishment than he would, if he had committed the same act in a sober state. Modern law does not accept drunkenness as an excuse or defence in a charge of crime. However, the situation will be different, if the intoxicating drink was administered to the accused by force or without his knowledge.

The law on this subject is contained in **Section 85 of Indian Penal Code** which reads as follows:

"Nothing is an offence which is done by a person who at the time of doing it is, by reason of intoxication, incapable of knowing the nature of the act, or that he is doing what is either wrong or contrary to law, provided that the thing which intoxicated him was administered to him without his knowledge or against his will." Hence it is clear that in order to sustain a valid defence on the ground of drunkenness, it should be proved that the drink was not taken voluntarily and that it was administered without his knowledge or against his will, and that he would not have committed the act but for the unwholesome influence of the drink. Voluntary drunkenness may be an extenuating circumstance, if the mind of the accused was so obscured by drink that he might not be able to form the criminal intention **(means rea)** if such intention formed an essential ingredient of the crime in question **(Section 86 IPC).**

### Drunkenness and Contract

According to the Indian Contract Act, 1872, a sane man who is delirious from fever or who is so drunk that he cannot understand the terms of a contract or form a rational judgement as to its effect on his interests cannot enter into a contract whilst such delirium or drunkenness lasts.

So it would appear that mere drunkenness does not invalidate a contract. To repudiate a contract on ground of drunkenness, it must be shown that the person was drunk to such a degree that he was not able to understand the terms of the contract or its natural consequence on his interests. It follows from the above provisions that a registered medical practitioner acting at the request of a subinspector of police may lawfully examine the arrested person without his consent, even using reasonable force.

### Drunkenness and Prohibition

Consumption of alcoholic beverages would be an offence in areas where the Prohibition Act is in force. It is necessary that the person should be under the influence of alcohol. However, medical opinion to this effect would offer corroborative evidence to the fact that the accused consumed a quantity of alcohol which is not ordinarily possible, if he has only consumed medical preparation containing alcohol. Conviction will follow, if the court is satisfied by medical and other evidence that the accused consumed prohibited liquor.

## MEDICAL EXAMINATION IN DRUNKENNESS

### Consent for Examination

It is a general proposition of procedural law that any subject could be physically examined only with his consent. Such consent may be expressed or implied. When an accused is to be medically examined, it is necessary that the nature and possible consequence of such examination should be explained to him and thereafter he should consent for examination. This is called "informed consent". It is likely that some persons might refuse medical examination and thus block a complete investigation. To avert this eventually, the Criminal Procedure Code (1973) has introduced Section 53 to facilitate effective investigation. Section 53 of Cr. PC provides as follows:

1. When a person is arrested on a charge of committing an offence of such a nature and alleged to have been committed under such circumstances that there are reasonable grounds for believing that an examination of his person will afford evidence as to the commission of an offence, it shall be lawful for a registered medical practitioner, acting at the request of a police officer not below the rank of a subinspector, and for any person acting in good faith in his aid and under his direction order to ascertain the facts which may afford such evidence, and to use such force as is reasonably necessary for that purpose.

2. Whenever the person of a female is to be examined under this section, the examination shall be made by, or under the supervision of a female registered medical practitioner.

*Explanation:* Examination shall include the examination of blood, blood stain, semen, swabs in the case of sexual offences, sputum and sweat, hair samples and finger nail clippings by the use of modern and scientific techniques including DNA profiling and such other tests which the registered medical practitioner thinks necessary in a particular case.

## Drunkenness Certification

After the physical examination, based on the clinical findings, a certificate is issued despite samples have been collected for chemical examination or not. It is customary not to wait for the chemical examiner's report. The opinion could be one of the three statements given below:
a. Has not consumed alcohol
b. Has consumed alcohol and is not under its influence.
c. Has consumed alcohol and is under its influence.

Apart from the smell of alcohol in the breath, there is no single sign or symptom which cannot be produced by some other conditions such as severe head injuries, low blood sugar (hypoglycemia) due to overdose of insulin, thyroid disorders, disorders of brain like disseminated sclerosis, epilepsy, Parkinson's disease, unusual reactions to certain drugs like antihistamines, barbiturates, morphine, etc. The doctor has to exclude these conditions by a proper history and physical examination. The following findings taken in combination would justify an opinion that the subject has "consumed alcohol and is under its influence".
1. Smell of alcohol in the breath
2. Congested eyes
3. Dilated and sluggishly reacting pupils
4. Thick and slurred speech
5. Unsteady gait
6. Defective muscular coordination.

If there is undoubted smell of alcohol in the breath with or without some eye signs, but muscular coordination is normal the person may be adjudged to have "consumed alcohol, but not under its influence". In the absence of all these signs, certify that he "has not consumed alcohol". In Norway and Sweden, blood examination is compulsory by law. In England, the accused has the right to refuse a blood examination, but such refusal would go to support the prosecution case. It is generally accepted that 150 mg% alcohol in blood can render a person invariably intoxicated. But there are variations from person to person. Even 50 mg% BAC may cause signs of drunkenness. This depends upon factors like habituation, idiosyncrasy, etc. In certain countries, it is an offence to drive a vehicle if the driver is having blood alcohol more than a particular statutory level. Clinical behaviour of the accused is more important than the blood levels. The point at issue is how the person responded to alcohol in his body at the material time and not the amount of alcohol in his system. (This is not applicable as far as the Motor Vehicle's Act is concerned.)

**Pathological intoxication** is a condition in which epileptic persons or persons who had sustained a head injury in the past may go into a psychotic phase after consuming a small quantity of alcohol. They may show destructive tendency and abnormal behaviour.

## CHRONIC ALCOHOLISM

Chronic alcoholism has become a worldwide social problem. Dependence on alcohol develops due to psychological and sociological causes. Chronic alcoholics develop increased tolerance to alcohol. Later they develop liver damage and will get intoxicated even after consuming a small quantity. Many physical disorders involving the skin, gastrointestinal, cardiovascular and nervous systems, may develop in chronic alcoholics. They will also develop various mental disorders, such as paranoia, hallucinations, delusions, psychoses etc. Alcohol can produce serious withdrawal symptoms. Alcoholic hallucinosis, alcoholic tremulousness, alcoholic seizures (rum fits), delirium tremens, etc. are some of the conditions seen in chronic alcoholisme. Of these, delirium tremens is medicolegally significant.

## DELIRIUM TREMENS

This is a condition precipitated by excessive drinking, abstinence of alcohol, acute febrile illness, injury or surgery. This condition is characterised by delirium, delusions, hallucinations and convulsions. Initially there will be irritability, insomnia, agitation, mild fever and sweating. Medicolegal importance of this psychological disorder occurring in chronic alcoholics is that they develop suicidal as well as homicidal tendencies. Death can occur from cerebral edema, cardiac failure and shock. Usually, the condition is short lived and person recovers fully. They need de-addiction and psychiatric treatment.

## Methyl Alcohol (Methanol)

Methyl alcohol is a colourless, volatile liquid having a peculiar smell and burning taste. It is produced by destructive distillation of wood or molasses. This is mainly used for industrial purposes and to denature ethyl alcohol. Methyl alcohol is mistakenly or purposely added to ethyl alcohol beverages for consumption. Consumption of 30 to 60 ml of methyl alcohol will result in death.

When methyl alcohol is consumed, it is converted in the body to deleterious substances such as fomaldehyde and formic acid. Retinal damage and consequent blindness will result as the retina is sensitive to these metabolic products. Other symptoms of methyl alcohol poisoning include severe abdominal pain, nausea, vomiting, headache, vertigo and visual disturbances. These are followed by convulsions and unconsciousness. Death occurs usually within 24 to 36 hours.

Persons who have consumed methyl alcohol require urgent hospitalisation. Treatment includes stomach wash, treatment of acidosis, protection of eyes, administration of ethyl alcohol common whisky, or brandy at a dose of 1 ml/kg body weight every 4 to 6 hours by mouth. Administration of ethyl alcohol will block the oxidation of methyl alcohol by competitive inhibition. Nowadays antidotes like fomepizole (4 methyl pyrazole), is available. In severe poisoning, hemodialysis can be done.

## DIRECTIONS TO THE INVESTIGATING OFFICER

Persons taken into custody U/S 52 of Police Act, should be subjected to medical examination for drunkenness without delay. As time passes, the blood alcohol level will fall and signs of intoxication may disappear. Similarly, the initial examination may not show positive signs of drunkenness as the blood alcohol level might not have reached the peak. In such cases, examination should be repeated at half an hour interval.

It should be borne in mind that many disease conditions may simulate drunkenness.

When a person who has consumed alcohol is examined, apart from the smell of alcohol in the breath, there is not a single sign which is absolutely diagnostic of drunkenness. Even the perception of the smell of alcohol is also a subjective one. Therefore, analysis of blood alone can substantiate the clinical findings and opinion. If the person is not under arrest, consent is needed for examination as well as collection of blood or other body fluids.

Death due to methyl alcohol poisoning is common. People consume ethyl alcohol adulterated with methyl alcohol (methylated spirit). Mass fatalities are common. People who adulterate ethyl alcohol with methyl alcohol and distribute it for consumption are liable for the death of persons and charged for murder.

Therefore, all deaths suspected to be due to consumption of liquor should be subjected to autopsy. The doctor should be requested to collect viscera, blood and urine, preserve them properly and despatch to the chemical examiner's laboratory for analysis.

Samples of liquor consumed, left overs in the bottles, vomitus found in the scene, stomach washings, etc. should be collected and sealed properly for chemical analysis. If the bottles are not closed and sealed airtight, alcohol may evaporate.

# 28

# Poisoning

Police officers may have to encounter cases of poisoning in the living and the dead. In recent years, the incidence of poisoning has increased considerably. Most of the cases of poisoning are due to intentional self-administration. Homicidal and accidental poisoning are also not uncommon. Insecticides, corrosives and vegetable irritants are commonly ingested for suicidal purpose, as they are freely available. Poisoning with hypnotics and tranquillisers are rare. The police officer should possess a basic knowledge of common poisons and be able to identify the signs and symptoms seen in human poisoning. Very often, the information given by the relatives or witnesses may be helpful. The features of poisoning are generally the following:

- Sudden onset of symptoms
- Increase in severity of the symptoms as time passes
- Peculiar or unusual smell of breath, vomitus, or froth at mouth and nostrils
- Signs of corrosion of hands, face, lips and oral mucosa in the case of acids and alkalies.

Acute poisoning can occur by routes other than oral. Insecticides will be absorbed through skin or by inhalation. Drugs like morphine may be injected. Onset of symptoms depends upon the quantity, solubility and route of administration of the poison. Some of the poisons can be identified by the colour and smell. Organophosphorus and organochloro insecticides have an aromatic smell or a smell similar to that of kerosene. Cyanides have a peculiar odour of crushed tapioca (cassava) leaves. Phenolic smell of carbolic acid can be easily identified. Some of the insecticides are coloured, e.g. ekalux has got a blue colour; dimecron violet; zinc phosphide black and carbofuran (furadan) is magenta. Corrosive acids have a pungent smell. Nitric acid will produce a yellow stain on the clothes and tissues. If vomitus is present in the scene, look for the presence of unusual colour or smell. Vomitus has to be collected and preserved for chemical analysis.

Constricted pupils may be seen in poisoning with morphine, phenol, organophosphorus compounds, etc. Dilated pupils are present in endrin, dhatura, cocaine, nicotine and amphetamine poisoning. Presence of erythematous blisters in an unconscious patient is highly suggestive of barbiturate poisoning. Flushing, sweating, tinnitus, deafness and hyperventilation are indicative of aspirin poisoning. Antidepressant drugs will produce loss of consciousness with widely dilated pupils and cardiac arrhythmias. Black or greyish discolouration of lips, chin or hands with dull white burns of mouth cavity indicate the consumption of acids or alkalies. The skin of the upper arms and front of elbows should be examined for needle puncture marks. In drug addicts, these puncture marks may be associated with infection.

# FIRST AID IN POISONING

If any person is found to be suffering from signs of poisoning, he should be immediately hospitalised. If the person has consumed poison orally, first aid measures can be tried to prevent the absorption of poison from the stomach. Poisons consumed orally may remain in the stomach for varying periods. Therefore, the unabsorbed portions have to be removed quickly. Evacuation of the stomach can be achieved by inducing vomiting.

Vomiting is induced only if the person is conscious. It is contraindicated in poisoning with volatile poisons and corrosives. The patient is to be placed in a left lateral position with his head lowered. The easiest method of inducing vomiting is to stimulate the pharynx by introducing a finger. Another method is to administer two teaspoonful of ground mustard in a glass of warm water. The best method is to give a stomach wash. But this should be done only in a hospital. This procedure has to be carried out carefully as it is associated with dangers like perforation of stomach, aspiration, etc. It must be remembered that the the vomitus and stomach washings should be preserved for chemical analysis.

At present, there are advanced methods of diagnosis and treatment of poisoning. In many hospitals, poison centres equipped with modern diagnostic equipment are functional. The poison consumed can be identified within minutes by analysing blood and urine. This will be very helpful in giving proper treatment without delay. Now effective antidotes are available for most of the poisons.

## Antidotes

These are substances which counteract the effects of poisons. They act in different ways. Some substances neutralise the poisons by forming unabsorbable or inert compounds which are excreted from the body. Antacids like milk of lime, aluminium hydroxide gel, etc. can be given as antidotes in corrosive acid poisoning. Weak acids like vinegar can be administered in poisoning with alkalies.

Oils, fats, milk, egg albumin, etc. have a demulcent action. They form a coating on the stomach mucosa. They prevent absorption of poison and protect the mucosa from the direct action of the poison. Activated charcoal absorbs alkaloids and chemicals. Potassium permanganate oxidises poisons like morphine, strychnine, cyanides, etc. Some antidotes reduce or inhibit the conversion of toxic metabolites. Ethyl alcohol is given as antidote in methyl alcohol poisoning as it will block its oxidation by competitive inhibition.

Other methods like forced diuresis, peritoneal dialysis, hemodialysis, etc. are done in hospitals to remove the poison from the body. Apart from these measures, symptomatic and supportive treatment are also given to save the life of the patient.

## Intimation to Police

All the cases of poisoning are not informed to the police. If the patient is conscious and gives a history of suicidal or accidental poisoning, it is not mandatory to inform the police. But the doctor will record the history, clinical findings, treatment given, prognosis, etc. carefully in detail. If the condition of the patient deteriorates or if he becomes unconscious, the matter is intimated immediately. All cases of death due to poisoning, whatever be the manner will be intimated to the police as per **Sec. 174 of Criminal Procedure Code.**

According to **Section 39 of Cr. PC,** a doctor is legally bound to inform all cases of homicides or homicidal attempts. Therefore, if the patient or the relatives give a history or raise a suspicion of homicidal poisoning, the matter has to be reported to the police. If the patient is unconscious, doctor should invariably inform the police, as he is not aware of the manner of poisoning. In such instances, he should not rely on the version of the relatives. Whatever be the history given by them, there is no option, but to inform police. Even though the doctor is not legally bound to inform cases of suicidal/accidental poisoning, he cannot withhold information regarding the case when he is questioned by the police. Under Section 161 of CrPC doctors have to provide all the information when they are questioned by a police officer. Withholding information in such instances is an offence. Head constables are also station house officers who can question medical officers.

# POISONS

A poison is any material which has fatal or deleterious effect upon a living organism. Poisons are liquid, solid, animal, mineral or vegetable. They may be consumed, inhaled or absorbed through the skin. Toxicology is the study of poisons. Forensic toxicology is a specialised area of analytical chemistry. Usually, poisons enter the body in a single massive dose. Many poisons in minute quantities can affect the body. A toxicologist detects poison from the body fluids and other samples. Sophisticated and sensitive instruments are needed for this purpose.

Toxic effects of a substance are the undesirable results of a direct effect of that substance. Deleterious effects are produced by the metabolic products of the poison. Toxicity of any substance is estimated by animal experiments. But humans are more vulnerable than animals and the calculations of lethal doses are conservative.

The poisons are classified according to their chemical properties and action as follows:

*Acids:* Sulphuric acid, nitric acid, hydrochloric acid, hydrofluoric acid, oxalic acid, carbolic acid, picric acid, salicylic acid, acetic acid, tartaric acid, citric acid, formic acid.

*Alkalies:* Sodium hydroxide, potassium hydroxide, ammonium hydroxide, ammonium carbonate, calcium hydroxide, potassium carbonate.

*Irritants (metallic):* Arsenic, antimony, mercury, copper, lead, zinc, silver.

*Nonmetallic:* Organo phosphorus compounds, chlorine, bromine, Iodine,

*Organic vegetables:* Castor oil, croton oil, abrus precatorius, colocynth, ergot, semecarpus anacardium, plumbago rosea, colchicum autumnale, gloriosa superba

*Animals:* Snakes, insects, cantharides, mechanical powdered glass, diamond powder, pins and needles, hair.

*Neurotics (somniferous):* Opium and its alkaloids

*Inebriant:* Ethyl alcohol, methyl chloride, ethylene glycol, amyl alcohol, isopropyl alcohol, amyl nitrite, formaldehyde, ether, ethyl chloride, chloroform, carbon tetrachloride, chloral hydrate, barbiturates, paraldehyde, thalidomide, tranqu-

ilizers, antihistamines, amphetamines, naphthaline, benzene, nitroglycerine, petroleum, turpentine, eucalyptus, ethylene glycol.

*Delirients:* Datura, belladona, cannabis, cocaine, camphor, mushrooms, lathyrussativa (kesari dal)

*Spinal:* Nux vomica (strychnine), brucine, physostigmine, gelsmium

*Cardiac:* Tobacco (nicotine), digitalis, quinine, aconite, nerium odorum (white or pink oleander), cerbera thevetia (yellow oleander), cerbera odollam (othalanga - in Malayalam), hydrocyanic acid (cyanides)

*Asphyxiants:* Carbon dioxide, carbon monoxide, nitrous oxide, sulphur dioxide, tear gases,

*Peripheral poisons:* Hemlock (conium maculatum), curare.

## Common Poisons

### Corrosive Acids and Alkalies

Strong corrosive acids and alkalies can damage or destroy tissues. The severity of the damage depends upon the strength of the substance. When stronger corrosives are consumed, the tissues of the alimentary tract are destroyed immediately and the victim cannot be saved. The substances can cause perforation of the stomach and intestines resulting in severe inflammation of the peritoneum. If the victim survives, strictures of the oesophagus, cardiac and pyloric sphincters can develop subsequently. Acids can be organic or inorganic. Common inorganic acids are sulphuric, hydrochloric, nitric and hydroflouric acids. Organic acids are carbolic, oxalic, formic and acetic acids. Fatal dose of concentrated sulphuric acid is 20–30 ml. Consumption of even 5 ml of strong acid can cause death.

**Vitriolage** is throwing acids or other corrosives on a person. Usually, acids are thrown on the face. This can cause severe acid burns and permanent scarring and disfigurement. Legally, this is classified as grievous hurt. If the corrosive falls on the eye, cornea will be destroyed leading to permanent blindness. Immediate treatment is irrigation of the area with plenty of water or soap solution followed by washing with 1% solution of sodium bicarbonate.

## Zinc Phosphide (Rat Poison)

Zinc phosphide is a fine crystalline greyish black powder with a garlicky smell, practically insoluble in water. It is used as a rat poison. It is a common suicidal poison. Accidental poisoning is rare. Zinc phosphide when consumed will react with the hydrochloric acid of stomach and phosphine ($PH_3$) gas is liberated. The gas is absorbed into the bloodstream. Zinc phosphide is not absorbed from the stomach. Aluminium phosphide having the same properties as that of zinc phosphide is also used as a rat poison. Phosphine will damage the blood vessels and membranes of RBCs. Clinical findings include anorexia, nausea, vomiting, abdominal colic, diarrhoea, lethargy, ataxia, dyspnoea, dysrrhythmias, convulsions and coma. Death is due to tissue anoxia. Medicolegal importance is that the poison is not absorbed from stomach and hence it will not be detected in blood, liver or kidneys during chemical analysis. Therefore, it is difficult to exclude postmortem administration of the poison.

## Arsenic

Arsenic is an extremely poisonous semi-metallic element. It has many industrial uses and is commonly used in the manufacture of glass and as a semiconductor in electronics. In the past, organic arsenic compounds like arsphenamine and acetarsone were used in the treatment of syphilis. Lead arsenate and calcium arsenate are used extensively as insecticides. Arsenious trioxide or white arsenic is the poisonous "arsenic" in detective stories. It is used as a pigment in pesticides and preservative of hides and wood. Arsenic pentoxide is also used in insecticides, herbicides, metal adhesives and pigments. Arsenic is poisonous in doses larger than 60 mg and the poisoning can arise from a sigle large dose or from repeated small doses. White arsenic is an odourless, tasteless white powder. When consumed, it is absorbed from the stomach and intestines. It is deposited in all internal organs and connective tissue including bones, hair and nail. Acute poisoning is characterised by abdominal pain, nausea, vomiting and diarrhoea. The vomitus and stools will be blood stained. Pain and weakness of muscles are characteristic symptoms. These are followed by circulatory collapse and death.

As arsenic has no colour, smell or bad taste and hence it is used as a homicidal poison. It is mixed with food and administered to the victim. As the symptoms resemble those of acute gastroenteritis or cholera, poisoning is usually not suspected. Consumption of 200 mg of arsenic can cause death within 24 hours. If the poison is administered in small doses for a longer period, death will be delayed. The symptoms of chronic poisoning will resemble debilitating natural disease. Examination of urine, stools, blood, hair, nails can reveal the presence of arsenic.

As the hair and nails grow at known rates, it is possible to find out when a person was poisoned by locating the presence of arsenic on a shaft of the hair of the poisoned victim. Hair grows at the rate of 0.37 mm per day, so a 2.5 cm long hair would provide a record of 60 days' growth. The shaft of hair is cut into lengths of 3 mm and analysed for arsenic. This will show poisoning during one week.

Even though there are several modern tests like atomic absorption spectroscopy, mass spectrometry and neutron activation analysis, the good old **Marsh test** is still used as a screening test.

## Carbon Monoxide

Carbon monoxide is a colourless, odourless gas, a chemical compound of carbon and oxygen. It is about 3% lighter than air, and is highly poisonous. Carbon monoxide is formed due to incomplete combustion of carbonaceous substances. Carbon monoxide is an important industrial fuel. It is a constituent of water gas, blast furnace gas, and coal gas. Automobile exhaust gases contain about 4–8% of carbon monoxide. Nowadays catalytic converters are fitted in cars to keep the level below one percent. Inhalation of air containing more than 1% of carbon monoxide may prove fatal in less than 30 minutes. Carbon monoxide is a major constituent of the air pollution in urban areas.

When inhaled, carbon monoxide combines with hemoglobin in the blood producing carboxy hemoglobin, preventing absorption of oxygen and causing anoxia. Affinity of carbon monoxide for hemoglobin is 250 times higher than oxygen. If the saturation of carboxyhemoglobin exceeds 50–60%

death will result. Old and debilitated people may die even at a 25% saturation. Cigarette smokers will have a level up to 10–15%. The symptoms of poisoning with carbon monoxide will have an insidious onset. At 30–40% concentration, it produces only mild symptoms of headache, nausea, fatigue, followed by unconsciousness. Above 40–50% levels, the victim will develop cardiorespiratory failure and death.

It is said that the driver and the occupants in a motor vehicle can get mild symptoms of poisoning, if there are leakages in the exhaust pipe and defects in the floor. If a car engine is running in a closed garage, the air in that place will become vitiated within a few minutes. Inhalation of exhaust gas is a method of committing suicide. Carbon monoxide is formed during house fires and can cause death of occupants apart from the effects of burns.

The striking external finding is the cherry pink colouration of the skin. In death due to carbon monoxide poisoning, the postmortem staining will be of the same colour. Internally, all the organs will be pink in colour.

### Carbon Dioxide

Carbon dioxide is an inert and non-poisonous gas. But it is an irrespirable gas and >3% concentration in the atmosphere can cause headache, drowsiness, giddiness and loss of muscle power. Concentration of 25–30% can be fatal. Carbon dioxide is heavier than oxygen and it will accumulate in the bottom of deep wells and tunnels. Persons getting into deep wells for cleaning can die. People trying to rescue the victim may also die. Death due to exposure to carbon dioxide can cause death very rapidly. There may not be any marked asphyxial changes. Death could be due to cardiac arrest.

To find out whether oxygen is deficient in the well, before entering, a lighted wick lamp can be placed in a bucket and slowly passed into the well with the help of a long cord. The lamp will be extinguished, if there is no oxygen. This can be used as a warning sign. Oxygen masks should be used by persons entering deep wells. Before rescuing a person, fresh air or oxygen should be pumped into the bottom of the well.

### Hydrogen Cyanide, Hydrocyanic Acid and Cyanides

Solution of hydrogen cyanide gas in water is hydrocyanic acid (prussic acid). It is a highly poisonous, colourless liquid with the smell of bitter almonds or crushed tapioca leaves. Hydrogen cyanide has many industrial uses, including the making of plastics and several important cyanide compounds. Important salts of hydrogen cyanide are potassium cyanide and sodium cyanide which are used in photography, metallurgy and electroplating. Characteristic smell of HCN and cyanides cannot be appreciated by all. The ability to identify the smell is presumed to be genetic. Liquid hydrocyanic acid can be absorbed through the mucus membrane and intact skin. Gaseous form is absorbed through respiratory system. Cyanide salts become poisonous when they are hydrolysed by water or hydrochloric acid in the stomach. Symptoms of cyanide poisoning are usually very rapid and death occurs within minutes. Some persons have survived for 15–20 minutes, even after taking large doses. There will be symptoms of difficulty in breathing, headache, vomiting, dizziness, coma and death.

Death can occur in 30 minutes with 150–300 mg of cyanide. During autopsy, the blood remains pink due to failure of uptake of oxygen. Postmortem staining will be purple red. Pinkish froth will be exuding from mouth and nostrils. Mucosa of the stomach will be congested, mildly corroded with prominent rugae. All internal organs will be congested and bright red with petechial haemorrhages in the surface. Cyanides are consumed to commit suicide. Homicidal administration is not uncommon. Cyanide is mixed with alcoholic beverages and given to the unsuspecting victim.

### PESTICIDES

As a part of green revolution, our country started importing highly toxic pesticides by the beginning of the 1950s. In 1958, a Bharat Sevak Samaj (BSS) youth camp was organised by the army personnel at a place called Sasthamkotta in Kollam district of Kerala. More than 100 campers who ate breakfast died. There were isolated deaths and illness in many parts of the state. Subsequent investigation revealed that Folidol E-605, a highly toxic organophosphorus compound kept in glass containers in the hold of a ship had broken and contaminated wheat flour and sugar bags kept in close proximity of the poison. We are still facing the adverse effects of the indiscriminate use of insecticides for the last half a century. All our ground water sources are contaminated with pesticides. Even the breast milk contains traces of these compounds!! The farmer consumes the insecticides to commit suicide easily!!

Pesticides include insecticides, rodenticides, ascaricides, avicide, molluscicides, virucides, insect repellants, nematicides, herbicides, fungicides, bird repellants, etc. Most common pesticides having medicolegal importance are organophosphorus compounds, organochloro compounds and carbamates.

## Organic Phosphates

*Brand names:* Parathion, malathion, diazinon, monocrotophos, phosphamidon, quinalphos, etc.

Organic phosphates are the most popular and widely used insecticides in the agriculture fields in our country. There are several brand names of these insecticides. Most of the compounds are available as concentrated liquids, the solvent being an aromatic compound having a disagreeable smell. Some solvents have a kerosene like smell. It is diluted with water and sprayed on the plants in the field. The toxin is absorbed through leaves and stem of the plants. The compounds are also available as powders and granules, which are mixed with soil. In that case, the insecticide is absorbed by the plant through the roots. Insects coming into contact with the residual poison are killed. The insects also die when they eat the leaves. Human poisoning occurs by inhalation of the vapours while spraying the insecticide or through the mucus membrane or skin while handling the toxin.

The symptoms of poisoning are constricted pupil, nausea, salivation, vomiting, abdominal colic, diarrhoea, sweating, lacrimation, bronchospasm, increased secretions, hypotension, muscle twitching, fasciculations, muscular weakness, paralysis, headache, dizziness, restlessness, tremor, delirium, ataxia and convulsions. Paralysis of the diaphragm and secretions in the air passages will produce anoxia. Death will be due to respiratory failure. Fatal dose varies considerably in different compounds. Parathion, phorate, diazinon, monocrotophos, quinalphos, etc. are highly toxic. Consumption of 100 mg can cause death. Malathion, primiphos, phanthoate are less toxic. Fatal dose is 3–30 gm. These compounds are mostly used as suicidal poisons and rarely used for homicidal administration as they have a pungent smell and bad taste.

## Organochloro Compounds

*Brand names:* DDT, endine, dieldrin, lindane, BHC, chlordane, endosulfan, aldrin, heptachlor.

Chlorinated hydrocarbons were popular insecticides once. Nowadays many of the old compounds are not marketed. DDT was the most popular insecticide among the group. Of these BHC, endrine, etc. are used as suicidal poisons. Fatal dose for endrine and dieldrine is 2–6 gm. DDT and BHC require a large dose to cause death (15–30 gm). Fatal dose of endosulfan is 3–30 gm.

Long-term exposure to compounds like endosulphan can produce deleterious effects on the body. Endosulphan spraying in the large cashew plantations is alleged to have caused many diseases in the local population. Homicidal administration of these compounds is rare as they have a pungent smell and bad taste.

## Carbamate Insecticides

*Brand names:* Furadan (carbofuran), carbaryl, carbosulfan, dimetan, propoxur.

Carbamate insecticides are also widely used in agriculture. Most of these insecticides are commonly sold in the market as powders and granules. The insecticide is added to the soil.

Carbofuran (furadan) is a popular suicidal poison in many agricultural areas. It is available as violet granules and gives a tell tale evidence on examining the hands and oral cavity of the person who has consumed the compound. Autopsy will reveal violet discolouration of the oesophagus and stomach mucosa. The other autopsy findings will be similar to those of poisoning with an OP compound. Fatal dose of furadan is 30 gm.

## PLANT POISONS

### Abrus Precatorius/Rosary Pea (Malayalam: Kunnikkuru)

These are seeds of a slender climber. The seeds are about 5–8 mm in diameter, round to oval in shape, red in colour with a black spot on one end. The seeds contain a poisonous principle 'abrin'. This can destroy red blood corpuscles of blood. The action of abrin resembles viper venom. The seeds are harmless if swallowed. Abrin will be liberated only if the seeds are chewed or crushed and the pericarp is broken. Boiling will also destroy the poison. When taken orally, there will be nausea, vomiting and haemorrhagic diarrhoea. Fall in blood pressure, convulsions and coma will develop soon. Death may be due to circulatory failure.

In villages of northern India, abrus seeds are used for poisoning cattle. The seeds are ground and made into the shape of needles known as **sui.** These are introduced under the skin of cattle. There will be severe local reaction simulating a snake bite. There will be erythema, edema, oozing of serum and necrosis of tissues. The affected animal dies soon and foul play is seldom suspected, as the symptoms will be those of snake bite. Abrus seeds cause accidental poisoning in children.

### Datura Stramonium/Fastuosa (Devil's apple) (Malayalam: Ummam)

Datura is a wild plant grown all over the country. There are two varieties; D. fastuosa and D. stramonium. D. fastuosa having white flowers is called D. alba and with purple flowers is called D. niger. All parts of the plant are poisonous. The fruit is spherical in shape, green in colour and covered with multiple thorns. It is known as **thorn apple.** The fruit contains more than 100 seeds resembling chilly seeds. The seeds contain mainly three toxic principles; **atropine, hyoscine** and **hyosciamine.** Consumption of 40–50 seeds can stupefy a person. Consumption of 40–50 seeds can cause death within 24 hours.

Datura seeds are consumed for committing suicide. Accidental poisoning occurs in children.

It is used as a stupefying agent for robbing and cheating people. Usual modus operandi in train robberies is to mix the datura seeds with sweets and given to the unsuspecting co-passengers. The drowsy or stupefied victim is robbed off his money or articles. Homicidal poisoning is also common in northern parts of India.

### Strychnos Nux Vomica (Strychnine tree) (Malayalam: Kanjiram)

This is a tree grown in India, Sri Lanka and Indonesia. It attains a height of 18–20 feet. The fruits of the plant when ripe, are red in colour and contains three or four seeds. The seeds are circular, disc shaped, 2 to 2.5 cm in diameter having a thickness of 0.5 cm. The seeds have a thick covering. The pulp, which is very bitter to taste, contains two highly poisonous principles; **strychnine** and **brucine.** All parts of the plant are poisonous. Consumption of 60–100 mg of strychnine (2 gm of powdered seed) can cause death in 2 hours. Symptoms of strychnine poisoning are similar to those of the disease tetanus. The onset of tetanus will be gradual with a history of injury and infection. Muscles of the neck and lower jaw (lock jaw) are affected first and between the contractions muscles will be rigid. Death due to tetanus will be delayed for few days.

Accidental poisoning is possible in children. Rodenticides and dog poisons containing strychnine are available in the market even though the sale of such drugs is prohibited. A brand called **Dogkill** containing strychnine, available in the market is being used by people to commit suicide. Pet dog poisoning and cattle poisoning are not uncommon.

### White/Red Oleander (Nerium Odoruml Indicum) (Malayalam: Chuvanna/Vella arali)

There are two varieties of oleanders, viz white/ red oleander and yellow oleander. These plants are widely cultivated as ornamental plant. Red/white oleander flowers are used in temples as an offering and to make floral garlands. This is a shrub grown in all warm regions. It has lanceolate thick leaves. The flowers have different colours; red, pink and white. They are seen in large clusters at the tip of the branches. All parts of the plant are poisonous.

Animals eating 50–100 gm of leaves of the plant can die. There are two active principles; **nerin** and **oleandrin**. The leaves and bark of the roots are used in some ayurvedic medicinal preparations.

The toxic principles act on the gastrointestinal tract and heart. Abdominal pain, vomiting, diarrhoea, difficulty in swallowing, salivation are the initial symptoms. Pulse becomes slow rapid and irregular. Rhythm of the heart is affected. Muscular twitchings and convulsions are also seen. Person will become drowsy and comatose. Fatal quantity is not certain; however 5–10 gm of the root can cause death. Roots of the plant are ground into a paste and consumed to commit suicide. Cattle will die if they eat the leaves; though not palatable. Even dry leaves are poisonous.

### Yellow Oleander (Cerbera Thevetia, Thevetia Nerifolia) (Malayalam: Manja Arali)

The leaves and flowers of yellow oleander are different from the red oleander. The plant has linear, lanceolate leaves with yellow bell-shaped flowers and green globular fruits. The fruit contains one to two nut like seeds. Plant stem exudes a milk-like sap, which can produce allergic reaction. All parts of the plant are highly poisonous. The active principles are two glycosides; **thevetin** and **cerberin**. Seeds contain another toxic principle; **thevetoxin**. Symptoms are similar to those of red oleander. Consumption of one seed can cause death of a child and 5 to 10 seeds can cause death to an adult. Usually, the root is consumed for committing suicide.

Death can occur within hours due to heart block and peripheral circulatory failure. Accidental poisoning is common among children who eat the nut. The roots are used for inducing abortion. It is also used as a cattle poison.

### Cerbera Odollum (Malayalam: Othalanga/ Chattanga)

Cerbera odollum is a tree seen in the coastal areas of India and Southern Asia. It grows in the swamps and marshy areas and is known as the 'suicide tree'. It grows to a height of 10–15 meters. The dark green leaves and fruits resemble those of mango tree. Leaves have a milky white latex sap. Unlike mango tree, it has large white flowers growing in clusters with a faint jasmine like smell. The dark green fruit has one or two dull white kernels inside. The kernel also resembles mango kernel. The kernel contains a higly toxic principle **cerberin** affects the conducting system of the heart.

The kernel has a very bitter taste. It is mixed with jaggery or sugar and consumed to commit suicide. Due to the bitter taste, it is difficult to administer the kernel in deceit for homicidal purpose. But cases of homicidal poisoning have been reported. Accidental poisoning is possible in children who eat the fruit kernel. On consumption, person develops nausea, vomiting, abdominal pain, diarrhoea, bradycardia, general weakness, irregular respiration and death due to cardiac failure. One kernel can cause death. Usually death occurs in a few hours. Sometimes it will be delayed for a day or two. In Kerala, the incidence of suicidal poisoning with odollum is very common. More than 50 deaths occur every year. The majority of the victims are women. The survivors will be double the number. Persons who develop severe vomiting on consumption may survive.

### Croton Tiglium (Purging Croton) (Malayalam: Neervalam)

This plant is grown in India, Indonesia, China and Philippine Islands. This is a small tree which can grow up to 5 to 6 meters in height. The fruit of this plant is a three celled capsule, each cell having a single seed which yields croton oil. In ayurvedic medicine, croton seed is an ingredient of a powerful purgative. The oil contains toxic principles; crotin, crotonoside, crotonol and crotonoleic acid. Root, bark and leaves also have the properties of the seeds.

The action of crotin is similar to that of abrin and ricin. After oral consumption, nausea, vomiting and purging with abdominal pain will develop immediately. Death will be due to circulatory failure. Croton oil is a vesicating agent and will produce erythema and blisters on the skin. Eating 4 to 5 seeds can cause death in few hours to 2 to 3 days. Accidental poisoning is possible due to the consumption of croton oil instead of castor oil. Suicides and homicides are rare with croton oil. In olden times, croton oil was used as an abortifacient.

### Ricinus Communis (Castor plant) (Malayalam: Avanakku)

The name 'ricinus communis' means 'common tick' because the seed of the plant resembles a tick. Castor plant is a shrub grown in many tropical and warm temperate regions of the world. It can grow up to 2 to 5 meters in height. The stems and leaves may have reddish and greenish colour. Flowers occur as terminal dense clusters. There will be clusters of red and green spiny fruits. A fruit may contain up to 3 seeds. The seeds of the plant known as castor beans are extremely poisonous. The oil extracted from the seeds was used to light lamps in ancient times. Castor oil has many industrial uses. It is used in making lubricating oils, soaps, inks, plastics, polishes, brake fluids. Castor oil is used as a good purgative.

The residue after extraction of the oil contains a potent toxin 'ricin' which is a highly poisonous principle. Ricin is many thousand times potent than cyanide or snake venom. One milligram of ricin or 5 to 10 crushed seeds can cause death of an adult. Ricin causes destruction of RBCs, bleeding in the gastro-intestinal tract and damage to liver and kidneys. On consumption, abdominal pain, vomiting and diarrhoea develop soon. These are followed by severe dehydration, reduced urine output and fall of blood pressure. Powder of the seed can cause irritation to the eye and respiratory passage. Accidental poisoning in children is not uncommon. Suicidal poisoning is rare. Castor oil is used as an abortifacient.

### Calotropis Gigantea/Procera Milkweed (Malayalam: Erukku)

Calotropis is a shrub grown as a wasteland weed in tropics and subtropic regions. The plant grows to a height of 8–10 feet. There are about 200 species in this group. Common species seen in India are C. Procera and C. gigantea. The plant has thick green leaves, white or purple flowers and small seeds. The leaves and the stem will exude a latex like sap. In Ayurveda and Homoeopathy, calotropis is used in many medicinal preparations. The calotropis juice is used as an abortifacient by quacks. The juice is used to anoint abortion sticks.

Calotropis contains the toxic principles; **calactin, calotropin, calotoxin, gigantin** and **uscharin.** The sap known as madar juice is a vesicant. It will cause irritation and blister formation of skin. If taken orally, there will be burning pain in the mouth and abdomen, salivation, nausea, vomiting and diarrhoea. Tetanic convulsions and dilated pupils are the characteristic features of calotropis poisoning. Fatal dose is not certain. If the sap has come into contact with skin, the area should be washed with plenty of water and soothening lotions may be applied. Suicidal poisoning with calotropis is rare. It is taken orally and applied on the mouth of uterus to induce abortion. It is used to produce artificial blisters to simulate injuries. It is used as a cattle poison. Both calotropis gigantea and procera have the same toxic properties.

### Semecarpus Anacardium/Marking Nut (Malayalam: Cherkkuru)

The fruit of this plant is known as 'marking nut' because the juice of the fruit is used by dhobies as a marking ink on the clothes. The active principles of the juice are **semecarpol** and **bhilawanol.** The juice when applied to the skin, irritation and painful blisters are produced. When taken internally, blisters will be caused in the mouth and throat. It is highly irritant to the gastrointestinal mucosa. Severe gastroenteritis is produced. The toxins cause dyspnoea, tachycardia, delirium and hypotension. Consumption of 5–10 gm can cause death in 12–24 hours.

The juice of the nut is used to produce artificial bruise. The blister produced by the juice will simulate a bruise. The fraud can be easily identified by examining the bruise carefully. These blisters will contain acrid serum. As the serum is irritant, will produce scratching and hence scratch marks in the surrounding area can be identified. The fabricated bruise will be seen in accessible areas only. A typical bruise will show colour changes due to the degradation of the blood elements. Semecarpus juice is applied to the mouth of the uterus (cervix) or used to anoint abortion sticks to produce abortion.

### Food Poisoning

Food poisoning is an acute illness caused by the consumption of food contaminated by bacteria, bacterial toxins, virus, mycotoxins, icthyotoxins, poisonous plants and chemical substances. Every year, 60–80 million people are affected worldwide. Death toll is about 6–8 million. Food poisoning can affect one person or as an outbreak in a group of people who ate the same food from a hotel, in a feast or picnic. Usually, the illness has a short incubation period with mild symptoms like nausea, vomiting, abdominal cramps, headache and prostration. Some cases can be serious with neurologic, hepatic and renal involvement leading to death. Infants, old people and persons suffering from diabetes, renal disease or a weakened immune system have a great risk for food poisoning.

Poor hygiene, unsafe food sources, inadequate cooking and improper storage of food are the common causes of food poisoning. Bacterial food poisoning is the commonest and about 20 organisms can cause illness. When food infected with bacteria is consumed, bacteria multiply in the stomach and intestine. Some bacteria liberate toxins when they multiply. As a result of this, the gastrointestinal symptoms develop. Some viral infections can also produce symptoms similar to food poisoning. Contamination of the food is mainly due to inadequate cooking and leaving prepared food at temperatures optimal for bacterial growth. Another source of infection is from the food handlers.

## Poisonous Fish

Poisoning from eating toxic fish is not uncommon. Outbreaks of poisoning due to the consumption of shell fish occurs seasonally. The oysters, mussels, clams, crabs, prawns, etc. feed on certain type of toxin producing marine algae which bloom seasonally. The sea water will be red in colour during those seasons and is called the **red tide**. The algae produce toxins and the fish concentrate the toxins in their body. The toxin is heat stable. The shell fish also acquires disease producing bacteria from the contaminated sea water. The toxin produces gastrointestinal and neurological symptoms which start within 30–60 minutes after consumption. Initial symptoms of paralytic shell fish poisoning include perioral, intraoral and limbs paresthesia, headache, ataxia, vertigo, cranial nerve palsies and paralysis of respiratory muscles. Symptoms of neurotoxic shellfish poisoning will be milder.

## Poisonous Mushrooms

Mushroom is the reproductive portion of an underlying vegetative portion of a fungus. There are many edible varieties, but some are poisonous. They contain potent toxins. Common poisonous varieties are Amanita phalloides, A. muscaria, A. virosa, Galerina autumnalis, G. marginata, Lepoita helviola, L. chlorophyllum, etc. Amanita phalloides contain the toxic principles **amanitin** and **phalloidin**. They inhibit cellular protein synthesis and cause damage to liver and kidneys.

## Cyanogenic Plants

Plants like tapioca, bitter almonds, choke cherry, bamboo shoots contain cyanide producing substances such as amygdalin, prunasin, linamarin, etc. These are hydrolysed to cyanides by an enzyme in the body. Animals are affected easily as their rumen (first stomach) does not contain acid. An animal weighing 100 kg can die by eating 100 gm of leaves which will yield 200 mg of cyanide.

## DETECTION OF POISON

Detection of poisons from the samples of stomach and intestinal contents, liver, kidney, blood, urine and cerebrospinal fluid is done by the forensic toxicologist. The human body metabolises various poisons and the toxicologist identifies the metabolites or derivatives. The analytical procedure has two steps. The identification stage is termed the screening or initial test. The second analytical test is the confirmatory test. The confirmatory test, also provides quantitative measure of the substance. In both tests, there should be analytical consistency. Apart from detecting the physical properties of the poison, the screening tests are crystal tests, chemical spot tests, chromatography (thin layer) and spectroscopy (ultraviolet). The confirmatory tests are enzyme multiplied immunoassay (EMIT), fluorescence polarisation immunoassay (FPIA), cloned enzyme donor immunoassay (CEDIA), radioimmunoassay (RIA), gas chromatography (GC), mass spectrometry (MS), high performance liquid chromatography (HPLC), atomic absorption spectroscopy (AAS), etc.

The common poisonous substances can be categorised into four classes: alcohols, illicit drugs, licit drugs and non-drug poisons.

Alcohols include generally ethanol and methanol. Illicit drugs include barbiturates, amphetamines, cocaine, opiates, cannabis, fentanyls, LSD, etc. Licit drugs are prescription drugs including pain killers, tranquilisers, anticonvulsants, antidepressants, etc. The non-drug poisons include insecticides like organic phosphates, carbamates, carbon monoxide, cyanide salts, plant poisons, etc.

## Chemical Examination

Chemical analysis of all the material objects are carried out in the chemical examiner's laboratory. The head of the institution is the chief chemical examiner to government and he is assisted by the joint chemical examiner and assistant chemical examiners. Toxicological analysis of viscera and body fluids, identification of biological stains, analysis of alcohol under the Abkari Act, etc. Are conducted by them. The certificate of analysis issued by the chemical examiner is used as evidence in any enquiry, trial or other proceedings under section 293 of the criminal procedure code. Under the ordinary circumstances, this certificate need not be proved in a court of law.

## Chemicolegal Examination Rules (1956 ! )

These rules regulate the transmission of materials for chemical analysis. Separate rules are laid down for the guidance of magisterial/police officers and medical officers. Substances for chemical analysis shall not ordinarily be forwarded by the medical officersto the chemical examiner except upon the written requisition of a magistrate or police officer. When a medical officer thinks it necessary to forward some articles for chemical analysis, he should inform the matter to the magistrate or police officer concerned for necessary authorisation. The magistrate/police officer shall invariably issue the requisition and depute a police constable promptly for transmitting the material objects. But if the articles are liable to decomposition rapidly, the medical officer can forward them to the chemical examiner in anticipation of the requisition from police officer/magistrate. In that case, the doctor should at once communicate the matter to the magistrate/police officer.

Police officer has to issue an authorisation to the medical officer and depute a police constable for transmission of articles. Material objects can be transmitted by post also. But the ideal and safe method is to send them through a police constable.

## Collection of Material Objects during Autopsy

The medical officer has to collect viscera and body fluids from the following medicolegal cases subjected to autopsy.

- All cases of suspected poisoning
- All cases of sudden death
- Dead bodies recovered from water when conclusive evidence of drowning is absent
- Traffic accidents and homicides when the stomach contents have smell of alcohol
- All cases of death where no definite cause of death is detected
- All cases of death where an unusual smell, colour or an unidentifiable material is detected in the stomach contents.
- Deaths due to hypersensitivity reaction to drugs/food
- Anaesthetic deaths.

The investigating Police Officer can also request the doctor to forward the viscera irrespective of the cause of death or opinion of the medical officer.

## Materials to be Collected

- Stomach with contents (entire stomach)
- Small intestine (first part of jejunum) 30 cm in length with contents
- 500 gm of liver and one kidney or one-half of each kidney (whole liver, if less than 500 gm)
- Blood — 30 ml
- Urine — 30 ml (if the bladder contains less than that, take as much as possible).

## Forwarding the Material Objects

Viscera, blood, urine and sample of the preservative are collected, preserved, labelled, and packed (see Figs 7.10 to 7.15). To identify each bottle the post-mortem number and bottle number are written on each packed bottle. These can be enclosed in a card board box and transmitted to the chemical examiner's laboratory. Medical officer has to address the chemical examiner advising him about the despatch of the materials. This letter should contain all the relevant details of the case.

The best method of forwarding the materials is through a police constable. The medical officer hands over the material objects to the constable when he reports with an authorisation from his superior police officer. The packed and sealed material objects are handed over to the constable along with the letter to the chemical examiner. The name and number of the constable are to be entered in the letter. Medical officer should keep a register regarding the despatch of these articles. The register should contain the reference number of the case, number of bottles, date of collection, date of despatch of the articles, name and number of the police constable and his signature when he receives the articles for transmission.

In many states the chemical analysis of viscera and body fluids is conducted in the chemistry division of the state forensic science laboratory. In some states like Kerala, chemical examiner's laboratory is an independent establishment under the home department. In Kerala state, the chief chemical examiner's laboratory is situated in the capital. There are regional laboratories at Ernakulam and Kozhikode district headquarters.

The material objects will be accepted by the chemical examiner's laboratory, only if the articles are well preserved, packed, labelled and sealed. If the seals are absent or found broken, the articles will be returned. Therefore, proper care should be taken in packing, labelling and sealing of the material objects. In order to obtain the result of the analysis in murder cases and other sensational cases, the investigating officer has to request the chemical examiner to give priority for the examination.

## Material Objects from Clinical Cases

When the invetsigating officer receives information that a case of poisoning is admitted and treated in the hospital, request the medical officer concerened has to collect materials for chemical analysis. They include the following:

1. Stomach wash
2. Vomitus
3. Faeces
4. Remnants of food, medicine, etc.

To all these materials, rectified spirit should be added as the preservative. If alcoholism is suspected, the preservative shall be saturated saline. Sometimes, the vomitus or purged matter may be mixed with earth as they are brought by the relatives or police. If they are dry and not offensive, preservative need not be added. Faecal matter is sent only when metallic poisoning like arsenic, etc. is suspected. Method of labelling, packing and sealing of these articles is similar to that followed in the case of the viscera.

## Forwarding Materials from Clinical Cases

Procedure of forwarding these articles is the same as that of the autopsy cases. In some hospitals, the medical officers entrust the work to their assistants. In major hospitals, the articles are sent to the office of the superintendent or the head of institution for despatching. Legally this is not correct and may invite criticism. There is a chance of tampering the material objects also. The whole procedure of collecting, preserving, labelling, packing, sealing and forwarding shall be done in the presence and under the direct supervision of the medical officer concerned.
* History of the case
* Interval between the time of consumption of poison and onset of symptoms.
* What were the first symptoms?
* Were any of the following symptoms present?
  – Vomiting and purging
  – Deep sleep
  – Tingling of the skin and throat
  – Convulsion and twitching muscles
  – Delirium and hallucinations
  – Any other symptom?
  – Any other information?

## Interpretation of Results

Chemical examiner will forward his report to the medical officer after analysis of the materials. If poison is detected in the materials, the medical officer will furnish a final opinion as to the cause of death. But sometimes the report will be negative. This can be due to several reasons. In a treated case of poisoning, entire poison might have been metabolised and eliminated from the system. The person could have died due to the complications. This is commonly seen in organophosphorus poisoning. The enzyme, cholinesterase is completely inhibited by the poison and elimination of the poison by treatment alone will not restore the cholinesterase activity and this can lead to death. Sometimes fatal complication like pneumonia will arise.

Because of improper preservation and delay in analysis, some poisons will be destroyed. Cyanides easily volatilise from the viscera and detection will be difficult if analysis is delayed. Drugs administered during treatment can sometimes cause interference to the analysis. If poison is detected only in the stomach, the interpretation is that it could be a case of postmortem administration, because contents of the stomach will be absorbed only during life.

In the case of zinc/aluminium phosphide (rat poison), the material will not be absorbed from the stomach or intestines. Death is due to the release of 'phosphene' produced by the interaction between the phosphide radical and gastric hydrochloric acid. Phosphene is a respiratory poison and is difficult to be detected by the common analytical methods. Usually poison will not enter the small intestine after death. But if the body is putrefied, the stomach contents pass to the intestines even after death. Hence the detection of poison in the small intestine cannot be accepted as a proof of antemortem consumption of poison. But the presence of poison in the liver, kidney, blood and urine indicates that the poison was absorbed, metabolised and excreted. The final opinion as to the cause of death along with a copy of the chemical examiner's report will be forwarded to the investigating officer. The investigation can be completed after obtaining these documents.

## Rules for the Guidance of Magisterial and Police Officers

Substance for chemicolegal examination shall not ordinarily be forwarded by medical officers to the chemical examiner except upon the the written requisition of a magistrate or police officer. Such requisition shall be issued invariably and with promptness if the medical officer considers it advisable to obtain the opinion of the chemical examiner. Conversely, the medical officer is bound to forward substances to the chemical examiner on receipt of a requisition to that effect from a magistrate or police officer, although in his opinion, analysis of viscera is not necessary.

When the substance with regard to which the medical officer considers it advisable to obtain the opinion of the chemical examiner, is one liable to rapid decomposition, he shall forward the substance to the chemical examiner in anticipation of the requisition of the magistrate or police officer. Viscera and other highly decomposable articles shall not be detained by the medical officer longer than 24 hours. In such cases the medical officer shall at once communicate the fact of despatch to the officer authorised under this rule to require an examination and such officer shall thereupon send the required requisition by the next post.

The magistrate or the police officer on instructing medical officers to forward articles for analysis to the chemical examiner shall at the same time, address the latter officer, quoting the number and date of their requisition to the medical officer and shall furnish the chemical examiner with a brief summary of the history of the case, together with the following information:

• Date and hour of crime.
• Date and time of collection of material objects
• They should also specifically mention the urgency, if any, for the certificate, and the return of the articles after examination, if required.
• If the articles are sent after charge sheet is laid in the case, the date of posting of the case should be specified.

*Note:* If the articles are bulky and cannot be conveniently returned by post, the messenger should be directed to wait and take back the articles, if the results are likely to be ready soon. The chemical examiner will give priority to such cases and return the articles through the same messenger. In cases of suspected poisoning, the principal points on which magistrates and police officers shall furnish information to the chemical examiner are as follows:

• What was the interval between the last eating or drinking and the first appearance of symptoms of poisoning?

- What was the interval between the last eating or drinking and death (if this occurred)?
- What were the first symptoms?
- Were any of the following symptoms present? if so, specify which?
  - Vomiting and purging
  - Deep sleep
  - Tingling of the skin and throat
  - Convulsions or twitching of the muscles
  - Delirium and clutching at imaginary objects
- Were any other symptoms noticed?
- Did any other persons partake of the suspected food and drink and did they also suffer from similar or other symptoms of poisoning? Any other information, likely to serve as a guide to the class of poison administered, shall also be furnished. In every case of suspected human or animal poisoning, it is desirable that all the substances requiring analysis shall be packed and forwarded to the chemical examiner by the nearest medical officer. But where veterinary dispensary exists, or where the officer of the veterinary department is available, the post-mortem or other examination of animals shall be conducted and substances transmitted by such officer.

## Suspected Blood or Seminal Stains

Articles requiring examination for the presence of blood or seminal stains may be forwarded direct to the chemical examiner, the following rules being strictly adhered to: When clothes are sent, they shall be sent as a whole and the stains need not be indicated by pencil marks, pins, etc. Stains on wall/floors/ground, or articles of furniture, etc. shall not be scraped off, but the stained area shall be carefully cut out. When the material is brittle, as in the case of earth or *chunam*, it should be carefully wrapped in cotton wool and packed in a box so that the surface may be preserved from damage. Articles of clothing, etc. if wet or moist, be carefully dried before being packed, otherwise the stains rapidly decompose and their nature cannot be determined. Each article requiring separate examination shall be packed separately and labelled. The labels shall be numbered consecutively and shall bear the signature of the forwarding officer, and the number and date of his letter of advice to the chemical examiner. All the packets belonging to one case shall then be enclosed in one box or outer cover unless disparity in the size of the various articles makes this inconvenient. Articles belonging to different cases shall never be forwarded in the same cover. Articles sent for examination must never be used as wrappers. Labels shall not be pasted over instruments suspected to contain any stains. All parcels shall be carefully sealed by the despatching officer and packed in such a manner that they cannot be opened without destroying the seals. The seal used shall be the same throughout, either a private seal or an official seal which is kept in safe custody. Impression of keys, weights, etc. shall not be used. A letter of advice shall be separately forwarded to the chemical examiner. This letter shall contain:

- An impression of the seal used in closing the packets and description thereof.
- A list of the articles forwarded and a statement as to how the articles have been forwarded. The numbers given to the articles on the lot must correspond to the number on the labels.
- Information as to whether any of the weapons, clothes, etc. are to be returned after examination.
- Information as to how many persons or animals were affected, how many died and section of the Indian penal code under which charge, is being brought.
- Crime number
- The date of posting, if any, of the case in the court.
- Information as to whether all or any of the stains were exposed to the sun or rain, and if so for how long?
- If exposed to rain, whether the downpour was heavy or light?
- If it is stained with soil, the nature of the soil, whether loose, porous or hard; whether barren or cultivated? In the case of stained leaves, name of the trees or plants to which the leaf belonged.

## Miscellaneous Examination

Estimation of morphine and other ingredients of opium, examination of ganja and other narcotic drugs, coins, documents, paints, firearms, bullets, etc. in shooting cases, gun barrel residues, fireworks and other explosives, incendiaries, articles involved in cases of explosion, bones, hairs, liquor, illicit arrack samples under the Abkari Act and blood specimens involved in offences in force are conducted by the chemical examiner. In forwarding any miscellaneous article such as mentioned herein before, the magistrates, police officers or excise officers as the case may be, shall include in their letter of advice to the chemical examiner, information as to the nature and object of the examination required, and to furnish any other information likely to assist the chemical examiner in making the required examination.

### Firearm/Ammunition

In the examination of firearm/ammunition, etc. the points on which expert opinion is normally needed are:
- Whether there are blood marks or fingerprints on a weapon;
- Whether a weapon shows signs of recent firing: and if so, the nature of the powder used;
- Whether there is blood or powder on clothing;
- What are the weight and measurement of the projectile; and
- Whether the projectile could have been (or actually was) fired from a particular weapon. All firearms and ammunition shall be handled and packed with special care to prevent surface marking being disturbed or obliterated. The mouth of a firearm barrel shall be corked up with a tight fitting cork.

### Clothing of an Injured Person

Clothing of an injured person shall be carefully examined for the powder or blood marks and signs of burning. When a projectile has passed through any clothing, the appearance of the part through which it has passed shall be carefully examined and described by the magistrate or police officer concerned. Clothing shall be handled with particular care to prevent any flakes of smokeless powder that adhere being shaken off. It shall be carefully preserved and sent for examination. A detailed and accurate observation and record of

every injury is essential for the subsequent inferences to be of value. If the wound is situated on a part of the body which is usually clothed, the examiner can insist on the production of the clothing before he ventures an opinion as to the range at which the shot was fired.

### Samples of Opium

Samples of opium seized in connection with illicit traffic shall in the first instance be sent to the chemical examiner by the excise department. The supply of samples to the united nations research laboratory in connection with the implementation of their scheme for scientific research on narcotics shall be made through the Chief Chemist, Central Revenue's Central Laboratory, New Delhi, to whom a full report of the tests carried out by the chemical examiner shall be supplied along with the samples. Excise officers shall forward the articles seized under the provisions of the abkari act in force through the magistrate within whose jurisdiction the offence has been committed.

### Tissues and Bones

In the examination of tissues and bones, the professors of pathology and anatomy of the medical colleges, may be consulted. The material shall pass through the professor of forensic medicine who shall obtain expert opinion from the specialists and pass on the information to the chemical examiner.

### Water Samples

Magistrates and police officers may send water samples by the public analyst or water analyst as neither of them is a chemical examiner for purposes of Section 293; code of criminal procedure.

## DIRECTIONS TO THE INVESTIGATING OFFICER

### Inquest in Death due to Poisoning

Irrespective of the manner of death, all deaths due to poisoning are reported to the police. The investigating officer has to conduct a detailed inquest before sending the body for autopsy. The main objective of the inquest is to find out the apparent cause of death.

When an unnatural death due to suspected poisoning is investigated, it is essential to find out the nature of poison which caused death. Secret homicides by administration of poison is not uncommon. Poisons like cyanides which cause sudden death can be administered by mixing them with food or drinks or by force. Forcible administration may leave some marks of violence on the body. Face, neck and limbs have to be examined for the presence of contusions and nail marks.

Signs of corrosion and discolouration of face, lips, oral mucosa and hands, if any, have to be noted. Smell of the oronasal froth has to be observed. Postmortem staining will have different hues in different types of poisoning. It will be cherry red in carbon monoxide poisoning and bright red in cyanide poisoning. Chlorates and nitrates will impart a brownish staining.

Even though homicidal poisoning is rare, quick acting poisons like cyanides can be administered forcibly or in deceit. Usually, poison is administered by mixing it with food or drinks. Poisons which have bad taste, foul smell and colour cannot be administered easily. When added to alcoholic beverages, they can be given easily, especially to intoxicated persons. Sometimes poison is administered homicidally, masquerading it as a drug. During inquest, remnants of food, drinks, utensils, vomitus, excreta, clothes worn by the deceased, etc. should be collected and preserved for chemical analysis.

Latent fingerprints should be developed from the containers of poison and utensils and glassware found in the scene. If the person was under treatment in the hospital, request the doctor to collect and preserve stomach washings, blood and urine for chemical analysis. When death is delayed, the poison and its metabolites might be excreted from the body and analysis of postmortem samples may not detect the poison.

After the inquest, the body is sent for autopsy. If the deceased had undergone treatment in a hospital prior to death, copy of the hospital case record may also be sent for the perusal of the autopsy surgeon. It is not proper to request a doctor to conduct autopsy on a person whom he had treated; even though the law does not object to it. In a case of poisoning, even if all the findings are suggestive of poisoning, definite opinion as to the cause of death can only be furnished after chemical analysis. But if the poison is not detected during chemical analysis, an inference as to the cause of death can only be formed from the clinical findings and autopsy findings. When the nature of the poison is identified, the source of poison should be found out. The manner of death is a material point which has to be ascertained by the investigating officer by a thorough field investigation.

Investigating officer should be cautious and diligent in the investigation of death due to alleged poisoning. Many cases which appear to be prima facie suicides, could be homicides. The following points are to be ascertained:

- Whether death was due to poisoning?
- If hospitalised, what were the clinical findings?
- Did the clinical findings indicate poisoning?
- Was the blood or urine of the patient analysed? If so what was the poison?
- What was the route of administration—oral/injection/inhalation?
- What was the last meal? When was it consumed?
- How long did the victim survive?
- Has the victim given any statement?
- What is the source of the poison? household? purchased?
- Who has purchased it? Bill? Other proof?
- Do the autopsy findings tally with the clinical findings of poisoning?
- What is the cause of death as per the autopsy report?
- Is there any evidence of violence or forcible administration?
- What is the result of chemical analysis?
- Does the result tally with the autopsy findings?
- What is the manner of death?

The following steps may be taken during inquest and subsequent investigation:
- Photographs of the scene, dead body, remnants of poison, bottles, vomitus, excreta, etc.
- Develop latent fingerprints on the bottles, utensils, etc.
- Collect, preserve and pack the remnants of food, poison, excreta, vomitus, etc. for analysis.

- Collect the clothes worn by the deceased for chemical analysis.
- Request the autopsy surgeon to collect viscera and body fluids for chemical analysis.
- Request the doctor to collect hair and finger/ toe nails for analysis, if heavy metal poisoning is suspected.
- Request the chemical examiner to conduct a quantitative estimation of the poison when, alcohol, narcotic drugs, etc. are suspected.
- Record the statement of the victim of poisoning undergoing treatment in the hospital.
- Request the treating doctor to preserve the stomach washings for chemical analysis.
- Request the treating doctor to collect blood and other body fluids for chemical analysis.
- Examine the treating doctor U/S 161 Cr.PC and obtain his opinion as to the possible nature of the poison inferred from the signs and symptoms.
- Send a request to the chemical examiner to expedite the analysis and furnish the result at the earliest.
- Examine the autopsy surgeon U/S 161 Cr. PC and obtain his opinion regarding the cause of death, nature of poison, the fatal dose and fatal period of the poison.
- Conduct a detailed inquiry into the circumstances of death by a thorough field investigation.
- In the case of suicides, a 'psychological autopsy' can be conducted !! (legally not required).
- Documentation of injuries especially those on *In cases of food poisoning:* Death due to food poisoning can become a medicolegal issue when

it happens under suspicious circumstances. Mass fatalities can also occur due to consumption of common food. A detailed inquest is to be held. A detailed history of the incident should be obtained from the witnesses. Vomitus, faeces, remnants of the food, vessels used for cooking, raw food materials, etc. should be collected and preserved for microbiological analysis. Help and guidance from the forensic pathologist and microbiologist may be obtained. Dead bodies should be sent for routine autopsy. The autopsy surgeon should be informed about the possibility of food poisoning so that he will give special attention should be given to the changes in the GI tract, liver and kidneys. He may be asked to collect samples of stomach and intestinal contents, blood, liver, spleen, etc. for chemical and microbiological analysis.

### Method of Collection of Samples for Microbiological Analysis

- Collect the specimens aseptically using sterile implements.
- Collect in sterile glass containers.
- Sterile swabs from the utensils used for keeping the food.
- Specimens should be kept at 2–8 °C.
- The containers should be labelled properly.
- No preservative need be added.
- Covering letter shall contain the details of the case.

**Outbreak of food poisoning should be reported to the health authorities immediately!!**

# Narcotic Drugs and Psychotropic Substances

**Narcotic Drugs and Psychotropic Substances Act 1985** consolidates and amends the old laws relating to narcotic drugs and makes stringent provisions for the control and regulation of operations relating to narcotic drugs, psychotropic substances and related matters. Another law called "Prevention of Illicit Traffic in Narcotic Drugs and Psychotropic Substances Act was enacted in 1988. This law provides for the detention of drug traffickers. NDPS Act was amended in 1988 incorporating certain new provisions to make the law more stringent.

**Narcotics Control Bureau (NCB)** is a central authority set up by the Government of India in 1988 to coordinate the functioning of the various state and central drug enforcement agencies. NCB is also engaged in the prevention and control of drug abuse and trafficking by enforcing the provisions of the NDPS Act.

**Central Bureau of Narcotics (CBN)** supervises the licit cultivation of opium in India. CBN is the competent authority to issue license for the manufacture, import and export of narcotic drugs. CBN also plays a major role in the survey, detection and destruction of illicit poppy cultivation and suppression of drug trafficking.

## NARCOTIC DRUGS AND PSYCHOTROPIC SUBSTANCES

Narcotic drugs include a variety of substances which when consumed will produce an altered state of consciousness. Most of the narcotic drugs are useful in the practice of medicine for the relief of pain. Some of them are used for suppressing cough. When narcotic drugs are used by a person for medical purposes, he will experience a state of euphoria for a short period. This will induce the person to use the drug again and again. A larger dose will induce sleep. But before that, other symptoms such as drowsiness, lethargy, decreased physical activity, etc. will develop. A high dose can cause respiratory depression and death. Psychotropics are substances which when consumed will produce hallucination, disorientation to time and space, uncontrolled emotions and psychotic reactions leading to violent behaviour

## Drug Addiction

Drug addiction is the repeated consumption of a drug resulting in physical and psychological dependence. Almost all narcotic drugs, psychotropic substances, alcohol and tobacco, if taken repeatedly will lead to addiction.

## Drug Abuse

Drug abuse is the improper and excessive use of therapeutic drugs. But usually the use of non-medical or illegal drugs is termed drug abuse even when the use is moderate and not harmful. Addiction will produce a physical dependence which is a biological phenomenon. When the use of drug is abruptly stopped, many unpleasant symptoms will develop. These are known as withdrawal symptoms, which are opposite to the effects of the drug itself. Psychological dependence is a compulsive need for a drug in order to maintain a state of well being or euphoria. This is the first stage of development of addiction. The present time terminology for addiction, habituation and abuse is 'drug dependence'.

## Drug Dependence

Dependence is a group of cognitive, behavioural and physiological symptoms that indicate that a person has impaired control of the use of a psychoactive substance and continues the use of that substance despite adverse consequences. Drug dependence is a major problem which has social, moral and ethical ramifications. Repeated use of drugs produces mental, physical and moral deterioration leading to sexual perversions and crimes. Continuous use of these drugs will produce **tolerance** and the user will consume progressively larger doses to get the desired effects.

Narcotic drugs are administered by oral route, sniffing, smoking and injections. The addicts will also suffer from malnutrition, infection and diseases. By using contaminated and non-sterile syringes and needles diseases like viral hepatitis, AIDS, etc. will be contracted. Many conditions and circumstances like slums, easy access, peddlers, organised crime, etc. have been blamed as the factors responsible for the drug problem. But no single cause or condition, leading to drug dependence has been found out as this problem is seen in all social and economic classes. Many persons are exposed to drugs by reason of medical use, but only a minority becomes addicts. Even though drugs are available easily, only a small percentage of individuals joins the rank of abusers. It is believed that persons having emotional instability or those who suffer from some psychiatric disorders become addicts. Addicts often reveal a history of broken families, childhood deprivation, over-protectivenes, etc. Anxiety, frustrations, inner conflicts, etc. are contributory factors.

## Drug Trafficking

The spread of drug abuse across the whole world is threatening the quality of human life in many ways. This menace not only destroys the individual, but also disrupts families and the social structures of the communities. The nations suffer from huge economic losses in terms of lost productivity, loss of life and property in narcotics-related crimes. Total number of drug users in the world at present is about 185 million, equivalent to 3% of world's population.

Drug abuse and trafficking have been slowly spreading across Indian sub-continent during the past decades. India is one of the countries where illicit cultivation of poppy and cannabis is rampant. India is also a transit point in the Middle East-South Asia illicit drug trafficking. To take effective action against this menace, old laws like opium laws are inadequate. Moreover, apart from the conventional drugs of addiction, many newer drugs have appeared on the scene. In order to have a deterrent effect, it has become necessary to award severe penalties to the habitual offenders engaged in the supply and trafficking of drugs.

## OPIUM

Opium is the best known source of many substances which relieve pain. The word opium is derived from the Greek word *"opos"* means juice. In Arabic, it is known as *"afyun"*. In Sanskrit, it is called *"aahi phenam"* meaning snake venom!! In Malayalam and Tamil, it is known as *"karuppu"* or *"aveen"* (Figs 29.1 and 29.2). The first recorded use of opium dates back to third century BC in the writings of Theophrastus. Chinese literature has described the use of opium as early as 2700 BC. Arab physicians were well versed in the use of opium. They introduced this drug into the orient. At that time, opium was used as a remedy to control diarrhoea. Even by the beginning of the Christian era, many segments of the world population were addicted to this drug.

Opium is consumed orally or by smoking. The effects include euphoria, drowsiness, nausea, itching, constipation and respiratory depression. Opium is believed to prolong the duration of the sex act and hence it is consumed by young persons who eventually become addicts. Opium will produce a state of excitement and increased sense of well-being immediately on consumption.

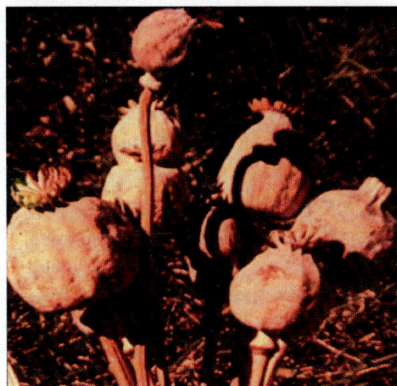

**Fig. 29.1:** Poppy capsules

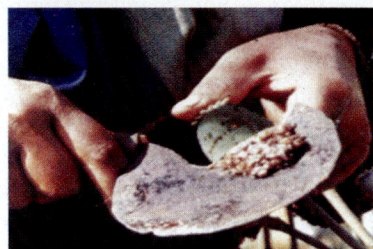

**Fig. 29.2:** Extraction of opium

This is followed by drowsiness and sleep. Symptoms of overdose are slow and shallow breathing, clammy skin, convulsions, and coma. One to two gramm of opium can cause death. Injections of morphine, heroin, codeine and other derivatives will also produce the same symptoms. Addicts will develop tolerance and can tolerate large quantities.

Withdrawal symptoms are watery eyes, running nose, loss of appetite, yawning, irritability, tremors, panic, chills, sweating and cramps. Opium is refined to yield about 20 alkaloids. Among these, majority are narcotics like morphine, codeine and thebaine which are depressants of central nervous system. The rest are smooth muscle relaxants like papaverine, narcotine, noscapine, etc. These are not addictive substances.

### Morphine(Brand names—morcontin, roxanol, dramorph)—(Slang terms—'M', white stuff, Miss Emma)

Morphine is the chief constituent of opium. Opium yields 15–20% of morphine on chemical processing.

It is a white powder or white shining crystals having a bitter taste. Morphine is ten times as potent as raw opium. It is a depressant of the central nervous system. Like opium, morphine also produces a state of excitement initially, followed by stages of stupor and unconsciousness, leading to death. Fatal dose is 200–250 mg orally or 50–100 mg by injection.

### Codeine (Brand Names—Tylenol, Robitussin) (Slang terms—clay, school boy)

Codeine is found in raw opium in concentrations ranging from 0.7 to 2.5%. Although it occurs naturally, it is manufactured from morphine. As compared to morphine, codeine produces less sedation, analgesia and respiratory depression. Usually, it is consumed by oral route or by injection. It is smoked by some addicts. Codeine is available as odourless white crystals, crystalline powder, tablets, capsules or in solution as in cough syrups. It is available in combination with other products. APC tablets contain aspirin, phenacetin and codeine. As codeine has central action to suppress cough, it is a main ingredient in cough syrups (e.g. linctus codeine). Codeine is also manufactured to a lesser extent in injectable form for the relief of pain. Addiction to codeine is not uncommon. Many addicts consume large quantity of cough syrups containing codeine. In large quantities it can produce euphoria and stupor. The other symptoms are respiratory depression, nausea, itching, constipation, etc. The action lasts for 3–6 hours. The addicts can be identified by the constricted pupils. Withdrawal symptoms include watery eyes, running nose, loss of appetite, yawning, irritability, tremors, panic, chills, sweating and cramps.

### Thebaine

Thebaine is a minor constituent of opium. Raw opium yields 0.5 to 1% thebaine. Thebaine is chemically close to codeine and morphine, but it is not a depressant of the central nervous system. It can produce tetanic spasms due to its convulsant action. Even though it is not a drug of abuse, it can be converted to therapeutically useful narcotic drugs. Hence thebaine also comes under the purview of NDPS Act. The allied products are papaverine and narcotine. Papaverine is an isoquinoline alkaloid, used as a smooth muscle relaxant used in medical practice. Narcotine has a toxic effect only in higher doses.

## SEMISYNTHETIC AND SYNTHETIC NARCOTICS

Substances which are derived by modification of the chemical constituents of opium are called semisynthetic narcotics. In contrast to the pharmaceutical substances produced directly from the narcotics of natural origin, synthetic narcotics are entirely produced in laboratories by chemical process. They are chemically related to opium alkaloids and are called opioid analogues. Research till today has not produced a drug which has analgesic properties of morphine, but without the dangers of tolerance and dependence or susceptible to abuse. Opioid analogues are mainly used for relief of moderate to severe pain. Some of them are used in anaesthesia. Adverse effects include nausea, vomiting, constipation and drowsiness. Larger doses can cause respiratory depression. Their euphoric effect has led to abuse. Dependence will develop after prolonged use. Several synthetic analogues called 'designer drugs' have been manufactured illicitly in clandestine laboratories for recreational use. They are highly potent and addictive. Most of them can cause respiratory depression and death.

### Heroin (Diacetyl morphine) Slang terms— Horse, Smack, Junk, Dope, Brown sugar

Heroin is the most popular drug of addiction synthesised from morphine. Pure heroin is a white powder with a bitter taste. Illicit heroin is brown in colour and hence the name 'brown sugar'. Many diluents like cocoa, starch, milk powder and brown sugar are added to increase the weight. It is manufactured in clandestine laboratories all over the world. It is four times powerful in action than morphine. It is usually injected, sniffed or smoked. The euphoria produced is higher than any other narcotic. The other symptoms are drowsiness, nausea and respiratory depression. Pupils will be constricted. Heroin will cause high physical psychological dependence.

Many new users begin by sniffing or smoking heroin. These methods are also addictive. For getting a rapid effect, regular users inject the drug subcutaneously or intravenously (main lining). The effect of heroin is felt within one minute after the injection. The intense euphoria lasts for several minutes followed by a period of sedation. There will be a sensation of warmth and intense pleasure. It is said to relieve feelings of despair and worthlessness. There is a saying that **'it is so good, don't even try it once'**. Once a person becomes an addict, withdrawal of the drug will cause painful physical symptoms. Symptoms include abdominal cramps, nausea, vomiting, sweating, restlessness, tremors, nasal congestion, changes in the heart rate and blood pressure, etc.

Many serious medical problems like hepatitis, cirrhosis, renal failure, retinal damage, endo- carditis, HIV/AIDS are associated with heroin addiction. Addicts can be identified from the physical signs and symptoms. There will be multi- ple venipuncture marks or thrombosed veins (tracks). The addicts tattoo the injection sites to mask the puncture marks. They will be possessing paraphernalia like spoons, syringes, needle, etc.

## PSYCHOTROPIC (PSYCHOACTIVE) SUBSTANCES

Psychotropic substance is a drug or substance which when ingested, affects mental process, cognition and affect. These include hallucinogens, stimulants, sedatives, and hypnotics. In the context of international drug control, this refers to substances controlled by the international conventions on psychotropic substances.

### Depressants

Depressants are substances which have a depressant effect on the central nervous system. Depressants are prescribed by the physicians for the treatment of sleeplessness, anxiety, irritability and tension. Among the depressants, the most commonly used are a broad range of barbiturates, benzodiazepines, methaqualone, meprobamate, glutethimide, chloral hydrate, etc.

If an excessive dose is taken, these drugs will produce a state of intoxication similar to that of alcohol. As in the case of alcohol, the effects may vary from person to person and from time to time in the same individual. Low doses will produce mild sedation; higher doses will produce euphoria. But sometimes they may produce depression of mood. In contrast to narcotics, high doses will invariably cause slurred speech, muscular incoordination, impaired judgement, drowsiness, sleep, stupor, coma and death. If an addict cease to take the drug, severe withdrawal symptoms will be precipitated. These symptoms are characterized by anxiety, agitation, apprehension, nausea, vomiting, palpitation, insomnia, fainting and muscle spasms. If the addict was using a large amount of the drug, delirium, psychotic behaviour, convulsions and death will occur.

### Barbiturates (Brand names —Amytal, Seconal, Pentothal, Luminal, etc.) Slang terms—barbs, yellows, yellow jackets, reds, red birds

Barbiturates are derivatives of barbituric acid. About 2500 derivatives of barbituric acid have been synthesised. Of these only a few remain in clinical use. They are mostly sedatives and hypnotics. In smaller doses, the drug will allay tension and anxiety. Larger doses will produce sleep. As in the case of alcohol, some persons may experience a state of excitement before sedation takes effect. If dosage is increased, the effects will progress through different stages of sedation, sleep, coma and death due to respiratory depression and cardiovascular complications. Reddish areas and blisters on the skin are characteristic features in unconscious victims.

Barbiturates are classified as ultra-short-acting, short-acting, intermediate-acting and long-acting. The ultra-short- acting barbiturates such as thiopental, thiamytal, methohexital, hexobarbital, etc. will produce anaesthesia within a minute after intravenous administration of the drug. The rapid onset and brief duration of action preclude the abuse of these drugs.

The short-acting and intermediate-acting barbiturates like pentobarbital, secobarbital, amobarbital, butabarbital, allobarbital, aprobarbital and vinbarbital are widely abused. Long-acting barbiturates are used in clinical practice as sedatives, hypnotics and anticonvulsants. Barbital, phenobarbital, methyl phenobarbital and metharbital belong to this group.

## Stimulants

Stimulants are chemicals which stimulate the central nervous system. The two most common stimulants are nicotine contained in tobacco, and caffeine contained in tea/coffee. When used in moderation, they produce effects of relief from fatigue and increased alertness. There are a wide variety of stimulants which produce mood elevation and a heightened sense of well-being. But almost all of them will eventually lead to physical dependence. The stimulants are available from medical stores only on prescription. But they are also clandestinely manufactured and available in the illicit market.

Abusers rely on stimulants to feel 'stronger and confident'. They always follow a pattern in the use of drugs. They take stimulants in the morning and depressants like alcohol or sleeping pills at night. This will affect the normal body processes and lead to many physical and mental illness. Young people consume stimulants in large quantities which will result in a state of exhilaration, hyperactivity and wakefulness. These effects are intense when the drugs are taken intravenously and known as **rush** or **flash**. This state is followed by a stage of depression called "crashing" which will be very unpleasant. This depressive state is counteracted by a further injection of stimulant. Heavy users may inject the drug every few hours. Common stimulants which are widely abused are cocaine, amphetamines, etc.

Tolerance will develop rapidly in these persons. Larger doses will also result in mental aberrations. Auditory and visual hallucinations with paranoia are the characteristic manifestations. Dizziness, tremor, agitation, panic, headache, flushed skin, sweating, vomiting and abdominal cramps are the symptoms of an overdose. The abuser who uses a high dose regularly, does not return to normal easily even if the drug is withdrawn. Severe apathy, mental depression, fatigue and disturbed sleep are the characteristic withdrawal symptoms. The thought process is also affected.

The psychological dependence caused by the prolonged use of stimulants is very strong leading to anxiety, tension and even suicidal tendency.

### Cocaine(Brand name—Surfacaine) Street Names—bernice, big C, blow, coke, dream, gold dust

Cocaine is the active principle of the South American cocoa plant, erythroxylum cocoa (Fig. 29.3). It is the strongest stimulant of natural origin. Cocoa plants have been cultivated from time immemorial in the Andean mountain ranges and high lands. Natives used to chew the leaves of the plant for refreshment and to relieve fatigue. Active ingredient is extracted as cocaine hydrochloride, which is a white crystalline powder (Fig.29.4). The de-cocainised leaves are used to produce flavouring agents for 'coca cola' type of beverages.

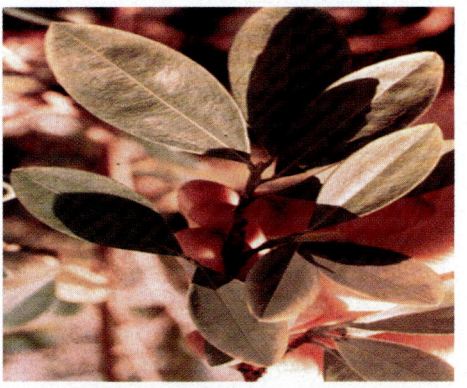

**Fig. 29.3:** Erythroxylon cocoa plant

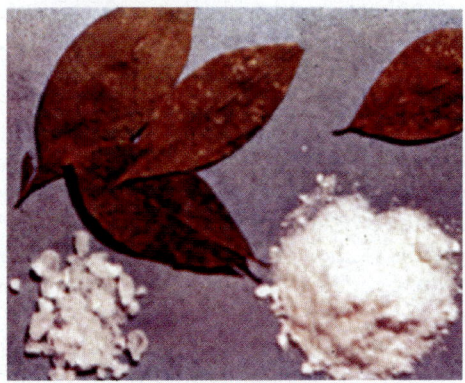

**Fig. 29.4:** Cocoa leaves and cocaine

Cocaine is illicitly manufactured and sold as white crystalline powder containing 5–10% of pure cocaine mixed with other substances like procaine, lidocaine and lactose. The drug is administered orally or by sniffing, snorting or smoking. For heightened effect, the drug is dissolved in water and injected intravenously. It is an extremely powerful stimulant that speeds up the heart rate, breathing and brain activity. It produces an intense euphoria with feeling of energy, confidence and mental alertness. Sometimes cocaine and heroin are taken together intravenously (speed ball). Overdosage will produce agitation, increase in body temperature, hallucinations, convulsions, loss of memory, extreme anorexia, respiratory failure, stroke, heart failure and death. Death can occur in few hours, if 1–1.5 gm of cocaine is taken orally.

Regular use will produce tolerance and will intensify the negative effects. There will be restlessness, irritability, agitation and paranoia. The intensity of the "high" feeling gradually diminishes and is replaced by a state of depression. This will result in stronger craving for more drug. Withdrawal symptoms include nasal discharge, apathy, long periods of sleep, irritability, depression, disorientation, suicidal tendency and tremors. Chronic users will develop degeneration of central nervous system resulting in hallucinations, delusions, delirium and insanity. The addict will have a feeling of insects crawling under the skin **(Cocaine bugs)**. This will give rise to itching sensation.

### Amphetamines (Brand names—Dexamine, Biphetamine) Street names—bennies, beans, black beauties

Amphetamine was first synthesised in 1887 and used clinically in 1935 to treat a rare sleep disorder, characterised by uncontrollable desire to sleep. Many similar compounds like dextro-amphetamine, methamphetamine were also synthesised later. Once they were sold without prescription. Amphetamine inhalers were also available in the market. Abuse of the inhalers became popular among the teenagers. People from all walks of life started using amphetamines orally. Abusers known as **speed freaks** who used to inject the drug exhibited bizarre and often violent behaviour. Physical symptoms like high blood pressure, increased heart rate, delirium and convulsions can develop. The amphetamines are widely abused nowadays. The main reasons are that the drug is cheap and the effects are similar to those of cocaine. Addicts may develop mental symptoms like hallucinations and delusions.

Commonly abused drugs are amphetamine sulphate, benzphetamine hydrochloride, dexamphetamine sulphate, amfepramone hydrochloride, fenethylline hydrochloride, phentermine, fenproporexhydrochloride, mefenorex hydrochloride, methylamphetamine hydrochloride, methylenedioxy methamphetamine, methylphenidate hydrochloride and tenamfetamine.

## HALLUCINOGENS

Hallucinogens are substances that distort the perception of reality. They produce sensory illusions which will make the abuser unable to distinguish between reality and fantasy. If large doses are taken, visual and auditory hallucinations will be experienced. Hallucination is the apparent perception of unreal sights and sounds. Under the influence of a hallucinogen, a user may speak of "hearing colours' and "seeing sounds". There will be disorientation of direction, distance and time. Restlessness and sleeplessness are also common symptoms. Recurrent use will result in tolerance, making the user to consume larger quantities more frequently.

The greatest hazard of hallucinogens is that the effects are not predictable every time. Sometimes toxic reactions and even death may occur. Suicidal and homicidal tendencies are likely to develop. There is no pattern of withdrawal symptoms and hence physical dependence is rare. Hallucinogens are natural and synthetic. The commonly abused hallucinogens are peyote, mescaline, psilocybin, psilocyn, LSD, dimethyl tryptamine (DMT), diethyl tryptamine (DET), dimethoxy amphetamine (DOM/ STP), phencyclidine (PCP), tenamfetamine (MDA), methylene dioxymethamphetamine (MDM).

### *Peyote (mescaline)* Street Names—beans, big chief, buttons, cactus, mescal, moon, mescal buttons

Peyote is a cactus which grows in the northern regions of Mexico (Fig. 29.5). The natives use the cactus for religious ceremonies. Peyote when taken orally will give a trance-like state. Mexican tribal dancers take this during religious functions. The top of the plant consists of round buttons, known as "mescal buttons". These are cut, dried and chewed to obtain the hallucinogenic effect. The effects last for 8–12 hours.

The active principle of the cactus is mescaline, a natural hallucinogen. Mescaline can be made synthetically. There are no medical uses and all the mescaline is manufactured in clandestine laboratories. Possible effects are similar to those caused by LSD. They include illusions, hallucinations, disorientation of time and space, impaired coordination of hand and eyes, chills, sweating, sleeplessness, psychosis, increased heart rate and blood pressure. Overdose will produce more intense effects, psychosis and death.

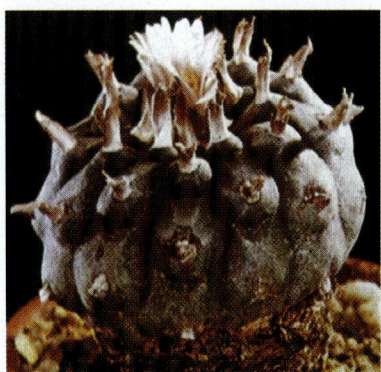

**Fig. 29.5:** Peyote cactus

### *Psilocybin/Psilocin* (Street names—shrooms, magic mushrooms, purple passion)

Psilocybin and psylocin are alkaloids present in the Mexican mushroom "psilocybe mexicana" (Fig. 29.6). It is also present in other varieties of mushrooms. Like mescaline, these mushrooms are used in Indian religious rites. Psilocybin and psilocyn have hallucinogenic properties. It is less potent than LSD. When consumed orally, these

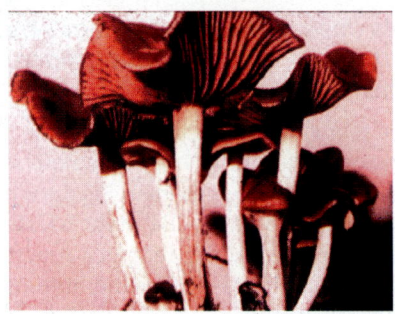

**Fig. 29.6:** Psilocybe mushroom

mushrooms cause physical and mental relaxation, fatigue, hallucinations, nausea and sensory cross over. In addition, these can cause liver damage and even death. Psilocybin is made synthetically in clandestine laboratories. The effects last for about 6 hours. Adverse side effects include disorientation of time and space, muscular incoordination, mental disturbances, increased heart rate and blood pressure. Overdose can cause longer and intense symptoms and death.

### Lysergic Acid Diethylamide (LSD)
### (Street Names—acid, microdot, cubes, blotter, boomers sugar, sunshine)

Lysergic acid diethylamide, popularly known as LSD is a semisynthetic compound produced from lysergic acid, a natural substance found in a fungus 'claviceps purpura'. Lysergic acid diethylamide (LSD) is the most potent and highly studied hallucinogen known to man. He noticed a sense of vertigo and restlessness. The objects and workers in the laboratory appeared to undergo optical changes. The light was intensified with bizarre visions and appearance of bright colours. This condition lasted for 2 hours. Users refer to their experience as a trip. The average effective oral dose is from 20 to 80 µm with the effects of higher doses lasting for 10 to 12 hours. LSD is usually sold in the form of impregnated paper (blotter acid), tablets (microdots), or thin squares of gelatin (window panes).

The amount of LSD per dosage unit varies. For a psychedelic trip, 100–250 µm are used. Overdose can cause psychosis and death. There is consi-

derable variation in individual reaction to the drug. Disorders of visual perception is the first effect. Subjects will become hypersensitive to sound. They will develop extreme alteration of mood, distortion of body image, disorders of thought, anxiety, panic, etc. Under the influence of the drug, the person may commit a crime. There will be recurrence of symptoms (**flash back**) induced by alcohol or other drugs many days after the ingestion of the drug. This can lead to suicide or homicide.

### Cannabis (Brand names—Marijuana/Ganja) Street Names—pot, grass, roach, joint, reefer, weed, mary jane

Cannabis sativa/indica/mexicana is a plant grown in temperate and tropical regions of the world. Its origin is in the orient. The plant was cultivated in China 5000 years ago for taking fibres from the stem. Some Hindu saints use cannabis for religious rites. They call it as 'sidhi' or 'Sivamooli'. The cultivation started in Western Asia in the 16th century and in Europe by 19th century. In USA, the cultivation and use of cannabis spread by the beginning of 20th century. Now the plant is grown extensively in Jamaica, Colombia, Mexico, Africa and India.

The plant is a shrub which grows to a height of 5–10 feet. The leaves consist of odd number of leaflets with serrated margins. Good climatic conditions produce better plants with dark green luxurious foliage (Fig. 29.7). The active substance in cannabis is delta-9-tetrahydrocannabinol (THC), known as dronabinol or marinol, a unique

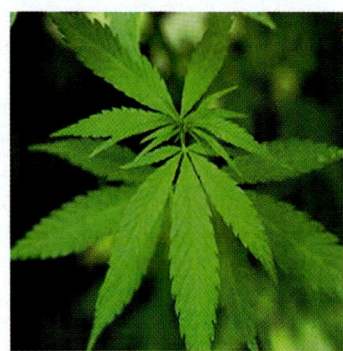

**Fig. 29.7:** Cannabis plant

chemical found now here else in the world. In addition to THC, cannabis contains cannabinol, cannabidiol, cannabinoleic acid and 400 other cannabinoids.

Ganja/marijuana is prepared from the flowering tops and dried tender leaves of cannabis plant in the form of a tobacco like material. This has a rustic green, brown or grey colour and a peculiar smell. This is mixed with tobacco; filled in a pipe or rolled into the form of a cigarette and smoked. The loosely rolled cigarettes are called 'reefers, pots or joints'. Cannabis is also filled into hollowed out commercial cigarettes or cigars (**blunts**) and smoked (Fig. 29.8). In India, cannabis is used by filling in country cigars known as 'beedi'. When cannabis is smoked, it is immediately absorbed from the lungs, producing an almost immediate effect. It is also consumed in the form of an infusion or beverage by mixing it with sugar, black pepper and water (**bhang, majun**). This is a favourite beverage of certain cults in northern India.

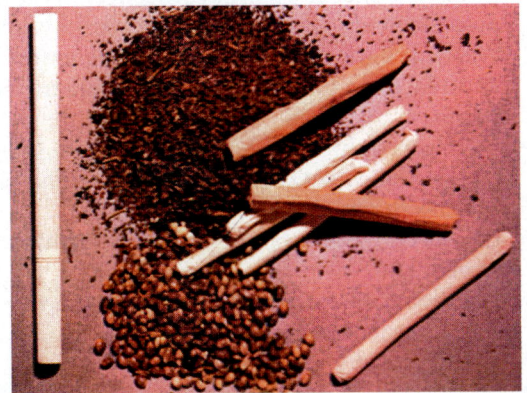

**Fig. 29.8:** Cannabis flowering tops, seed and cigarette filled with the same

The dried resinous secretion from the flowers, leaves and stem of the cannabis plant is known as **hashish/charas**. This is richer in cannabinols. This is smoked in a pipe. A concentrate of cannabis, produced by repeated extraction to yield a dark viscous liquid is called **hashish oil**. One or two drops of hashish oil is added to the tobacco of a cigarette and smoked. Cannabis is the most widely abused substance for its psychoactive or psychedelic effects. Soon after smoking cannabis,

symptoms appear. There are two stages; a stage of excitement and later a stage of sleep. Initially, it produces an increased sense of well-being, followed by a dreamy carefree state of relaxation.

There will be alteration of sensory perception with complete disorientation of time and space. The sense of touch, sight, smell, and sound becomes more vivid. Hunger, craving for sweets with changes in the thought process and expression are also experienced. Moderate doses may result in a state of intoxication. The person may experience rapidly changing emotions, frightful hallucinations, wild delirium, fear of death, suicidal and homicidal tendencies. In ancient times, soldiers were given cannabis to **run amok** a condition characterised by a frenzy to kill. Impaired memory, dulling of attention, distortion of body image, loss of personal identity, fantasies and psychotic symptoms resembling schizophrenia and paranoia will also occur. Later the person will feel giddy, ataxic and suffers from muscular weakness. This stage will pass on to the stage of sleep with dilated pupils. Recovery usually occurs after a deep sleep.

Apart from the psychological effects, cannabis will produce increased heart rate, elevation of blood pressure, deterioration of muscular coordination, nausea, conjunctival congestion and vomiting. Rarely death can occur from respiratory depression. Prolonged heavy use can lead to tolerance and psychic dependence. Physical dependence is rare; but withdrawal symptoms like insomnia, anorexia, irritability, anxiety, sweating, headache and gastrointestinal disturbances occur when the drug is withdrawn.

There is a school of thought that cannabis is not a dangerous drug as it does not produce physical dependence. In some states of USA, there was a move to legalise cannabis use. Scientific studies and observations prove beyond doubt that cannabis is a dangerous substance. It will impair the mental faculties to such an extent that even in smaller doses it will affect the behaviour and performance of the user. Because of the disorientation, muscular incoordination and visual disturbances, driving a vehicle under the influence of cannabis is highly dangerous. Suicidal and homicidal tendencies can develop even in a casual smoker of cannabis. Many of the motiveless suicides and homicides can be attributed to the use of cannabis. Addicts can develop mental disease (**ganja psychosis**). No doubt, cannabis produces moral and mental deterioration. Addicts become mental wrecks, lethargic, indifferent and unenergic (**amotivational syndrome**).

## INHALANTS

Some persons are addicted to inhalation of the vapours of different substances like glue. Thy are called **glue sniffers**. Many of the glues contain volatile solvents. Other volatile solvents are paint thinners, nail polish removers, lighter fluid, etc. Hair sprays and other aerosols are also used by the addicts. Anaesthetic agents like ether, chloroform and nitrous oxide are also abused. Amyl nitrite and butyl nitrite vapours are inhaled to get a strong orgasm during intercourse. Inhalation of vapours give a 'kick' to the addict. Chronic use can produce toxic effects, tolerance and withdrawal symptoms.

## MEDICAL EXAMINATION OF A DRUG ADDICT

Possession and use of narcotic drugs and psychotropic substance is an offence. Investigating officers may have to encounter a person who has consumed or who is in the habit of consuming such drugs and substances. In general, the drug addicts fall into four main groups.

*I Group:* These persons use drugs for a specific purpose or during a special situation. For example, some students take amphetamines during the time of examinations to keep them awake. Drivers take these drugs to keep them awake during night-driving. They never develop dependence.

*II Group:* The members of this group are usually students of schools and colleges. Drugs are used to get some kick or just for an experience. They are called **"spree users"**. They use the drugs in groups or during some functions.

*III Group:* This group is formed by the hard-core addicts. The activities of the hard core addict is entirely concerned about procuring and using drugs. He exhibits physical and psychological dependence. Spree users can become hard core addicts.

*IV Group:* This group consists of persons who considers drug addiction as a way of life, e.g. hippies. Drugs are an integral part of their lives. They are hard core addicts who have usually come from higher strata of the society.

### Identification of a Drug Addict

- The addict will have in his possession the drugs, syringes, needles, etc.
- Usually, the person will appear to be drowsy or sleepy.
- Sudden changes in the behaviour pattern.
- Sudden changes in discipline and performance of jobs.
- Sudden outbursts of temper, emotion and irrational flare ups.
- Indifferent attitude in the general demeanour, dress and appearance.
- Personal hygiene and habits will be below standard and poor.
- Furtive behaviour regarding actions and possessions.
- Wearing dark glasses at inappropriate times and places to hide the dilated or constricted pupils.
- Full sleeved shirts are worn to hide the injection marks. Some may tattoo the elbows and hands to mask the needle puncture marks.
- Presence in shady places and in the company of peddlers.
- Borrowing or stealing money or selling articles such as watches, ornaments, etc.
- Staggering or stumbling gait.
- Narcotic addict will have constricted pupils which poorly respond to light.
- The addict who uses stimulant drugs will have dilated pupils.
- The ganja addict will be very animated or hysterical. Loud and rapid talking and laughing are common. They may possess cigarettes, beedies or packets of ganja. Typical smell can be noticed in the breath and clothes.

The person suspected to have consumed a nacotic drug can be sent to a medical officer for examination and certification. There is no prescribed proforma for the certificate. The one used for drunkenness certification is used with modification. Blood and urine of the suspect have to be collected for chemical analysis. The paraphernelia, if any found in the possesion of the suspect may also be seized and sent for analysis.

## DEATH DUE TO DRUG ABUSE

Drug addicts usually die due to infections like hepatitis, tetanus and allied complications. AIDS, malaria, syphilis, etc. are also contracted by contamination of syringes, needles and other paraphernalia used by the addicts.

A careful examination of the scene of occurrence will yield valuable evidence. Death due to drug overdosage is rare but not uncommon.

During inquest, the dead body should be examined carefully for stains on the fingers, needle puncture marks on the elbows, forearms, back of hands and legs. Sometimes abscesses will be seen in these areas. The clothes may contain stains and remnants of the drugs. Clothes, syringes, needles, empty vials and other materials should also be subjected to chemical analysis. The medical officer may be requested to collect viscera, blood, urine and tissues from the sites of injection for chemical analysis.

## Narcotic Drugs and Psychotropic Substances Act 1985

Narcotic Drugs and Psychotropic Substances Act 1985 is to consolidate and amend the old laws relating to narcotic drugs and to make stringent provisions for the control and regulation of operations relating to narcotic drugs, psychotropic substances and related matters. Drug abuse and trafficking have been slowly spreading across the nation during the past decades. India is one of the countries where illicit cultivation of poppy and ganja is rampant.

India is a transit point in the Middle East-South Asia illicit drug trafficking. To take effective action against this menace, the old laws like Opium Act, etc. were inadequate. Moreover, apart from the conventional drugs of addiction such as opium and ganja, newer drugs of addiction have appeared in the scene. Awarding severe penalties was also necessary to have a deterrent effect on the habitual offenders and traffickers of drugs. Another law called 'Prevention of Illicit traffic in narcotic drugs and psychotropic substances Act

was enacted in 1988. This law provides for the detention of drug traffickers.

NDPS Act was amended in 1988, incorporating certain new provisions to make the law more stringent. NDPS (amendment) Act came into force in May 1989. Government of India has constituted a central authority, viz Narcotic Control Bureau in March 1986 to coordinate the functioning of various state and central drug enforcement authorities. Other objectives were prevention and control of drug abuse and trafficking by enforcing relevant provisions of the NDPS Act.

The Act was further amended in the year 2001 to iron out the anomalies and to remove the technical snags, almost recasting the entire statute. New sections were added and many sections were amended. Punishment was enhanced for the offenders involved in dealing with commercial quantity. Small quantity has also been defined (Table 29.1).

Punishment has been provided for the consumption of any narcotic drugs or psychotropic substance. Drug addicts volunteering treatment may have immunity from prosecution. For the purpose of speedy trial of offences under NDPS Act, government may constitute special courts consisting of a single judge not below the rank of a sessions judge or additional sessions judge. Punishment for offences related to possession, sale, purchase, transport, import, export or use of any narcotic drugs or psychotropic substances shall be rigorous imprisonment for a term which shall not be less than 10 years, but which may extend to 20 years and shall also be liable to fine which shall not be less than one lakh rupees but which may extend to two lakh rupees.

If any person who has been convicted of the commission of any of the offences punishable under the Act is subsequently convicted for any offence, enhanced punishment with imprisonment which may extend to one-half of the minimum term of imprisonment and with one-half the maximum amount of fine.

Death penalty will be given to persons who have been convicted for offences U/S 19, 24, 27 A and offences involving commercial quantity of any narcotic drug or psychotropic substance. All the

**Table 29.1:** List of narcotic drugs and psychotropic substances (Notification specifying small quantity and commercial quantity)

| | Proprietary name | Chemical name | Small quantity | Commercial quantity |
|---|---|---|---|---|
| 1. | Acetorphine (3-0-acetyltetrahydro-7-alpha-(1-hydroxy-1-methylbutyl)-6,14-endo ethano-oripavine) | | 2 | 50 |
| 2. | Acetyl alpha methyl fentanyl (N-[1-(alpha-methylphenethyl)-4-piperidyl]acetanilide | | 0.005 | 0.1 |
| 3. | Acetyl dihydro codeine (acetyl dihydrocodeine) | | 5 | 100 |
| 4. | Acetyl methadol (3-acetoxy-6-dimethylamino-4,4-diphenyl heptane) | | 2 | 50 |
| 5. | Alfentanil(N-[1-[2-(4-ethyl-4, 5-dihydro-5-oxo-1H-tetrazol-1-yl)ethyl-1]-4-(methoxymethyl)-4-piperidinyl]-N-phenyl propanamide | | 0.005 | 0.1 |
| 6. | Allyprodine (3-allyl-1 methyl-4-phenyl-4-propionoxy piperidine) | | 2 | 50 |
| 7. | Alphacetyl methadol (alpha-3-acetoxy-6-dimethylamino-4, 4-diphenyl heptane) | | 5 | 100 |
| 8. | Alpha meprodine (alpha-3-ethyl-1-methyl-4-phenyl-4-propionoxy piperidine | | 2 | 50 |
| 9. | Alpha methadol (alpha-6-dimethylamino-4, 4-diphenyl-3-heptanol) | | 2 | 50 |
| 10. | Alpha methyl fentanyl (N-[1(alpha-methyl phenethyl)4-piperidyl] propionanilide | | 0.005 | 0.1 |
| 11. | Alpha methyl thio fentanyl (N-[1-[1-methyl-2-(2-thienyl)ethyl]-4-piperidyl]propionanilide) | | 0.005 | 0.1 |
| 12. | Alpha prodine (alpha-1, 3-dimethyl-4-phenyl-4-propionoxypiperidine) | | 5 | 100 |
| 13. | Anileridine (1-para-aminophenethyl-4-phenylpiperidine-4- carboxylic acid ethyl ester) | | 2 | 50 |
| 14. | Benzethidine (1-(2-benzyloxyethyl)-4-phenylpiperidine-4-carboxylic acid ethyl ester) | | 5 | 100 |
| 15. | Benzylmorphine (3-0-benzylmorphine) | | 2 | 50 |
| 16. | Beta acetylmethadol (Beta-3-acetoxy-6-dimethylamino-4, 4-diphenylheptane) | | 2 | 50 |
| 17. | Betahydroxyfentanyl (N-[1-(beta-hydroxyphenethyl)-4-piperidyl] propionanilide) | | 0.005 | 0.1 |
| 18. | Beta hydroxy 3 Methyl fentanyl (N-[1-(beta-hydroxyphenethyl) -3-methyl-4-piperidyl] propionanilide) | | 0.005 | 0.1 |
| 19. | Beta meprodine (beta-3-ethyl-1-methyl-4-phenyl-4-propionoxypiperidien) | | 5 | 100 |
| 20. | Beta methadol (beta-6-dimethylamino-4, 4-diphenyl-3-heptanol) | | 2 | 50 |
| 21. | Beta prodine (beta-1, 3-dimethyl-4-phenyl-4-propionoxypiperidine) | | 5 | 100 |
| 22. | Bezitramide 1-(3-cyano-3, 3-diphenylpropyl) -4-(2-oxo-3-propionyl-1-benzimidazolinyl)-piperidine) | | 5 | 100 |
| 23. | Cannabis and Cannabis resin (charas, hashish )—Extracts and tinctures of cannabis | | 100 | 1kg |
| 24. | Clonitazene (2-para-chlorobenzyl-1-diethylaminoethyl-5-nitrobenzimidazole) | | 2 | 50 |
| 25. | Coca derivatives (excluding cocaine) and its salts | | 2 | 50 |
| 26. | Coca leaf | | 100 | 2kg |
| 27. | Cocaine (methyl ester of benzoyl ecgonine) | | 2 | 100 |
| 28. | Codeine (3-0-methylmorphine) | | 10 | 1 kg |
| 29. | Codoxime (dihydrocodienone-6-carboxymethyloxime) | | 5 | 100 |
| 30. | PEPAP (1-phenethyl-4-phenyl-4-piperidinol acetate (ester) | | 2 | 50 |
| 31. | Pethidine (1-methyl-4-phenylpiperidine-4-carboxylic acid ethyl ester) | | 10 | 200 |
| 32. | Pethidine intermediate A (4-cyano-1-methyl-4-phenylpiperidine) | | 10 | 200 |
| 33. | Pethidine intermediate B (4-phenylpiperidine-4-carboxylic acid ethyl ester) | | 10 | 00 |
| 34. | Pethidine intermediate C(1-methyl-4-phenylpiperidine-4-carboxylic acid) | | 10 | 200 |
| 35. | Phenadoxone (6 morpholino-4, 4-diphenyl-3-heptanone) | | 5 | 100 |
| 36. | Phenampromide (N-(1-methyl-2-piperidinoethyl)-propionanilide) | | 5 | 100 |
| 37. | Phenazocine (2-hydroxy-5,9-dimethyl-2-phenethyl-6, 7-benzomorphan) | | 1 | 20 |
| 38. | Phenomorphan (3-hydroxy-N-phenethyl morphinan) | | 5 | 100 |
| 39. | Phenoperidine (1-(3-hydroxy-3-phenylpropyl) -4-phenylpiperidine-4-carboxylic acid ethyl ester) | | 2 | 50 |
| 40. | Pholcodine (nomocodeine, hybernil-morpholinylethylmorphine) | | 5 | 100 |
| 41. | Piminodine (4-phenyl-1-(3-phenylaminopropyl)-piperidine-4-carboxylic acid ethyl ester) | | 5 | 100 |
| 42. | Piritramide (1-(3-cyano-3, 3-diphenylpropyl)-4-(1-piperidino)-piperidine-4-carboxylic acid amide) | | 2 | 50 |
| 43. | Poppy straw | | 1000 | 50 kg |
| 44. | Preparations made from the extract of tincture of Indian Hemp | | 5 | 100 |
| 45. | Proheptazine (1,3-dimethyl-4-phenyl-4-propionoxy azacycloheptane) | | 2 | 50 |
| 46. | Properidine (1-methyl-4-phenylpiperidine-4-carboxylic acid isopropyl ester) | | 2 | 50 |
| 47. | Propiram (N-(1-methyl-2-piperidinoethyl)-N-2- pyridyl propionamide) | | 10 | 200 |
| 48. | Racemethorphan (+-)-3-methoxy-N-methylmorphinan) | | 2 | 50 |

*Contd...*

*Contd...*

| Proprietary name | Chemical name | Small quantity gm | Commercial quantity gm |
|---|---|---|---|
| 49. | Racemoramide (+-)-4-[2-methyl-4-oxo-3, 3-diphenyl-4-(1-pyrrolidinyl)-butyl]-morpholine) | 2 | 50 |
| 50. | Racemorphan (+-)-3-hydroxy-N-methylmorphinan) | 2 | 50 |
| 51. | Sufentanil (N-[4-(methoxymethyl)-1-[2-(2-thienyl)-ethyl]-4-piperidyl]propionanilide) | 0.005 | 0.1 |
| 52. | Thebacon(acetyldihydrocodeinone) | 2 | 50 |
| 53. | Thebaine (3, 6-dimethoxy-4, 5-epoxy-9a-methylmorphine-6, 8-diene) | 2 | 100 |
| 54. | Thiofentanyl (N-[1-[2-(2-thienyl)ethyl]-4-piperidyl]propionanilide) | 0.005 | 0.1 |
| 55. | Tilidine (++)-ethyl-trans-2-(dimethylamino)-1-phenyl-3-cyclohexene-1-carboxylate) | 10 | 200 |
| 56. | Trimeperidine (1, 2, 5-trimethyl-4-phenyl-4-propionoxypiperidine) | 10 | 200 |
| 57. | Brolamfetamine (DOB)(+-4)-4-bromo-2, 5-dimethoxy-alpha-methyl phenethylamine) | 0.5 | 10 |
| 58. | Cathinone (x)-(s)-2-aminopropiophenone) | 2 | 50 |
| 59. | DET (3-[2-(diethylamino)ethyl]indole, N, N, diethyltryptamine) | 0.1 | 2 |
| 60. | DMA (+)-2, 5-dimethoxy-alpha-methylphenethylamine) | 0.5 | 10 |
| 61. | DMHP (3-(1, 2-dimethylheptyl)-7, 8,9,10-tetrahydro-6, 6,9-trimethyl-6H-dibenzo[b,d]pyran-1-0l) | 2 | 50 |
| 62. | DMT(3-[2-(dimethylamino)ethyl]indole,N,N, Dimethyltryptamine) | 0.1 | 2 |
| 63. | DOET (+)-4-ethyl-2, 5-dimethoxy-alpha-phenethylamine) | 0.5 | 10 |
| 64. | Eticyclidine (PCE) N-ethyl-l-phenylcyclohexylamine) | 2 | 50 |
| 65. | Etryptamine (3-(2-aminobutyl) indole) | 2 | 50 |
| 66. | (+) Lysergide (LSD, LSD-25) 9,10-didehydro-N,N-diethyl-6-methylergoline-8 Beta -carboxamide) | 0.002 | 0.1 |
| 67. | MDMA, Ecstacy (+)-N, alpha-dimethyl-3, 4-(methylene-dioxy)phenethylamine) | 0.5 | 10 |
| 68. | Mescaline (3,4,5,-trimethoxyphenethylamine) | 5 | 100 |
| 69. | Methcathinone (2-(methylamino)-1-phenylpropan-l-one) | 2 | 50 |
| 70. | 4-methylaminorex (+)-cis-2-amino-4-methyl-5-phenyl-2-oxazoline) | 0.5 | 10 |
| 71. | MMDA, Ecstacy (2-methoxy-alpha-methyl-4, 5-(methylenedioxy) phenethylamine) | 0.5 | 10 |
| 72. | 4-MTA (alpha-methyl-4-methyl thiophenethylamine) | 0.5 | 10 |
| 73. | N-ethyl MDA (+/-)-N-ethyl-alpha-methyl-3, 4-(methylenedioxy)phenethylamine) | 0.5 | 10 |
| 74. | N-hydroxy MDA (+/-)-N-[alpha-methyl-3, 4-(methylenedioxy)phenethyl]hydroxylamine) | 0.5 | 10 |
| 75. | Parahexyl (3-hexyl-7, 8, 9, 10-tetrahydro-6, 6, 9-trimethyl-6H-dibenzo[b,d]pyran-1-0) | 2 | 50 |
| 76. | PMA (p-methoxy -alpha-methylphenethylamine) | 0.5 | 10 |
| 77. | Psilocine, Psilotsin (3-[2-(dimethylamino)ethyl]indol-4-ol) | 2 | 50 |
| 78. | Psilocybine (3-[2- (dimethylamino)ethyl]indol-4-dihydrogen phosphate) | 2 | 50 |
| 79. | Rolicyclidine (PHP, PCPY)1-(l-phenylcyclohexyl)pyrrolidine) | 2 | 50 |
| 80. | STP, DOM (2, 5-dimethoxy-alpha, 4-dimethyl phenethylamine) | 0.5 | 10 |
| 81. | Tenamfetamine (MDA) Alpha-methyl-3, 4-(methylenedioxy) phenethylamine) | 0.5 | 10 |
| 82. | Tenocyclidine (TCP)1-[l-(2-thienyl) cyclohexyl]piperidine) | 2 | 50 |
| 83. | Tetrahydrocannabinol—their isomers and stereochemical variants | 2 | 50 |
| 84. | TMA (+)-3, 4, 5-trimethoxy-alpha-methyl phenethylamine) | 0.5 | 10 |
| 85. | Amfetamine (Amphetamine)(+/-)-alpha-methyl phenethylamine) | 2 | 50 |
| 86. | 2 C-B (4-bromo-2, 5-dimethoxy phenethylamine) | 0.5 | 10 |
| 87. | Dexamfetamine (dexamphetamine)(+)-alpha-methyl phenethylamine) | 2 | 50 |
| 88. | Fentylline (fenethylline) 7-2-[(alpha-methyl phenethyl)amino]ethyl]theophylline) | 0.5 | 10 |
| 89. | Levamfetamine (levamfetamine(x)-(R)-alpha-methylphenethylamine) | 2 | 50 |
| 90. | Levomethamphetamine (x)-N, alpha-dimethyl phenethylamine) | 2 | 50 |
| 91. | Mecloqualone (3-(0-chlorophenyl)-2-methyl-4(3H)-quinazolinone) | 20 | 500 |
| 92. | Methamfetamine (+/-)-(S)-N, alpha-dimethyl phenethylamine, (+) 2methylamino-1-Phenylpropane | 2 | 50 |
| 93. | Methamfetamine racemate (+/-)-N, alpha-dimethyl phenethylamine) | 2 | 50 |
| 94. | Methaqualone (2-methyl-3-0-tolyl-4(3H)-quinazolinone) | 20 | 500 |
| 95. | Methyl phenidate (Methyl alpha-phenyl-2-piperidine acetate) | 2 | 50 |
| 96. | Phencyclidine (P.C.P.)1-(1-phenylcyclohexyl)piperidine) | 2 | 5 0 |
| 97. | Phenmetrazine (3-methyl-2-phenyl morpholine) | 5 | 100 |
| 98. | Secobarbital (5-allyl-5-(1-methyl butyl)barbituric acid) | 20 | 500 |
| 99. | Dronabinol (Delta-9-tetrahydro-cannabinol and its stereochemical variants) (6aR,10aR)- 6a, 7,8, 10a-tetrahydro-6,6,9-trimethyl-3-pentyl-6H-dibenzo{b,d}pyran-1-ol | 2 | 50 |

*Contd...*

| Proprietary name | Chemical name | Small quantity gm | Commercial quantity gm |
|---|---|---|---|
| 100. | Zipeprol (Alpha-(alpha-methoxybenzyl)-4-(beta methoxyphenethyl)-1-piperazine ethanol) | 5 | 100 |
| 101. | Amobarbital (5-ethyl-5-isopentyl barbituric acid) | 20 | 500 |
| 102. | Buprenorphine [21-cyclopropyl -7-alpha-(S)-l-hydroxy-1, 2, 2,-trimethylpropyl]-6, 14, endo-ethano- 6, 7, 8, 14-tetrahydro oripavine | 1 | 20 |
| 103. | Butalbital (5-allyl-5-isobutyl barbituric acid) | 20 | 500 |
| 104. | Cathine (+)-nor pseudoephedrine) (+)-(R)-alpha-[(R)-1-amino ethyl]benzyl alcohol) | 2 | 50 |
| 105. | Cyclobarbital (5-(1-cyclohexen-1-yl)-5-ethyl barbituric acid) | 20 | 500 |
| 106. | Flunitrazepam (5-(0-fluorophenyl)-!, 3-dihydro-1-methyl-7-Nitro-2H-1, 4-benzodiazepin-2-one) | 5 | 100 |
| 107. | Glutethimide (2-ethyl-2-phenylglutarioide | 20 | 500 |
| 108. | Pentazocine (2R, 6R, 11R)-1, 2, 3 ,4, 5, 6,-hexahydro-6, 11-dimethyl-3-(3-methyl-2-butenyl)-2, 6,-methano-3-benzazocin-8-ol) | 20 | 500 |
| 109. | Pentobarbital (5-ethyl-5-(1-methylbutyl)barbituric acid) | 20 | 500 |
| 110. | Allobarbital (5, 5-diallyl barbituric acid) | 20 | 500 |
| 111. | Alprazolam (8-chloro-1-methyl-6-phenyl-4H-s-triazolo [4, 3-a] [1, 4]benzodiazepine) | 5 | 100 |
| 112. | Amfepramone (diethylpropion)2-(diethylamino)propiophenone) | 10 | 250 |
| 113. | Aminorex (2-amino-5-phenyl-2-oxazoline) | 5 | 100 |
| 114. | Barbital (5, 5-diathyl barbituric acid) | 20 | 500 |
| 115. | Benzfetamine (benzphetamine) N-benzyl-N, alpha-dimethyl phenethylamine) | 20 | 500 |
| 116. | Bromazepam (7-bromo-1, 3-dihydro-5-(2-pyridyl)-2H-1, 4-benodiazepin-2-one) | 20 | 500 |
| 117. | Butobarbital (5-butyl-5-ethyl barbituric acid) | 20 | 500 |
| 118. | Brotizolam (2-bromo-4-(0-chlorophenyl)-9-methyl-6H-thieno[3, 2-f]-s-triazolo[4, 3-a][1,4]diazepine) | 5 | 100 |
| 119. | Camazepam (7-chloro-1, 3-dihydro-3-hydroxy-1-methyl-5-phenyl-2H-1, 4-benzodiazepin-2-one dimethyl carbamate (ester) | 20 | 500 |
| 120. | Chlordiazepoxide (7-chloro-2-(methylamino)-5-phenyl-3H-1, 4-benzodiazepine-4-oxide) | 20 | 500 |
| 121. | Clobazam (7-chloro-1-methyl-5-phenyl-1H-1, 5-benzodiazepine-2, 4(3H, 5H)-dione) | 10 | 250 |
| 122. | Clonazepam (5-(0-chlorophenyl)-1, 3-dihydro-7-nitro-2H-1, 4-benzodiazepin-2-one) | 5 | 100 |
| 123. | Clorazepate (7-chloro-2, 3-dihydro-2-oxo-5-phenyl-1H-1, 4-benzodiazepine-3-carboxylic acid) | 10 | 250 |
| 124. | Clotiazepam (5-(0-chlorophenyl)-7-ethyl-1, 3-dihydro-1-methyl-2H-thieno[2, 3-e]-1,4-diazepin-2-one) | 10 | 250 |
| 125. | Cloxazolam (10-chloro-11b-(0-chlorophenyl)-2,3,7,11b- tetrahydroxazolo-[3,2-d][1,4 benzodiazepin-6(5H)-one) | 5 | 100 |
| 126. | Delorazepam (7-chloro-5-(0-chlorophenyl)-1, 3-dihydro-2H-1,4-benzodiazepin-2-one) | 5 | 100 |
| 127. | Diazepam(7-chloro-1, 3-dihydro-1-methyl-5-phenyl-2H-1, 4-benzodiazepin-2-one) | 20 | 500 |
| 128. | Estazolam (8-chloro-6-phenyl-4 H-s-triazolo[4, 3-a][1, 4]benzodiazepine) | 5 | 100 |
| 129. | Ethchlorvynol (1-chloro-3-ethyl-1-penten-4-yn-3-ol) | 20 | 500 |
| 130. | Ethinamate (1-ethynyl cyclohexanol carbamate) | 20 | 500 |
| 131. | Ethyl loflazepate (Ethyl 7- chloro-5-(0-fluorophenyl)-2, 3-dihydro-2-oxo-1H -1, 4-benzodiazepine-3-carboxylate) | 10 | 250 |
| 132. | Etilamfetamine (N- ethylamphetamine)N-ethyl-alpha-methyl phenethylamine) | 2 | 50 |
| 133. | Fencamfamin (N-ethyl-3-phenyl-2-nor borananamine) | 2 | 50 |
| 134. | Fenproporex (+/-)-3-[(alpha-methylphenethyl)amino]propionitrile) | 2 | 50 |
| 135. | Fludiazepam (7-chloro-5-(0-flurophenyl)-1,3-dihydro-1-;methyl-2H-1,4-benzodiazepin-2-one) | 5 | 100 |
| 136. | Flurazepam (7-chloro-1-[2-(diethylamino)ethyl]-5-(0-flurophenyl)-1,3-dihydro-2H-1, 4-benzodiazepin-2-one) | 5 | 100 |
| 137. | GHB (y-Hydroxybutyric Acid) | 10 | 250 |
| 138. | Halazepam (7-chloro-1, 3-dihydro-5-phenyl -1-1-(2,2,2-trifluroethyl)-2H-1,4-benzodiazepin-2-one) | 20 | 500 |
| 139. | Haloxazolam (10-bromo-11b-(0-flurophenyl)-2,3,7,11b-tetrahydro oazolo[3,2-d][1,4] benzodiazepin-6(5H) | 10 | 500 |
| 140. | Ketazolam (11-chloro-8,12b-dihydro-2,8-dimethyl-12b-phenyl-4H-[1,3]oxazino[3,2-d] [1,4] Benzodiazepine-4,7(6H)-dione | 10 | 250 |
| 141. | Lefetamine (SPA)(x)-N, N-dimethyl-1, 2-diphenyl ethylamine) | 10 | 250 |

Contd...

| Proprietary name | Chemical name | Small quantity gm | Commercial quantity gm |
|---|---|---|---|
| 142. | Loprazolam (6-(0-chlorophenyl)-2,4-dihydro-2-[(4-methyl-1-piperazinyl)methylene]-8-nitro-1 H-imidazo[1, 2-a][1,4]benzodiazepin-1-one | 5 | 100 |
| 143. | Lorazepam (7-chloro-5-(0-chlorophenyl)-1, 3-dihydro-3-hydroxy-2H-1,4-benzodiazepin-2-one) | 10 | 250 |
| 144. | Lormetazepam (7-chloro-5-(0-chlorophenyl)-1, 3-dihydro-3-hydroxy-1-methyl-2H-1, 4-benzodiazepin-2-one) | 10 | 250 |
| 145. | Mazindol (5-(p-chlorophenyl)-2,5-dihydro-3H-imidazo[2,1-a]isindol-5-ol) | 10 | 250 |
| 146. | Medazepam (7-chloro-2, 3-dihydro-1-methyl-5-phenyl-1H-1, 4-benzodiazepine) | 20 | 500 |
| 147. | Mefenorex (N-(3-chloropropyl)-alpha-methyl phenethylamine) | 2 | 50 |
| 148. | Meprobamate (2-methyl-2propyl -1, 3-propanedio dicarbamate) | 20 | 500 |
| 149. | Mesocarb (3-(alpha-methyl phenethyl)-N-(phenyl carbamoyl) sydnone imine) | 5 | 100 |
| 150. | Methyl phenobarbital (5-ethyl-1-methyl-5-phenylbarbituric acid) | 20 | 500 |
| 160. | Methyprylon (3, 3-diethyl 1-5-methyl-2, 4-piperidinedione) | 20 | 500 |
| 161. | Midazolam (8-chloro-6-(0-fluorophenyl)-1-methyl-4H-imidazol[1, 5-a][1,4]benzodiazepine) | 20 | 500 |
| 162. | Nimetazepam (1, 3-dihydro-1-methyl-7-nitro-5-phenyl-2H-1, 4-benzodiazepin-2-one) | 10 | 250 |
| 163. | Nitrazepam (13-dihydro-7-nitro-5-phenyl-2H-1, 4-benzodiazepine-2-one) | 20 | 500 |
| 164. | Nordazepam (7-chloro-1, 3-dihydro-5-phenyl-2H-1, 4-benzodiazepin-2-one) | 20 | 500 |
| 165. | Oxazepam (7-chloro-1, 3-dihydro-3-hydroxy-5-phenyl-2H-1, 4-benzodiazepin -2-one) | 20 | 500 |
| 166. | Oxazolam (10-chloro-2, 3, 7, 11b-tetrahydro-2-methyl-11b-phenyloxazolo[3, 2-d][1,4]benzodiazepin-6 (5H)-one) | 20 | 500 |
| 167. | Pemoline (2-amino-5-phenyl-2-oxazolin-4-one(-2-imino-5-phenyl-4-oxazolidinone) | 2 | 50 |
| 168. | Phendimetrazine (+)-(2S, 3S)-3, 4-dimethyl-2-phenyl morpholine) | 20 | 500 |
| 169. | Phenobarbital (5-ethyl-5-phenyl barbituric acid ) | 20 | 500 |
| 170. | Phentermine (Alpha, alpha-dimethyl phenethylamine) | 20 | 500 |
| 171. | Pinazepam (7-chloro-1, 3-dihydro-5-phenyl-1(2-propynyl)-2H-1, 4-benzodiazepin-2-one) | 10 | 250 |
| 172. | Pipradrol (1,1-diphenyl-1-(2 piperidyl)-methanol) | 20 | 500 |
| 173. | Prazepam (7-chloro-1(cyclo propylmethyl)-1, 3-dihydro-5-phenyl-2H-1,4-benzodiazepin-2-one) | 20 | 500 |
| 174. | Pyrovalerone (4-methyl-2-(1-pyrrolidinyl) valerophenone) | 2 | 50 |
| 175. | Secbutabarbital (5-sec-butyl-5-ethylbarbituric acid) | 20 | 500 |
| 176. | Temazepam (7-chloro-1, 3,dihydro-3-hydroxy-1-methyl-5-phenyl-2H-1, 4-benzodiazepin-2-one) | 20 | 500 |
| 177. | Tetrazepam (7-chloro-5 (1-cyclohexen-1-yl)-1, 3, dihydro-1-methyl-2H-1, 4-benzodiazepin-2-one) | 20 | 500 |
| 178. | Triazolam (8-chloro-6(0-chlorophenyl)-1 methyl -4H-s-triazolo[4,3-a][1,4] benzodiazepin) | 5 | 100 |
| 179. | Vinylbital (5-(1-methylbutyl)-5-vinyl barbituric acid) | 20 | 500 |
| 180. | Zolpidem (N, N, 6-trimethyl-2-p-tolylimidazo[1, 2-alpha]pyridine-3-acetamide) | 10 | 250 |
| 181. | Any mixture or preparation that of with or without a natural material, of any of the above drugs. | * | ** |

* Lesser of the small quantity between the quantities given against the respective narcotic drugs or psychotropic substances mentioned above forming part of the mixture.

**Lesser of the commercial quantity between the quantities given against the respective narcotic drugs or psychotropic substances mentioned above forming part of the mixture.

1. The small quantity and the commercial quantity given against the respective drugs listed above apply to isomers, within specific chemical designation, the esters, ethers and salts of these drugs, including salts of esters, ethers and isomers; whenever existence of such substance is possible.

2. The quantities shown against the respective drugs listed above also apply to the preparations of the drug and preparations of substances of note 1.

3. Small quantity and commercial quantity with respect to cultivation of opium/poppy is not specified separately as the offence in this regard is covered under clause (c) of Sec 18 of the NDPS Act.

offences under this Act are cognisable and normally non-bailable for the offences mentioned above.

## DIRECTIONS TO THE INVESTIGATING OFFICER

- All narcotic drugs, psychotropic substances and related materials or any other articles seized in connection with an offence have to be sent for chemical analysis after packing, labelling and sealing along with a forwarding note.
- The samples must be sent through special messenger or by insured post within 72 hours of seizure of the drug addict should be seize and sent for chemical analysis.
- The offender/drug addict may be subjected to medical examination.

- Request the doctor to collect blood and urine of the subject for chemical analysis.
- In deaths due to drug abuse, detailed examination of the dead body and the scene may be conducted.
- Look for the presence of stains/injection marks on the elbows and hands of the deceased.
- Look for the presence of syringes, needles, vials ampoules, etc. in the possession of the addict.
- Preserve the clothes of the deceased for the detection of traces of the drugs.
- Request the doctor who conduct autopsy to preserve viscera, blood, urine and tissues from the sites of injection marks for chemical analysis.

# 30

# Sudden Natural Death

## SUDDEN DEATH

Sometimes police may have to investigate death due to natural causes when death was sudden, unexpected and occurred under suspicious circumstances. For example, a person is found dead in a hotel room. The deceased might have been suffereing from chronic heart disease and the pre-existing disease condition might not have been diagnosed earlier and the person was apparently normal till he died suddenly. Sometimes the person dies on the way to hospital or dies in the hospital before the attending physicians could arrive at a diagnosis. In all these cases, lesions responsible for death can only be detected during the autopsy. But in a small percentage of cases, there may not be any obvious cause of death. The cause may be dysfunction of the glands, biochemical disturbances, viral infections, etc.

A case of natural death may present itself as an unnatural one. A person who suddenly dies may fall and sustain injuries. Similarly, a person dying suddenly can involve in a vehicular, domestic or industrial accident. For example, a person while driving a car can suddenly die due to occlusion of the coronary artery, the car may crash and the case is notified as a traffic accident.

When death is associated with an accident, investigation is necessary to find out whether the disease/condition was responsible for the cause of death and thereby the accident or; whether it was the cause of the accident and not the cause of death. Sometimes, the natural disease may only

be an incidental finding. In any case, a detailed inquest has to be conducted to establish the apparent cause of death and send the dead body to a medicolegal expert for a detailed autopsy. Microscopical, biochemical and other laboratory investigations may be necessary to confirm the autopsy findings.

Majority of sudden unexpected deaths are due to disease of the heart. Eighty percent of sudden deaths are due to coronary artery disease of the heart. Sudden death due to high blood pressure disease is also often unrecognised, especially in the absence of a history of hypertension.

## Sudden Death due to Disease of the Heart

There are several diseases of the heart which can cause sudden death. In majority of cases, the cause is related to the disease of the two coronary arteries, which supply blood to the heart. The lumen of the coronary arteries become narrow due to disease (atherosclerosis). Blood clot (thrombus) can form in those areas which will cause occlusion. If the occlusion of a major vessel is total, sudden death may occur. If the occlusion is partial or gradual, the heart muscle will be damaged (myocardial infarction).

Myocardial infarction is the necrosis (death) of the heart muscle. Usually, the walls of the heart are involved. After the occlusion of the artery, the changes in the heart muscle occur gradually. In sudden deaths due to complete occlusion, there will not be any visible change in the heart muscle.

## Injuries and Heart Attack

Injuries can either precipitate or hasten death of a person who is already suffering from diseases. For example, trivial injuries may precipitate death in a person having diseases of the heart like coronary arteriosclerosis. The reaction of the body to injuries includes increased coagulability of blood, increased secretion of adrenaline, raised blood pressure, etc. which can initiate formation of blood clots (thrombosis) in an already narrow blood vessel.

A blood clot (thrombus) occluding the main coronary arteries or proximal portions of major branches can cause sudden death. In this instance, the proximate cause of death is coronary thrombosis. Scientific reasoning and logical presumption is that assault/injuries could have precipitated death. But it is not possible to establish this fact with autopsy data. But blunt impacts on the chest can cause cardiac arrest (**commotio cordis**). Many athletes have died a sudden death following blunt impacts on the chest.

## Vagal Inhibition

Vagus is a nerve which originates from the brain. Its branches supply many internal organs including heart. Pressure on the neck, blow on the larynx, hit in the pit of stomach, kick in the scrotum, dilatation of mouth of uterus, etc. can precipitate a reflex cardiac arrest due to the inhibitory action of the vagus nerve. There will not be any specific changes detectable in the organs during autopsy.

## Holiday Heart Syndrome

This condition is characterised by the development of irregulr rhythm of heart following the consumption of alcohol. This is often seen in holiday makers and hence the name. Sudden death has also been reported in persons consuming a large quantity of alcohol. Structural disease of the heart can be a contributory factor for sudden death.

Death can occur due to irregularity in the functioning of heart (atrial fibrillation, atrial flutter and ventricular ectopy). Several mechanisms play a part when alcohol is consumed. They include an increased secretion of adrenaline, noradrenaline, and a rise in plasma free fatty acids.

Acetaldehyde, a primary metabolite of ethyl alcohol exerts a direct action on the conducting system of heart. Mortality is rare in persons without any organic disease of the heart.

## Broken Heart Syndrome

This is a condition in which intense emotional stress results in rapid weakness of heart muscle, arrhythmia, fall of blood pressure, shock and death. During stress, body produces large quantities of adrenaline and noradrenaline. These hormones have a direct effect on the heart and coronary arteries. The arteries are constricted and the heart muscle becomes dysfunctional. Even though the condition is usually reversible, it can cause death in persons with pre-existing heart disease. Emotional stresses like grief (death of a loved one), anger, fear, surprise, detention in police custody, etc. can precipitate this condition.

## Myocarditis

Myocarditis is inflammation of the heart muscle (myocardium). Many infective agents like bacteria, virus, fungi, protozoa and worms can cause inflammation of the myocardium. The primary disease may be sometimes mild. For example, a mild viral fever can have a fatal termination due to viral myocarditis. Clinical symptoms will be chest pain, dyspnoea and signs of cardiac failure. Death will be due to shock and heart failure. The conducting system can be affected resulting in irregular rhythm (arrhythmia) and death. Autopsy diagnosis is by microscopic examination of the heart muscle.

## SUDDEN DEATH DUE TO DISEASES OF THE CENTRAL NERVOUS SYSTEM

### Cerebrovascular Accidents

#### Cerebral Haemorrhage

Stroke is a 'brain attack' due to deficiency of blood supply to the brain (ischemic stroke) resulting in neurologic disorders. Stroke due to bleeding in the brain is called haemorrhagic stroke. The main cause for ischemic stroke is the narrowing of the lumen of the arteries due to atherosclerosis or blood clots. Haemorrhagic stroke is due to increased blood pressure causing rupture of the arteries. It can also occur due to rupture of an aneurysm of the artery. Aneurysm is the formation of a sac due to a weakness in the wall of the artery. Bleeding can occur under the coverings of brain or in its substance (intracerebral). If the bleeding in the brain is massive, sudden death will occur. Thirty percent of persons who develop haemorrhagic stroke die.

### Berry Aneurysms

Congenital aneurysms of the arteries of the brain can spontaneously rupture. This is one of the causes of sudden death in a young adult. There may be forewarning symptoms of headache and sudden unconsciousness. Many persons die after physical exertion or emotional stress. Autopsy will reveal massive bleeding under the subarachnoid covering of brain.

## SUDDEN DEATH DUE TO DISEASES OF THE RESPIRATORY SYSTEM

### Bronchial Asthma

Persons suffering from bronchial asthma can die suddenly. Death can occur even if there is no acute asthmatic episode. The exact cause of death is still unknown. It may probably due to irritability of heart muscle caused by reduced oxygenation and respiratory acidosis. Drugs like aminophylline, theophylline used in asthma can also affect heart (ventricular fibrillation). Autopsy will reveal enlarged lungs with a pale spongy appearance. The bronchi will be filled with thick clear mucus.

### Acute Respiratory Distress Syndrome (ARDS)

ARDS is a sudden life-threatening lung failure. A variety of conditions such as blood-borne infections, injuries, shock, inhalation of irrespirable gases, ingestion of certain drugs, etc. can precipitate the condition. The exact causes for the lung damage is not clear. ARDS develops within 24–48 hours after initial injury or illness. If the condition is not diagnosed and treated, death will occur in 90% of patients.

## MISCELLANEOUS CONDITIONS

### Anaphylactic Deaths

Sudden deaths usually occur in drug sensitivity reactions. Any substance can be allergic to the human body and can result in an allergic reaction. The symptoms will be sudden and alarming. In severe allergic reaction (anaphylaxis), death will be sudden. Usually antibiotics like penicillin can bring about fatal anaphylactic reaction immediately after an injection. Milder symptoms will be skin rashes, fever, etc. Fatal reactions include swelling of larynx, glottis and lungs (pulmonary edema). Even a test dose can produce severe anaphylaxis and cause sudden death. To prevent this, test dose should be given in the skin (intradermal) in very low dilution.

When injections of drugs like penicillin are given to patients, sufficient precautions should be not taken by the medical personnel to counteract allergic reactions. Not giving a test dose and not taking adequate precautions to prevent death will amount to medical negligence.

## SUDDEN UNEXPECTED DEATHS IN EPILEPSY (SUDEP)

Sudden unexpected deaths occur in persons suffering from epilepsy. Incidence is higher in young patients (20–40 years). In majority of the cases, death is preceded by a convulsive attack. Death is often due to respiratory arrest. There may be sudden heart failure due to development of abnormal rhythm (cardiac arrhythmia) of heart. Sometimes death can occur during sleep also. Autopsy will not reveal the underlying cause of death. The respiratory and cardiac arrests are believed to be due to the massive cerebral electric discharge affecting the vasomotor centres in the brain.

Epileptics can also die due to accidental drowning, fall from heights and other accidents. when they become unconscious at the time of an epileptic fits. Epileptics can die suddenly following a convulsive episode or status epilepticus. Toxicological analysis and histopathological examination should be conducted in all negative autopsies to rule out other conditions.

### Obstructive Sleep Apnoea

This condition is seen in those who have diminished tone of the muscles of pharynx and thickening of the soft tissues of neck. Usually, obese persons with short fat neck suffer from this condition. Apnoea means lack of airflow past the nostrils and mouth. Apnoea occurs several times during sleep at night. This will lead to sleep arousal and irritability of heart. These conditions can lead to death.

## Acute Pancreatitis

Pancreatitis is the inflammation of the pancreas. It is associated with alcohol abuse, gallstones, abdominal injuries, viral infections and drugs such as steroids, thiazide, diuretics, etc. Pancreas will show inflammation, swelling, bleeding and destruction (necrosis). Cysts and abscesses are also formed. Acute pancreatitis is not considered as a cause of sudden death. But sometimes the illness develops rapidly in less than 24–48 hours, leading to complications and death.

## Intravenous Narcotism

Drug addicts die due to administration of a high dose of a narcotic drug through the veins. As a consequence of chronic drug use, addicts develop infections like bronchopneumonia, hepatitis B, HIV infection, etc. These conditions can cause sudden death.

## HIV Infection and AIDS

HIV infection is usually transmitted through sexual contact with an infected person, by receiving infected blood transfusion and intravenous drug abuse. Serious diseases of internal organs developing in HIV infection can lead to sudden death.

## Senile Myocardial Degeneration

Autopsy on the body of an old person may not reveal any specific finding. Most of the organs may show changes of atrophy. The heart will be small; but dilated in persons with high blood pressure. The heart muscle will be flabby and soft. The coronary vessels will be tortuous due to shrinkage of heart muscle. Microscopically there will be degeneration and fibrosis of the muscle fibres of heart. These changes of the heart muscle are known as senile myocardial degeneration. The changes are due to ageing. Ultimately, these conditions blow out the candle of life.

## DIRECTIONS TO THE INVESTIGATING OFFICER

When no apparent cause of death is revealed from the external examination of the body, from the examination of the scene or from the statements of witnesses, death due to natural causes should be suspected. In that case, body has to be sent to a forensic expert for a detailed autopsy. Sometimes, gross autopsy findings may not provide the cause of death. Organs or bits of tissues from organs have to be preserved for microscopical examination. A peripheral blood smear should be taken for examination. In all cases of sudden death, viscera, blood and urine have to be collected and preserved in saturated saline and despatched for chemical analysis. Sample of blood has to be collected for biochemical, hematological and microbiological examinations.

In all suspected natural deaths, examine the dead body thoroughly for signs of violence. Even trivial violence could have precipitated the death. If injuries are present on the body, they should be examined and details recorded. If the injuries are sustained at the time of death or just after death (perimortem), they will not be showing much vital reaction. Well-defined contusions, large hematomas, regenerative changes etc. will indicate that the injuries have been sustained earlier to death. However, effort should be taken to find out the causation of injuries found on the body by examination of the scene, examination of witnesses, etc.

In all cases of sudden unexpected deaths, a detailed past medical history of the deceased should be obtained from the relatives. The prescriptions of drugs, medical records, remnants of drugs, etc. are to be examined with the help of a doctor. The doctor who attended the person last should be questioned to elicit details of the ailment and its prognosis. It is also possible for a person to die suddenly due to natural causes without exhibiting symptoms preceding death. The deceased might have been suffering from chronic disease of the heart; without exhibiting any symptoms.

# Investigation of Hospital Deaths

At present, due to the advancements in the technology and availability of modern equipment, incidence of hospital deaths have come down considerably. However, unpredicted deaths occurring during treatment pose medicolegal problems. In some circumstances, risk of death can be predicted. There will be an increased risk of mortality in the case of complicated procedures, aged patients, persons with pre-existing diseases like coronary artery disease, diabetes, hypertension, endocrine diseases, immunological disorders, etc. Emergency procedures have a greater risk than those conducted electively.

The past few years have seen a steady increase in civil and criminal litigations alleging medical negligence. These malpractice actions are likely to rise in future for the following reasons:

- Bringing medical service under the purview of Consumer Protection Act.
- Awareness of the public of their legal and civil rights with the advent of consumer movements and laws of compensation.
- Deterioration of the traditional doctor – patient relationship.
- Existence of a certain degree of negligence due to deficiencies in many areas and overcrowding in hospitals.

Medical negligence is a part of the law of torts. A tort is a civil wrong for which the sufferer can seek compensation through legal action. Negligence itself is not a criminal act; but an act of commission or omission can also constitute a criminal act

separately. Lack of exercising reasonable skill and care in the treatment can constitute an offence of negligence. Death or damage occurring due to unforeseen complications does not imply liability on the part of the doctor. Performance of a surgical operation, administration of anaesthetic and conducting delivery of a child are never without risk to the life of the patient.

## ANAESTHETIC DEATHS

A variety of untoward and unexpected events may lead to complications during anaesthesia. The calamities can vary from a minor mishap to a fatal outcome or cerebral death. In the past, anaesthesiology was confined to pain relief for the surgical patient and best operating conditions for the surgeon. Functioning of life support systems, circulatory and respiratory control, maintenance of fluids, blood and electrolyte balance form an important aspect of this speciality. Now the scope has widened further to include extra operating room functions like intensive care, resuscitation, chronic pain relief, palliative care, etc.

Anaesthetic deaths can be due to the direct result of administration of an anaesthetic. Deaths can occur during the administration of an anaesthetic, but which are not due to the anaesthetic. The fatalities depend upon the types of anaesthesia, nature of surgical interference and physical status of the patient.

Local anaesthesia is the injection of an anaesthetic drug in the skin to make that are numb and painless. Excessive dosage, concentrated solutions, accidental injection into blood vessels, rapid absorption, etc. can produce alarming symptoms, especially in debilitated persons. Allergic reactions, depression of heart and brain resulting in low blood pressure, circulatory collapse, unconsciousness and death are some of the complications.

Spinal anaesthesia is the injection of an anaesthetic drug under the coverings of the spinal cord (epidural space) to produce anlgesia of body below the area of injection. Lowering of blood pressure is the common complication. Persons with occlusive coronary artery disease can develop myocardial infarction. High spinal anaesthesia can result in cardiac arrest. Muscle paralysis due to damage of nerve roots, epidural abscess, meningitis, subarachnoid bleeding, injury to spinal ligaments, osteomyelitis of vertebra are some rare complications.

General anaesthesia is the administration of gaseous anaesthetic drugs through inhalation. This type of anaesthesia may cause paralysis of intercostal muscles and diaphragm. Mechanical and functional obstruction of air passages will cause asphyxia. Misplaced endotracheal tube into one of the bronchi, passage of laryngoscope or endotracheal tube, etc. can cause laryngospasm and bronchospasm. Aspiration of secretions from throat, blood from the operation site, pus from an abscess, gastric contents, etc. can enter respiratory tract especially during the recovery phase unless precautionary measures are not taken. Gastric contents when aspirated can cause bronchospasm due to chemical irritation. Almost all the inhalant anaesthetic drugs like nitrous oxide, ethyl ether, etc. will cause lowering of blood pressure and anoxia to heart muscle.

## OPERATIVE DEATHS

Deaths occurring during surgical procedures are classified as preoperative, operative and postoperative deaths. Preoperative period extends from the time of admission to the beginning of surgery. Operative period is the duration of actual surgical procedure and period of recovery from anaesthesia. At present, 30 days after the surgery is considered as the postoperative period. However, death due to delayed complications can occur after many days. Investigative and interventional procedures also carry risk of mortality during the procedures. Angiography, balloon angioplasty, intra-arterial thrombolysis, embolisation, interventional neurovascular radiology, etc. are associated with the risk of mortality. In most of the fatalities, there will be associated systemic diseases. Common causes of operative deaths are related to the patient, anaesthesia, surgical procedure and postoperative complications. Patient factors such as advanced age, cardiovascular diseases, respiratory diseases, metabolic disorders, endocrine diseases, hepatic and renal dysfunctions, etc. can contribute to death.

Emergency operations are immediate life saving procedures conducted usually within one hour of the incident. Examples are injuries due to homicidal attempts, domestic, industrial and vehicular accidents, etc. Urgent surgical procedures are done after resuscitating the patient and stabilising him. Procedures done within 24 hours of the precipitating cause are included in this group. Elective surgery is done after conducting the necessary investigations and assessment of the patient at the convenience of the surgeon and the patient. Risk of mortality is higher in the case of emergency and urgent surgical procedures. Prolonged and extensive procedures, increased blood loss, malignancy, peritoneal soiling, etc. are factors attributable to surgical mortality.

## MATERNAL DEATHS

Maternal death is the death of a woman while pregnant or within 42 days of termination of pregnancy irrespective of the duration and site of pregnancy, from any cause related to or aggravated by its management; but not from accidental or incidental causes. Sudden, unexpected and unexplained maternal deaths often attract public attention because of the accusations and allegations of negligence levelled against the medical personnel by the relatives of the deceased. Majority of the cases are subjected to medicolegal investigations and end up in civil and criminal litigations. Deaths can occur during pregnancy, delivery or within 6 weeks after delivery from interventions, omissions or incorrect treatment or complications arising from any of these. Some pre-existing disease, or diseases developed during pregnancy are aggravated by pregnancy and cause death. Bleeding during delivery is the major direct cause of maternal death. Abnormalities of the placenta can cause severe haemorrhage. With the advent of advanced methods of ultrasound diagnosis, placental abnormalities can be detected early. Death due to bleeding after delivery occurs only in centres not equipped with facilities for blood transfusion or surgical interventions. Bleeding after delivery should be anticipated in every delivery. If proper precautionery measures are not taken, it will amount to negligence.

Amniotic fluid embolism, pulmonary thrombo-embolism, cerebral thrombosis, sepsis, hypertensive disease of pregnancy, cardiac conditions, CNS diseases, malignancies, chronic respiratory diseases, aneurysms, metabolic disorders like diabetes, etc. are some of the conditions which can complicate pregnancy and cause death during advanced pregnancy or delivery. Diagnosis, proper antenatal care and treatment can prevent death. After delivery, some women may develop psychosis characterised by depression and suicidal tendency. Intensive psychiatric treatment and care should be given to the persons to prevent suicide.

## DEATHS DUE TO ADMINISTRATION OF DRUGS

Deaths following the administration of drugs have been dealt within the previous chapter. Drugs like penicillin can cause sudden death following an injection of the drug. A very small dose of the drug should be injected in the skin as a test dose. If the person is sensitive to penicillin, there will be local reactions like itching redness and swelling. But even a test dose can cause fatal reaction. Therefore, injections of drugs should be given to patients after having taken all precautionary measures to treat allergic reactions if any arise. For example, necessary drugs and equipment for resuscitation should be made available before giving the injection. The services of a doctor should also be at hand. If all these measures are taken, there will not be any liability even if death occurs.

## DEATH FOLLOWING ANAESTHESIA/SURGERY/DELIVERY

Doctors and hospital authorities should be report to the police all unexpected and unexplained deaths occurring during the course of anaesthesia, surgery, child birth or other forms of treatment within reasonable time afterwards as those cannot be regarded as natural deaths (Sec. 39 and 174 of CrPC.). It is always proper and safe to report the matter to the police because an inquest and subsequent autopsy can find out what really has caused death and save the doctor from unnecessary litigations.

### Liability

Apportioning responsibility between the anaesthesiologist and surgeon may be difficult. Both have contractual obligations to the patient to exercise reasonable skill and care. Each one is responsible for his own negligent act and not that of the other. Surgeon has vicarious liability regarding his assistants and nurses only. Anaesthesiologist is an independent contractor liable for his acts of omissions and commissions. He is not responsible for an error of judgement unless it is so gross as to be inconsistent with the skill expected of every anaesthetist. Liability and negligence cannot be avoided by pleading that one anaesthetist was engaged in administering anaesthesia to two or more patients simultaneously.

### Medical Negligence

Medical negligence is defined as lack of reasonable skill and care or wilful negligence on the part of the doctor resulting in the bodily damage or death of the patient. The ingredients of negligence are duty of care, dereliction of duty, direct causation and damage/death. In all cases of negligence, the plaintiff has to prove that there existed a duty of care because of the contractual obligation, which was breached by the defendant doctor, resulting in damage.

The damage should have been reasonably fore-seeable. For example, a doctor has to take all the precautions in reducing a fracture and immobilising it. He should check X-ray to verify that the fractured ends of the bones are properly aligned.

If not, resulting malunion could be a ground for civil litigation as it amounts to negligence.

To constitute a case, the following conditions are necessary.

- The nature of damage is solely due to the negligent action. This may be based on the evidence given by experts in the medical field or the evidence which may speak for itself (res ipsa loquitur). A swab or instrument left in the abdomen by the carelessness of the surgeon is an example.

- A plaintiff/patient should not have contributed to his own damage (contributory negligence). A patient also has certain duties while undergoing treatment. He should not withhold any facts regarding his ailment from the physician. He should obey all the instructions scrupulously.

- The defendant doctor should be solely responsible for the damage. There should not be any new intervening incident which caused the damage.

- Civil litigation is initiated by the patient against the doctor in a civil court. The limitation period is 2 years.

## Criminal Negligence

Law really enables the doctor to perform any method of treatment and protects him from a criminal charge even if the treatment results in any harm to the patient. According to Sec. 88 of IPC "Nothing, which is not intended to cause death, is an offence by reason of any harm which it may cause, or be intended by the doer to cause, or be known by the doer to be likely to cause, to any person for whose benefit it is done in good faith and who has given a consent whether express or implied to suffer that harm, or to take the risk of that harm."

The above section should be read with Sec. 52 of IPC which states that "Nothing is said to be done or believed in good faith which is done or believed without due care and attention." A surgeon knowing that a particular operation is likely to cause the death of a person who suffers from a disease, performs that operation in good faith for the benefit of the patient with his consent. If the person dies or sustains any damage, the surgeon is not liable.

When the death of a patient is attributed to the negligence or undue interference of the doctor, the police charges a case in the criminal court under Sec. 304 A of IPC. The section of law states as follows: "Whoever causes the death of any person by doing any rash or negligent act not amounting to culpable homicide, shall be punished with imprisonment for a term which may extend to 2 years, or with fine or with both." In such cases, there is a presumption of absence of intention. The prosecution should prove that death was due to gross carelessness, negligence and ignorance or the doctor acted under the influence of alcohol or drugs. If the death of the patient occurred due to sensitivity reaction following the parenteral use of an antibiotic, doctor is liable if he has not given a prior test dose. Before charging a case, police will collect the evidence including the opinion of the experts.

## Litigations

Proof of negligence is established in several ways. Most commonly the court will adduce evidence from expert testimony. But very often the experts in the field are reluctant to testify against colleagues. Therefore, the law has to depend upon the doctrine of **Res ipsa Loquitur** the "act speaks for itself". This has been applied in situations in which harm could not have occurred except by negligence and the technique or treatment causing the harm was solely under the control of the doctor. The main reason for the malpractice litigations is the failure on the part of the doctor to establish rapport with the patient and relatives. The majority of the doctors are frequently unconcerned in this regard. They do not closely identify with their patients. There is very little opportunity for the patient to acquaint himself with the doctor during the brief period of medical treatment. Therefore, the doctors have to take sufficient precautions to avoid such an action in every case they deal with. No speciality can be practiced without accident or complications. Most of the patients and relatives are understanding and satisfied by frank discussion of problems. If the doctor belittles or ignores a complication or fails to impart sympathetic understanding, the stage is set for a suit for damage. The best protection against medicolegal action lies in the thorough and up-to-date practice of the profession coupled with sympathetic interest in the patient and maintenance of proper records of the treatment and therapeutic procedures.

## DIRECTIONS TO THE INVESTIGATING OFFICER

Hon. Supreme Court is of opinion that doctors should be protected from frivolous or unjust prosecutions (Crl Appeal-144-145/2004). Supreme Court has issued guidelines regarding prosecuting medical professionals for offences of which criminal rashness or negligence is an ingredient. A private complaint may not be entertained unless the complainant has produced prima facie evidence before the court in the form of a credible opinion given by another competent doctor to support the charge of rashness or negligence on the part of the accused doctor. Similarly, an investigating officer, before proceeding against the doctor accused of rash or negligent act or omission, should obtain an independent and competent medical opinion preferably from a doctor in government service qualified in that branch of medical practice, who can normally be expected to give an impartial and unbiased opinion.

When a complaint is received alleging death due to medical negligence, it has to be registered initially U/S 174 CrPC. Before proceeding with the inquest, the entire case records of the patient should be obtained from the hospital concerned. In all such deaths, a medicolegal autopsy is highly indicated to find out the reasons for death. A doctor accused of rashness or negligence may not be arrested in a routine manner simply because a charge has been levelled against him. Unless his arrest is necessary for furthering the investigation or for collecting evidence or unless the investigating officer feels satisfied that the doctor proceeded against, would not make himself available, to face the prosecution unless arrested, the arrest may be withheld.

In the State of Kerala, an allegation of medical negligence can be investigated only by a deputy superintendent of police. After registering the case, the Dy.S. P will refer the case to an expert panel consisting of the district medical officer of health (convener), district govt. pleader, a senior govt. doctor in the speciality concerned and a forensic expert. The investigating officer should consider the view expressed by the expert panel. **(vide Circular memorandum No 54608/SSB 3/2004/ Home dated 18-12-2006).**

# Recent Advances in Crime Investigation

Forensic medicine and forensic science have developed considerably in the past few decades. The scientific methods in crime investigation is keeping in pace with those advancements. The investigating officers should possess basic knowledge of the recent advances in science and technology and be able to apply them in crime investigation.

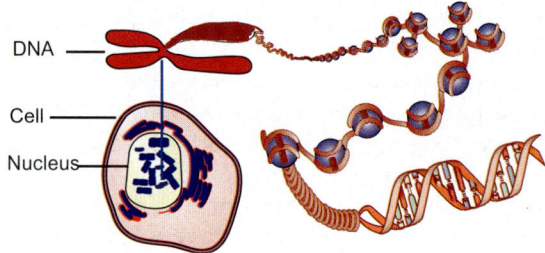

**Fig. 32.1:** DNA in the cell

## DNA ANALYSIS

DNA analysis, popularly known as DNA fingerprinting is an epoch making discovery in the field of molecular biology. The technique of DNA fingerprinting was developed in 1985 by Sir. Alec Jeffrey of the Department of Genetics in the University of Leicester. It is a revolutionary technique developed in criminology ever since the introduction of the method of fingerprinting in 1901. Nucleus of each cell in the human body contains 46 chromosomes. Of these, 23 are contributed by the father and the other 23 by the mother at the time of fertilisation of the ovum by the sperm. The building block of a chromosome is deoxyribonucleic acid (DNA). DNA contains genes which carry instructions that enable the cell to make a particular protein which performs a particular function. DNA is a double helix structure, which looks like a double-stranded spiral ladder (Fig. 32.1). The two strands are made up of nucleotides such as adenine (A), thymine (T), guanine (G) and cytosine (C), deoxy ribose sugar and a phosphate group. The strands are held

together by hydrogen bonds between pairs of the phosphate-sugar bases like the rungs of a ladder. Each chromosome is a continuous thread of DNA. The whole DNA constituent of a single cell is called genome. Human genome contains nearly three billion nucleotides.

DNA molecule is composed of two very long strands of As, Ts, Gs and Cs, which are tightly paired with each other. An A of one strand is always paired with a T of the other strand and G pairs with C. This means that if the sequence of nucleotides of one strand is known, the sequence of the other strand can be found out. One strand of DNA is like a negative photograph of the other (Fig. 32.2).

Sequence of nucleotides in a gene gives it meaning by storing instructions to build the other molecules for life. These instructions are read as a string of As, Ts, Gs and Cs such as ACGGTAACT. cAs there are 26 letters in English alphabet, there are four letters in the alphabet of

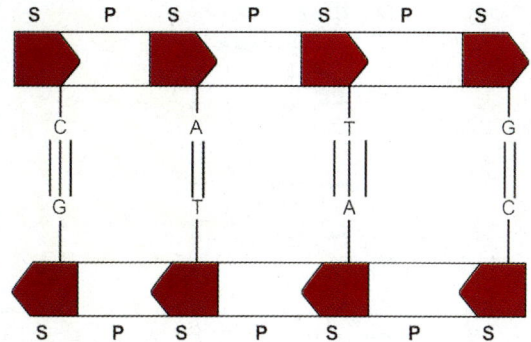

**Fig. 32.2:** Structure of DNA S = Deoxyribose sugar, P= Phosphate, A = Adenine, T = Thymine, C = Cytosine, G = Guanine

DNA. The letters of the genetic alphabet A, T, G and C are meaningless on their own, but they are combined into useful instructions in genes. Some genes carry enough information for one complete characteristic of an organism, but most characteristics result from combination of genes. Genome is like a library of instructions. Genes are like chapters in the books that fill the library of the genome.

Sequence of letters within a gene is like the letters in a book of instructions. Deciphering the enormously long sequence of As, Ts, Gs and Cs in an organism's genome reveals useful information. A difference in the gene sequence that codes for hemoglobin will result in a genetic disorder, **sickle cell anemia**. This is like a spelling mistake in a word which will alter its meaning.

The human genomic DNA may code for less than 35000 genes while the remainder is non-coding DNA known as **junk DNA**. DNA sequences which code for proteins make up approximately 3% of the human genome. The rest of the regions do not code for proteins. Much of this non-coding DNA contain areas in which sequences of the bases repeat very frequently. These repeated sequences account for 50% of the genome. Many different types of repetitive polymorphism such as short tandem repeats (**STR**), variable number tandem repeats (**VNTR**), single nucleotide polymorphism (**SNP**) and amplified fragment length polymorphism (Amp FLP). The number of these repeating units is highly variable. Thus the length of the repetitive DNA also varies. Using suitable techniques, the STRs and VNTRs can be analysed. This technique is applied in identifying individuals.

## ISOLATION OF DNA

DNA can be extracted from the nucleus of any cell in the body. It is usually extracted from blood, semen, bone, hair, buccal epithelial cells and other tissues. In a human cell, there are 46 chromosomes composed of millions of nucleotide pairs. These long DNA molecules are susceptible to degradation into fragments. But using new techniques (polymerase chain reaction), DNA fragments can be amplified.

### Detection Methods

There are several methods of DNA analysis: Restriction fragment length polymorphism (RFLP) analysis, VNTR analysis, polymerase chain reaction (PCR-STR), reverse dot blot analysis, and amplified fragment length polymorphism (Amp-FLP). RFLP analysis is time consuming and requires high quality and quantity samples. The other methods for DNA analysis are faster.

### RFLP Analysis

The hypervariable DNA sequences are detected by means of the 'southern blotting technique'. In this method, DNA fragments are visualised as bands on an autoradiogram. Unique patterns of nearly 40 bands resembling a bar code are produced (Figs 32.3 and 32. 4). The pattern of the bands is highly individualistic. Two persons having the same pattern of the variable bands is in the order of 1 in $10^{14}$ to $10^{30}$. The world's population is only $6 \times 10^9$. Therefore the DNA typing can be considered as highly unique except in the case of identical twins (uniovular).

### Polymerase Chain Reaction

In this method, DNA is replicated when a limited quantity of sample is available. In the first cycle, one DNA strand is replicated into two. After 30 cycles, more than a billion copies of the original DNA molecule are produced. The amplified DNA fragments are detected by a machine which converts the data into a graph. This method requires costly equipment. In western countries, chemical kits for DNA isolation, amplification and identification are available. New electronic DNA analysing techniques which can yield results within one hour are being developed.

### Mitochondrial DNA

Mitochondrial DNA is distributed throughout the cytoplasm of the cell, confined to the mitochondria. Mitochondrial DNA is inherited from the mother. So all members of a maternal lineage will share the same mitochondrial DNA sequence. Even though the mitochondrial DNA is a small molecule, some regions of the molecule are highly variable and it is easy to differentiate two samples. One disadvantage is that more than one mitochondrial DNA sequence is found in one individual.

### APPLICATIONS OF DNA TYPING

#### Disputed Paternity

In case of disputed paternity, DNA typing is done from the samples of blood collected from the child, mother and the putative father. Most of the laboratories perform RFLP analysis. The chance of an unrelated man matching the paternal bands of the child will be one in a million. This test conclusively proves/disproves paternity (Fig.32.3).

#### Criminal Investigation

DNA typing done from blood stains, seminal stains, hair, bits of tissues, etc. found in a crime scene can identify the criminal and connect him with the crime (Fig. 32.4). This can be applied in cases of murder, rape, etc.

#### Y Chromosome—DNA Typing

Of the X and Y sex chromosomes, Y chromosome usually retains its genetic makeup during cell division and is passed from fathers to sons only. Typing of the Y chromosome is becoming popular in solving cases of sexual assault. The vaginal swab of the victim will contain epithelial cells as well as the sperms of the accused. Testing of Y chromosome can sift through all the female DNA to locate the male DNA. This testing can detect the DNA type of different males also.

**Fig. 32.3:** Paternity testing: DNA profiles of mother (M), child (C)and two males (F1 and F2). The oblique lines indicate the paternally inherited bands in the child which are present in the F1. Therefore, F1 is the biological father of the child

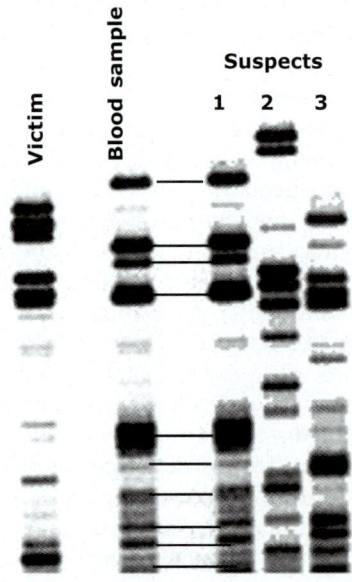

**Fig. 32.4:** DNA fingerprinting of blood stains. Comparison of the DNA pattern of blood sample in the crime scene with the blood of the suspects. DNA profile of the suspect 1 matches with the DNA pattern of the blood sample. Matching bands are indicated by lines in between them

## Identification of Human Remains

Identity can be established in the case of unidentified human remains by conducting typing of the tissues and comparing the pattern with those of close relatives.

## Other Applications

DNA typing can be utilized for blood typing, species identification, sexing of biological materials, tracing pedigree, family lineage, etc.

## Collection of Samples

Any human material which will yield high molecular weight DNA can be used for DNA typing. Body fluids and their stains, hair, bones and tissues are suitable for DNA analysis. Care should be taken to prevent contamination of samples while collecting them. The sample has to be preserved properly to prevent degradation of DNA.

### Blood, Semen and Salivary Stains

If the stains are present on small objects or clothes, the entire object should be forwarded after drying the stains. The materials have to be collected in paper bags after protecting the stained area with blotting papers. Then the entire samples have to be put in polythene bags, sealed and despatched.

If the stains are present on a large object, wet a sterile cotton swab with distilled water and swab the stained area. The swab is dried well in the air, packed in paper bags and despatched in sealed polythene bags. A control (unused swab) must also be packed separately. DNA will not degrade if the specimen is well dried.

### Liquid Blood

A blood sample of 10 ml should be collectedunder aseptic precautions in a sterile, screw capped container. Heparin or EDTA is added as preservative. Blood should be thoroughly mixed with the preservative and the bottle is placed in a thermos flask containing crushed ice. A label showing all the relevant details should be affixed on the bottle. If there is delay in transmitting the sample to the laboratory, it may be kept in a refrigerator. Blood should not be collected from persons who have received blood transfusion or bone marrow

transplantation within three months preceding the date of collection of sample to prevent vitiation of results due to unrelated genomic DNA in the blood received.

### Tissues/Bones/Teeth

Tissues such as skin, skeletal muscles, sternum, spleen, etc. are good sources of DNA. About 10 to 100 gm of tissues are put in a clean glass bottle. The ideal preservative for tissues is a 20% solution of Dimethyl sulphoxide in water. If it is not available, saturated solution of sodium chloride can be used. The bottles should be closed with bakelite screw cap, packed carefully and despatched. Ideal method is to send the tissues in a frozen state in an ice box. Dry bones can be packed in clean paper and put in polythene bags. There is no need to add any preservative to dry bones. Molar teeth are the ideal ones for analysis. Teeth are detached from the jaws and placed as such in clean polythene bags and packed.

### Vaginal Swab

Sterile cotton swabs are used for collecting the sample. The swabs have to be dried well in air and despatched in clean sterile bottles or paper bags. If there is delay in sending the swabs, the same may be kept in a refrigerator at 4 °C.

### Hair

The sample of hair with intact roots should be collected with a clean sterile forceps into a clean polythene bag. Control samples should also be sent.

### Disputed Paternity

DNA analysis is carried out by collecting blood from the mother, putative father and the child. Intravenous blood samples (10 ml) in a clean glass vial or bottle to which preservative such as EDTA, heparin or sodium citrate is added. The blood samples have to be kept in a thermos flask containing ice and despatched to the laboratory immediately.

## Forwarding

The DNA analysis is being conducted at the centre for DNA fingerprinting and diagnostics (CDFD),

Hyderabad and in many forensic science laboratories of the country. CDFD is a national centre for DNA fingerprinting and diagnostics set up by the Government of India to cater to the needs of the nation. In the state of Kerala, Rajeev Gandhi Institute of Biotechnology, Thiruvananthapuram is undertaking DNA analysis.

Any material for DNA analysis should be forwarded by a responsible authority like a judicial or investigating officer. The samples along with the control, should be properly packed, labelled and sealed before forwarding. The detailed facts of the sample and examination required should be furnished along with the exhibits. In the case of disputed paternity, the blood has to be collected by a government doctor who has to fill in an identification card. A signed photograph of the donor, attested by the medical officer in the presence of the investigating officer or a gazetted officer is to be affixed on the identification card. An extra copy of the photograph is also to be attached.

In criminal cases, investigating officer has to submit a forwarding note along with the material objects. The forwarding note shall contain details about the nature of crime, list of exhibits, nature of examination required, particulars of persons in custody and a certificate from the court concerned. The proformas of the identification card and forwarding note are given Proformas 32.1 and 32.2.

### Officers Authorised to Send Samples to a Govt. Laboratory for DNA Typing

- Judicial officers
- Police officers above the rank of a sub-Inspector of Police
- Medical officers of a government hospital
- Executive Magistrates.

## PROBLEMS CONCERNING DNA ANALYSIS

Improper preservation and storage of samples can result in the fragmentation of DNA molecule and can lead to problems in the analysis. When the sample is contaminated with bacteria, DNA will be degraded. Contamination of samples can happen during collection of samples and examination in the laboratory.

Contamination is defined as addition of individual's physiological material including DNA during or after collection of the sample as evidence. Most significant contamination is from a human source. Stringent measures should be taken in the laboratory to prevent contamination. Equipment and reagents should be kept in such a way to prevent contamination. Laboratory personnel should wear gloves and barrier clothing.

Mutation of the genes (non-inherited germline) in a child can give rise to wrong results in paternity testing. This should be taken into account when inconsistent results are obtained.

Recent DNA typing methods do not discriminate monozygotic (uniovular) twins. In such cases, DNA sequence of bone marrow derived B lymphocytes have to be studied. The B lymphocytes can be isolated from the blood.

Laboratory errors like mixing of samples can give wrong results. A challenge to DNA test results may be statistical. If there is no population database, one cannot say whether a DNA profile is common or rare. However, the statistical probability of two persons having the same DNA profile is almost nil !!!

## ADMISSIBILITY OF DNA FINGERPRINTING EVIDENCE

The Indian Evidence Act (IEA), though drafted in 1892 suits to the requirements of the present day in the light of the recent advances and developments in science. Under Section 45 of IEA, when the court has to form an opinion in any legal proceeding involving matters of science like DNA fingerprinting, it may resort to expert testimony on such facts. Many Indian courts have accepted the evidence of DNA analysis.

In the light of the stipulation laid down by the Supreme Court of India (*Kathikahoghad v/s State of Bombay*), the following observations will strengthen the credibility of DNA fingerprinting.

1. Court must be convinced that DNA analysis is capable of producing accurate and credible results so that it can be safely relied upon.
2. The court must be convinced that the tests were conducted in well-equipped laboratories by experienced persons.

**Proforma 32.1:** Identification Card

(Place a tickmark (a) in the appropriate boxes where provided)

| Affix signed photograph of the donor attested by the medical officer in the presence of the Investigating Officer or a gazetted officer (attach an extra copy) |
|---|

A. Particulars of the donor/source

    1. Name (Block letters) ......................................................

    2. Father/guardian's name ................................................

    3. Age: Months ......Years.......Sex:  M/F

    4. Address ...........................................................

    5. Medical history:    Normal ☐    General disorder ☐    Chronic disease ☐

    6. Regimental No:    Army ☐    Navy ☐    Air force ☐

       (if for defence record)

B. Purpose of test

    Paternity ☐    Maternity ☐   Both ☐

    Murder ☐    Rape ☐    Burglary ☐    Violence ☐    Other ☐

    Identity of deceased ☐    Inheritance ☐    Immigration ☐    Defence record ☐

    Medical screening ☐    Other ☐

C.

    1.  Case No. ☐    Police Station ☐

    2.  Blood samples of suspected accused ☐    Victim ☐    Relative ☐ (mention relation)

D. Blood collection:

Preferably 10 ml. blood should be collected in sterilised capped bottle using EDTA/Heparin anticoagulant. Ensure that donor did not receive transfusion during the last three months.

    1. Volume ☐

    2. Date of collection : Day ☐    Month ☐    Year ☐

E. Rape cases

    Swab No . ☐    Semen stain ☐    Blood stain ☐    Hair ☐

F. Specimen seal used on samples:

G. Name of examining doctor               Name of Investigating Officer/Judicial Officer

    Signature                                    Signature

    Designation                                  Designation

    Date                                          Date

    Witness- Name and address ........................................................

    Signature with date:........................................................

    Declaration of blood donor:

I, ...........................hereby certify that the blood in the bottle, signed by me and sealed in my presence, is my blood given on ........................ and I did not receive a blood transfusion within the last three months.

For CDFD use

CDFD No. ☐          Date: ☐

Case taken up ☐        Name of Examiner ☐

Date of report ☐

## Proforma 32.2: Forwarding Note

In all cases where examination of any material is required at the laboratory, a copy of this form duly filled in should accompany the exhibit.

Case No. .................................................    Police station ........................................

Section in Law .....................................    District .................................................

Date .....................................................    State ..................................................

### I. Nature of crime
(This should cover nature of charge, brief history and any relevant details)

..................................................................................................................................................

..................................................................................................................................................

..................................................................................................................................................

### II. List of Exhibits sent for examination

| S. No. | Description of exhibits | How, when & by whom found | Source of exhibit | Remarks |
|---|---|---|---|---|
| 1. | | | | |
| 2. | | | | |
| 3. | | | | |

### III. Nature of examination required

1. ............................................................................................................................................

2. ............................................................................................................................................

3. ............................................................................................................................................

### IV. Particulars of persons in custody

| S. No. | Full Name | Occupation | Age | Sex | Date & time of arrest | Whether on bail or in custody |
|---|---|---|---|---|---|---|
| 1. | | | | 2. | | |

Rank and signature of the Investigating Officer

Date:

No. ..................................................................

Forwarded to the Director, .........................................................................................................

Signature & designation of forwarding officer

Specimen(s) Seal (s) Impression(s) on Exhibit(s) Parcel(s)

### Certificate of Authority

Certified that the Director ................................... has the authority to examine the exhibits sent to him in connection with the case No.................. P.S ........................... under section ........................... dated ...................... State versus ............................... and for collection of blood from the individual involved in the case and if necessary to take the exhibits to pieces or remove portions for the purpose of the said examination.

Signature & Designation of forwarding authority

Date

Place:

If properly carried out by a well-experienced scientist, DNA analysis is a highly reliable method in solving many a civil and criminal matter. At present, DNA analysis is done in less than 20 centres in the whole country. The analytical equipment are very costly and hence the cost of the testing is also high.

## BRAIN FINGERPRINTING

Brain fingerprinting is a marvellous aid in scientific criminal investigation. The technique which is superior to polygraph was invented by Dr. Lawrence A Farwell (USA). It is a computer-based technology to identify the perpetrator of a crime accurately and scientifically by measuring brain wave responses to crime relevant words or pictures presented on a computer screen. Brain fingerprinting has proven accurate in tests on real life situations including actual crimes.

Brain fingerprinting is based on the cognitive functions of the brain. In a criminal act, the brain plans, executes and records the crime. The fundamental difference between a perpetrator and a falsely accused innocent person is that, the perpetrator, having committed the crime, has the details of the crime stored in his brain, and the innocent suspect does not. Brain fingerprint detects the evidence stored in the brain. Brain fingerprinting is similar to fingerprinting or DNA typing. It matches evidence from a crime scene with evidence stored in the brain of the perpetrator.

### Technique

In brain fingerprinting technique, words or pictures relevant to a crime are projected on a computer screen before the suspect along with other irrelevant words or pictures. Electrical brain responses of the suspect are measured non invasively through a head band equipped with sensors. A specific wave response called a **MERMER** (memory and encoding-related multi-faceted electroencephalographic response) is elicited when the brain processes the relevant information it recognises (Figs 32.5A to C). This pattern occurs within about a second after the stimulus presentation, and can readily be detected using EEG amplifiers and a programmed computer. When the details of the crime that the perpetrator would know are presented, an MERMER is emitted by the brain of a perpetrator but not by the brain of an innocent suspect. In brain fingerprinting, a computer analyses the brain responses to detect the MERMER and thus determines scientifically whether or not the crime relevant information is stored in the brain of the suspect.

For a subject with knowledge of the investigated situation ('information present') stored in the brain, the probes are noteworthy due to that knowledge, and therefore probes elicit a brain MERMER. For a subject lacking this knowledge ('information absent') not stored in the brain, probes are indistinguishable from the irrelevant, and thus probes do not elicit an MERMER. When the information tested is crime relevant and known only to the perpetrator and investigators then 'information present' implies guilt and 'information absent' implies innocence. Similarly, when the information tested is information known only to members of a particular organization/group (e.g. intelligence agency or a terrorist group), the information present indicates affiliation with the group in question.

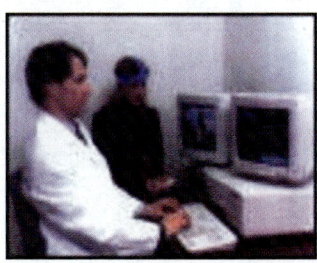 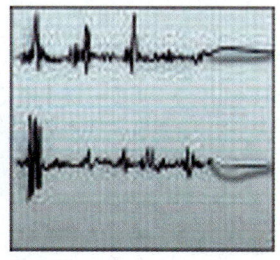 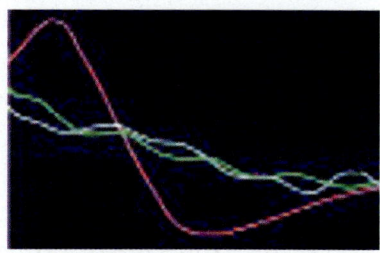

A       B       C

**Figs 32.5A to C:** Brain fingerprinting: A. Interviewing, B. Brain waves, C. MERMER

Conventional fingerprinting and DNA finger-printing match physical evidence from a crime scene with evidence on the person of the perpetrator. Similarly, brain fingerprinting matches informational evidence from the crime scene with evidence stored in the brain. Brain fingerprinting helps the investigator to determine if the suspect has committed a specific crime. Unlike polygraphy, no questions are asked and no answers are given during brain fingerprinting.

By providing an accurate, scientific means of identifying the perpetrator of a crime and clearing innocent suspects, brain fingerprinting will provide substantial result immediately for the law enforcement organization. Once the authorities know with certainty who has committed a crime, the resource can be devoted to bring the perpetrator to justice, rather than to seeking additional leads or pursuing innocent suspects. Because of its accuracy and non-invasive nature, brain finger-printing technique has superseded other methods of interrogation.

In the first phase, the crime scene is examined and evidence connected with the crime are collected. The details such as photographs of the victim, crime scene, weapon, etc. are collected. The brain evidence collection is conducted to determine whether or not the evidence from the crime scene matches with the evidence stored in the brain of the suspect. In the computer evidence analysis, the system makes a mathematical determination as to whether or not this specific evidence is in the brain and then the evidence is analysed. The result can be either "information present", i.e. the details of the crime are stored in the brains of the suspect — or "information absent", i.e. the details of the crime are not stored in the brains of the suspect.

### Advantages of the Technique

- Identifies the accused quickly and scientifically.
- Has 100% accuracy
- Excludes the innocent
- Provides immediate scientific result
- Discovers criminal espionage, and terrorists plots against individuals, corporations, governments and society
- Does not violate human rights.

## POLYGRAPH TECHNIQUE

Polygraph is an equipment which measures and graphically records the blood pressure, pulse, respiration, galvanic resistance of skin and muscular movements of an individual. This is based on the principle that if a person willfully utters a lie, it will produce physiological changes in his body. The blood pressure will rise, pulse rate will increase, respiration becomes shallow, galvanic resistance of skin lowers and there will be involuntary muscular movements. The blood pressure/pulse is measured by a cuff tied around the upper arm. Pneumographs tied across the chest and abdomen measure the respiratory movements of chest and abdomen. Two electrodes attached to the forefinger and third finger measure the variations in electrical conductance. Transducers fixed in the chair will pick up the muscular movements (Fig. 32.6).

To find out whether a suspect in a crime is deliberately telling a lie or not, he can be subjected to the polygraph test. The transducers of the equipment are attached to the body of the subject and preframed questions, both relevant and irrelevant are asked. The questions are prepared with the help of the investigating officer. Police officers will not be present during testing. A willful lie will produce notable changes in the graphic recordings of the various physiological parameters (Fig. 32.7).

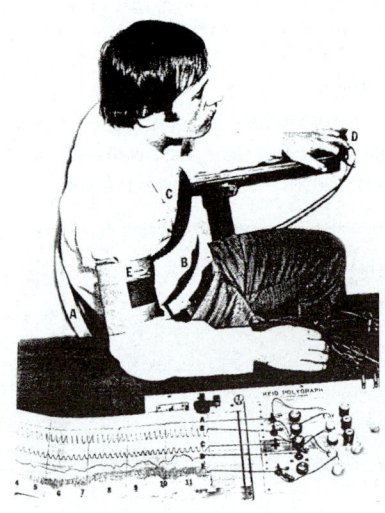

**Fig. 32.6:** Polygraph test

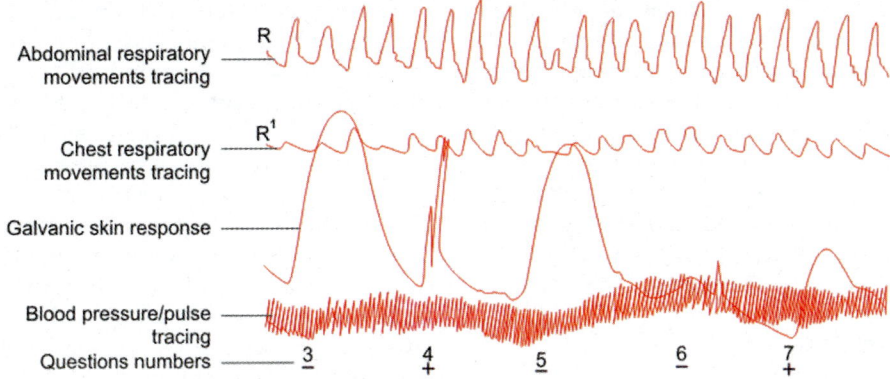

**Fig. 32.7:** Polygraph Test—Deceptive response can be seen when question numbers 3 and 5 were put to the subject. (Note the changes in respiratory rate, GSR and BP/pulse tracings)

Polygraph test is very useful in detecting deception provided the questions are framed carefully. The expert who performs the test is usually a psychologist or sociologist trained in polygraph technique. The investigating officer should discuss the case with him and frame the questions, both relevant and irrelevant, prior to the test.

## Changes Noted in Deception

Normal rate of respiration is 12–18/minute. In the case of deceptive response, many changes are noted in the tracings. There will be respiratory blocks during inhalation and expiration, suppression of respiration, change in the rate; faster, slower or heavier, erratic breathing, etc. Heavier breathing is noted after deception (sigh of relief). The blood pressure/pulse tracings will also show many abnormalities after a deceptive response. The graphs will show raise in the base level with or without reduction in the amplitude, raise in the baseline before a relevant question and fall after answering (anticipatory tension and relief thereafter).

The skin resistance is lowered due to increased activity of sweat glands resulting in quantitative changes in perspiration on the surface layers of skin. The deception response is an increase in the amplitude of the current passing between the electrode and it is shown by a higher amplitude in the tracings. Muscular movements and unobserved muscular pressure are detected in deception. These are picked up by the transducers in the bellows and hollow tubings fixed in the chair and indicated in the tracings.

Polygraph results are not infallible. Emotional stress can cause false positive responses. A **pathological liar** may not show any positive response when lying. Nervousness, individual physical or mental abnormalities, previous excessive interrogation and indifference to a question can affect the accuracy of the test. However, the polygraph can find out whether the answers of the subject are truthful or not. The test will be helpful in exonerating an innocent person accused of a crime.

## NARCO ANALYSIS

There are several methods of criminal interrogation to detect lying and deception of suspects and accused. Most of the techniques are founded on torture, either physical or mental. But modern techniques like polygraph and brain fingerprinting are non-invasive methods which will detect deception without causing physical or mental injury to the subject. Psychiatrists used to perform psycho-analysis by inducing a hypnotic state by injecting narcotics in their patients. During the trance, the patient will recall repressed facts and events which will be helpful for the doctor for further treatment. This is done with the assistance of qualified anaesthetists in a well-equipped hospital because fatal adverse reactions are possible with the narcotic drug.

Experts are of opinion that this method is risky and does not yield correct results. The subject will fabricate and confabulate due to the hallucinatory effect of the drug. Moreover the drug can cause serious adverse reactions like cardiac arrest, respiratory depression, etc. The tests are found effective on persons who, if they had been properly interrogated, would have disclosed the truth anyway. The person who is determined to lie will continue the deception even under the effects of the drug.

## Medical Aspects

The drug used for narcoanalysis is sodium Pentothal, also known as sodium thiopental. It belongs to the category of the narcotic barbiturates, listed in the schedule III of controlled substances under the NDPS Act 1985. It directly acts on the inhibitory channels which decreases the neuronal activity of the brain. It has anaesthetic, sedative and hypnotic properties. Thiopental is an ultra-short-acting barbiturate and hence used in the induction phase of anaesthesia and as a general anaesthetic in minor surgical procedures.

Intravenous injection of 20 ml of 2.5% solution of the drug can cause unconsciousness in 15–30 seconds which lasts for 5–10 minutes. If the drug is given in half the strength, the person enters into a **twilight stage**: a state between consciousness and unconsciousness. Some believe that the drug will relax the individual's defenses to the point that he will unknowingly tell the truth which he has been concealing and hence the name **truth serum**. The drug will remove inhibitions, but not self-control. Therefore, the subject may be able to tell lies, fabricate or confabulate. The reliability of the confessions is dubious.

The drug is a depressant of the central nervous system and myocardium (heart muscle). The drug can cause adverse effects like fall of blood pressure, cardiac arrest, laryngospasm, bronchospasm, respiratory arrest, etc. Shock and anaphylactic (fatal allergic reaction) reactions have been reported. It is absolutely contraindicated in persons with pre-existing natural diseases. Lethal dose of the drug varies from person to person and cannot be stated with certainty. It can be as low as 1 mg/100 ml or still less in combination with other depressants like alcohol.

The manufacturers of the drug caution that this drug should be administered by competent persons and resuscitative equipment, oxygen, etc. are to be kept readily available. If cardiac or respiratory arrest develops during anaesthesia, immediate resuscitative measures should be taken. If cardiac or respiratory arrest is prolonged, person may die due to cerebral anoxia or go into a persistent vegetative state. This is the reason why the drug is administered in a well-equipped hospital with ventilator facility by specialist doctors for anaesthetic purposes taking all measures to counteract adverse effects.

## Legal Aspects

### Consent of the Subject

Consent obtained from the person subjected to narco analysis is invalid as it does not conform to Section 88 of Indian Penal Code. The main ingredient of this section is that the act is one which is done for the benefit of the person, as in the case of a surgical operation to remove appendix from any patient suffering from acute appendicitis. Injection of the dangerous narcotic drug is not for the benefit of the person and hence the consent is invalid. Pentothal sodium, an anesthetic drug is to be administered in a well-equipped hospital; instead the procedure is conduted in a forensic laboratory. This cannot be considered as an act done in good faith as defined in **Sec 52 of IPC.** which states that *"Nothing is said to be done or believed in "good faith" which is done or believed* **without due care and attention."**

### Section 53 of Criminal Procedure Code

One of the arguments in favour of narco analysis is that it is conducted as per the provisions of Sec. 53 CrPC. As per this section, a doctor can physically examine an accused under arrest, without his consent and using sufficient force, if he resists examination. His body fluids and other samples from his person can also be collected without his consent for conducting tests like DNA profiling or other tests the doctor thinks necessary. The purpose of this section is to examine the body of the accused and collect materials which will yield evidence indicating the commission of an offence. Narco analysis cannot be considered as a physical examination for collection of samples. It is not a test using samples taken from the body of the accused.

## Article 20 (3) of Constitution of India

Privilege against self-incrimination is a fundamental principle enunciated in Article 20 which states as follows: *"No person accused of any offence shall be compelled to be a witness against himself."* No one should be compelled to give testimony which may expose him to prosecution for crime. (AIR 1954 Sc 300 & Sc.132 of Indin Evidence Act—M.P Sharma Vs Satish Chandra). One argument put forward in favour of narco analysis is that the suspect is not entitled to get protection under Art 20 (3) as he is not an accused against whom a formal accusation relating to the commission of an offence has not been leveled. In Nandini Satpathy v P L Dani, the Supreme Court has considerably widened the scope of clause 3 of Article 20. The Court has held that the prohibitive scope of Art 20 (3) goes back to the stage of police interrogation. This means that the protection to avoid questions, the answers to which incriminate him is available when police examines the accused during investigation U/S 161 CrPC.

As per this Article, protection is against compulsion to be a witness also. Supreme Court interpreted the expression "to be a witness" very widely so as to include oral, documentary and testimonial evidence. It covers not only testimonial compulsion in a court, but also compelled testimony previously obtained. The phrase 'compelled testimony' must be read as evidence procured not merely by physical threats or violence but by psychic (mental) torture, atmospheric pressure, environmental coercion, tiring interrogatives and the like. Therefore, it extends also to techniques of psychological interrogation which cause mental torture in a person subjected to such interrogation. Narco analysis is nothing but psychological interrogation of the subject in a drugged state that amounts to torture.

## Article 21 of Constitution

Article 21 of the Constitution says that *"No person shall be deprived of his life or personal liberty except according to procedure established by law."* Protagonists of human rights hold the view that a suspect is not an accused and he is not liable for detention in any form. If the person subjected to narco analysis is not an accused, he is a common citizen who has the right to life and liberty, and protection against the arbitrary action of the executive. State could interfere with the liberty of citizens, if it could support its action by a valid law. There is no enabling law and there is no procedure to subject a citizen to a life-threatening technique like narco analysis where a dangerous narcotic is introduced into his body.

## Section 161(1) and (2) of Criminal Procedure Code

Narco analysis is done as a part of investigation under the provisions of Sec 161 CrPC. In that case, the interrogation has to be done by the investigating police officer or his subordinate (Sec.2(h)and Sec. 156 of CrPC). In narco analysis, the interrogation of the subject is done by the forensic scientists. The revelations made during the 'narcotic interrogation' are recorded both in video and audio tapes. There is no legal sanctity for these documents. They are not admissible as evidence. If the interrogation is done under Sec. 161 Cr.PC, the subject is entitled for protection under Article 20(3) also.

## Nemo Tenetur se Ipsum Accusare

"No man, not even the accused himself can be compelled to answer any question, which may tend to prove him guilty of a crime, he has been accused of." It is quite possible for the subject to develop hallucinations and delusions due to the effect of these drugs. The revelations can be confabulations misleading the investigators. Narco analysis is another form of sophisticated torture where a dangerous narcotic drug is administered to relax the mind before interrogation. This method is gross violation of human rights. This method cannot be considered as a scientific method of interrogation like polygraph test or brain fingerprinting, which are non-invasive and not harmful to the subject.

## Amnesty International

The human rights group, Amnesty International condemns narco analysis by stating that the use of drugs in interrogation was outlawed under international standards and is a breech of medical ethics. It constitutes cruel, inhuman and degrading treatment amounting to torture as per the Declaration of Tokyo 1975.

## UN Principles of Medical Ethics

Doctors participate in the narco analysis procedure. The subject is examined by a doctor who performs various investigations like X-ray chest, ECG, etc and certifies that he is fit to undergo narco analysis. An anesthetist doctor injects the narcotic into the veins. These doctors are doing an unethical act as per the International Code of Medical Ethics which stipulates as follows: *"It is a contravention of medical ethics for health personnel, particularly physicians to apply their knowledge and skills in order to assist in the interrogation of prisoners and detainees in a manner that may adversely affect the physical or mental health or condition of such prisoners or detainees and which is not in accordance with the relevant international instruments."* **(see Annexation XV–Supreme Court Order)**

## FORENSIC ODONTOLOGY

Application of the principles of dentistry for the purpose of law is known as forensic odontology. The speciality plays a key role in the investigation of crimes. Clinical dentistry has advanced very much like other medical specialities. Doctors qualified in dentistry are competent to practise forensic odontology. In many dental colleges, forensic odontology wings exist. The specific areas of forensic odontology are the following:
- Identification of the deceased/human remains by the dentition
- Comparison of the bite marks with the dentition of the suspect
- Analysis of alleged negligence in dental practice.

## Dental Identification

Enamel of the teeth is the hardest substance of the human body which will resist putrefactive changes, moderately high temperature and physical injuries. Therefore, data from the examination of teeth will be very helpful in identifying the deceased. There are 32 teeth in the adults and a tooth has five surfaces. The changes and appearance of the 160 surfaces form the basis for identification. Apart from these, findings in the adjacent tissues, root canals, etc. will provide additional information helpful to fix the identity. Nowadays, most of the dentists keep detailed dental records of their patients. These records include charts, diagrams, X-rays, and dental casts. The postmortem dental data is compared with the antemortem records.

If antemortem dental records are not available or traceable, information can be obtained from relatives and friends of the deceased. Information regarding prominent dental peculiarities, dental work like fillings, artificial dentures, etc. will be helpful in comparing the findings. Dentists may be able to identify the dental work they have done like an artisan identifying his handicraft.

During a medicolegal autopsy or while examining human remains, forensic pathologist will examine the dentition. But in mass disasters like air crash, the investigating officer should obtain the services of a forensic odontologist also to examine the victims/human remains.

In decomposed bodies, teeth will become loosened and may be found in the oral cavity or in the surroundings. These teeth have to be retrieved (as many as possible), labelled and preserved for future identification. If a tooth is lost due to decomposition of periodontal tissues, the socket will be open and the rim of the alveolus will be sharp (Fig. 32.8). When a tooth is extracted from a living person, the socket will be immediately filled with blood clot. Due to repair process, there will be resorption of bone and obliteration of the socket. The alveolar rim becomes rounded. Within 6 months to one year, the alveolus will be completely obliterated with complete remodelling of the socket. If the tooth was lost due to recent trauma, fracture of alveolar margin can be noted.

In charred dead bodies, the anterior teeth will be involved more than the posterior ones. Enamel or sometimes the crown will be lost leaving the root in the socket. Dental amalgams or ceramic can withstand higher temperatures. Acrylic material will be destroyed in fire. During autopsy, the following points are noted during the examination of dentition:

- Total number of teeth in each jaw
- Postmortem loss, extractions, unerupted teeth
- Deformities and diseases like caries
- Artificial denture/prostheses/restorative work, etc.
- Diseases of the gums and oral mucosa.
- Dental X-ray to detect root canal treatment.

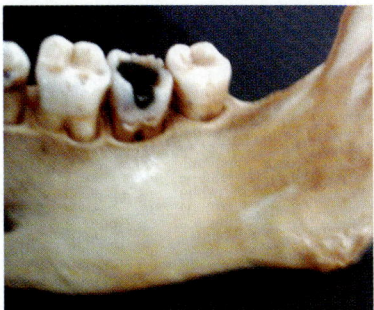

**Fig. 32.9:** Mandible showing amalgam filling of teeth No 18 (lower left 2nd Molar)

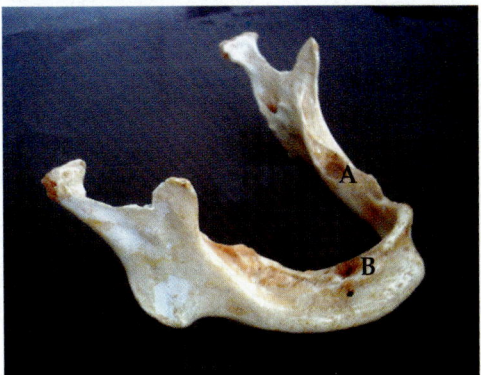

**Fig. 32.8:** Edentulous mandible (old age) A and B postmortem loss of teeth. Sockets are empty. In other areas there is complete resorption of bone indicating old loss

These pieces of informations are to be recorded in a dental chart and compared with the antemortem data obtained from the dental records of the deceased/missing person. The jaws are to be X-rayed and compared with antemortem X-rays if available. The jaws can be resected and preserved for future identification.

Sometimes even the close relatives may not be able to identify a deceased from dentition. They may not be aware of the dental diseases of the deceased or dental restorative work if any done. But gross peculiarities and deformities will be known to the parents or spouse. Dental restorative work (Fig. 32.9), artificial dentures, etc. can be helpful in establishing identity. At present, most of the dentists and dental clinics maintain dental records of their patients. If dental records are available, the antemortem and postmortem data can be compared. Comparison is to be done tooth by tooth. Similarities as well as the discrepancies

have to be noted. Discrepancies can be sometimes explained by collecting information from the relatives or dentist of the decedent. Unexplained discrepancies will rule out a positive identification.

## Determination of Age

Age can be determined more or less accurately from birth to 14 years by the examination of dentition. Estimation is based on the formation of tooth germ, formation of crown, eruption of teeth and calcification of root. Apart from visual examination, X-ray of the jaws is essential for a proper examination of the development of the structures of the teeth.

Germination of deciduous teeth starts during the 4th–5th month of intrauterine life. Germs of permanent teeth appear before birth. The first deciduous tooth to appear is the lower central incisor at sixth month. By 20–24 months, all the 20 deciduous teeth might have erupted. In the deciduous set, there will be two central incisors, two lateral incisors, two canines and two molars in each jaw.

The first permanent tooth to appear is the first molar behind the temporary second molar at the age of 6–7 years. This is followed by central incisors at the age of 7–8 years and then lateral incisors at the age of 8–9 years. The next teeth to appear are the first premolars at 9–11 years. Canines appear next at the age of 11–12 years. Recent studies show that canines erupt before the second premolars. At 10–12 years, the second premolars appear. Second molars appear by 12–14 years. At 14 years, there will be 28 permanent teeth; 14 in each jaw. From 14 to 17 years, estimation of age is based on the calcification of the second molar and development of the third molar. Usually the third molar erupts from 17 to 25 years. Sometimes the eruption may be as late as 30 years. Rarely third molars may not erupt at all. This may be due to inadequate space in the jaw. The condition is called 'impacted third molars'. This should be taken into account in the determination of age.

Secondary changes occur in the dental tissues as age advances. The changes are attrition, periodontosis, secondary dentine formation, cementum apposition, root transparency, root resorption, etc. Dr. Gosta Gustafson, a Swedish dentist has evolved a method of estimating the age from noting these changes in the teeth. The method is known as **Gustafson's technique.** For this, one of the incisor teeth is removed, ground; and a thin section made is examined microscopically. The tooth can be sent to the forensic odontology section of the oral pathology department of dental colleges or the department of forensic medicine in the medical colleges of the state for estimating the age by Gustafson's method.

## Personal Habits and Occupational Marks

Personal habits of a person are reflected in his dentition. Smoker's teeth will be stained yellow or blackish brown with nicotine. The stain found adjacent to the gum margin on the lingual aspect will be blackish brown in colour. On the labial aspect, the colour of the stain will be yellow. Pipe smokers and those who use cigarette holders will develop irregular gaps in the anterior teeth of both jaws. Persons who chew betel leaves with lime, arecanut and spices (pan) will have reddish brown staining of the entire teeth. The remnants of the pan can be found in the teeth. Chronic chewers may develop submucus fibrosis and leucoplakic patches in the oral cavity.

Carpenters and electricians are in the habit of holding nails in between the anterior teeth of the jaws. Similarly tailors and upholsterers hold needles in between the teeth. They will develop notches in the teeth edges. Poor oral hygiene, multiple caries, absence of dental restorations or prostheses indicate low socioeconomic status of the individual. On the other hand, costly ceramic restorations, bridgework, dental implantations, etc. indicate that the deceased was rich.

## Bite Marks

Bite mark is a patterned injury caused by the biting edges of the teeth. The injury could be an abrasion, contusion or superficial laceration depending upon the force applied. Bite marks are seen on the body of the victims of murder, sexual assault, child abuse, etc. Bite marks may be seen on fruits, cheese and other food articles recovered from the scene of crime, caused by the perpetrator of the crime. The shape of the dental arch will be imprinted in a well-defined mark. But sometimes a well defined mark may not be available for accurate comparison. Many objects like bangles, shoe heels, watch straps, etc. can produce injuries simulating a bite mark. Bites by animals such as dogs and cats should also be differentiated. The victim may inflict bite injuries on the body of the accused during a scuffle.

Comparison of the bite mark found on the victim with the dentition of the suspect is a very vital aspect in crime investigation. This work should be undertaken by a competent dental surgeon knowledgeable in all the aspects of forensic odontology. Examination of the bite mark should be done before the autopsy. Putrefactive changes will also alter the features of the bite mark.

A bite mark will invariably contain saliva of the biter. The saliva may contain blood group substances as 80% of people are secretors of blood group antigens in the saliva. Buccal epithelial cells and leucocytes of the gingival fluid present in the saliva can be utilised for DNA typing. Sterile swabs moistened with sterile saline or distilled water can be used to recover the saliva and cells from the bitten area for these tests. Priority should be given for DNA typing and the first swabs should be preserved for that purpose. Help from a forensic serologist may be obtained for collecting and preserving the trace evidence.

Bite mark can be compared with the dentition of the suspect by photographic or impression method (Fig. 32.10). The bite mark is photographed with a scale and life size enlargement of the bite mark is taken. This is to be compared with the dental models of the suspects. Full upper and lower dental impressions should be obtained using suitable impression material. Low or medium viscosity polyvinylsiloxane (PVS) is a good impression material. As it requires more time for setting, alginate impression material is a better choice. Two dental casts should be prepared. One should be kept as an untouched record. The second one is used for bite mark analysis. Wax exemplars of the bite impressions can also be taken from the suspect. This can be used for photographic comparison. These bite impressions can be photographed with a scale.

When bite marks are found on the dead body of a murder victim, the bite mark area can be dissected and preserved as a piece of evidence. This should be done after conducting the necessary examination by the forensic odontologist and serologist. From the colour changes of a bite bruise, age can be assessed. But there can be variations in the findings. Age of the bite injury can be determined by histological examination of the bite mark.

## FORENSIC RADIOLOGY

Radiology is the branch of medicine employing ionizing radiation in the diagnosis and treatment of diseases. Diagnostic radiology is the study of the images of the internal structures of the human body. Forensic radiology is the application of radiology for the purpose of law. Application of radiology for medicolegal investigation dates back

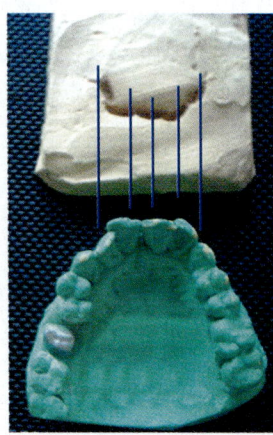

**Fig. 32.10**: Bitemark comparison (Photo by: Dr. Roopa Ramanathan)

to the last part of 19th century. In 1896, a bullet lodged in the leg of a gun shot victim was located by X-rays in the McGill University, Montreal. The X-ray plate produced before the court was the material evidence. Autopsy surgeons use X-rays to locate foreign bodies in the dead bodies prior to autopsy. X-rays are used to detect fractures sustained during assaults, presence of projectiles and sharpnels in gunshot injuries and explosions, to develop latent fingerprints and to determine age by assessing the ossification of long bones.

### Radiography

The epoch making discovery of an unknown (X) ray by Sir Wilhelm Roentgen (1845–1923) in 1895 paved the way for radiography and other imaging techniques. X-ray is a penetrating electromagnetic radiation produced by bombarding a target, usually made of tungsten, with high speed electrons. These radiations have a shorter wavelength than light. Absorption of X-rays by any substance depends upon its density and atomic weight. If the atomic weight of the material is low, it will be more transparent to X-rays. X-rays affect a photographic emulsion in the same way as light does and therefore cast dark shadows on a photographic plate. These are technically called **'roentgenograms'** or **radiographs**. When the human body is X-rayed, the bones, which are composed of elements of higher atomic weight than the surrounding flesh, absorb the radiation more effectively and the image will appear as a darker shadow in the photographic plate.

### Computed Tomography (CT)

Computed axial tomography, popularly known as CAT scan or CT scan is a technique where rays emitted by a rotating X-ray tube, pass through the body over multiple pathways in the cross-sectional plane. X-rays are absorbed according to the radiographic density of tissues. The radiation not absorbed by the tissues, reach the photo-receptors in the equipment. The differences in the attenuation of the rays is detected by the receptors and create an absorption profile. With the help of a computer, a series of axial images of the organs are produced.

## Magnetic Resonance Imaging (MRI)

Magnetic resonance imaging uses strong magnetic fields to generate electromagnetic signal from the elements in the body fluids and tissues. Human body is filled with the protons in the nucleus of hydrogen atoms which have got magnetic properties. The patient is placed in a cylindrical magnet which produces a magnetic field that is 30,000 times stronger than the earth's magnetic field. Then MRI stimulates the body with radio waves to change the steady-state orientation of protons. It then stops the radio waves and "listens" to the body's electromagnetic transmissions at a selected frequency. The transmitted signal is used to construct internal images of the body using principles similar to that of a CT scanner.

MRI scanners (Fig. 32.10) provide multiplanar, multidirectional sectional images or slices. MRI scanners provide good anatomical details, superior contrast and resolution when compared to a CT scanner. MRI can distinguish soft tissue in both normal and diseased states. Positron emission tomography **(PET)**, interventional radiology, ultrasound scanning, echocardiography, Micro CT, digital imaging, X-ray diffraction and crystall ography are the other radiological techniques used in forensic medicine and sciences.

## FORENSIC APPLICATIONS OF IMAGING TECHNIQUES

### Identification

Unknown dead bodies can be identified by radiological examination of the skeleton and matching it with premortem data if available. Postmortem evidence of a specific injury, congenital anomaly or disease, known to have been present in the deceased will provide positive identification. In mass casualties, this will be very helpful in identifying the victims.

Comparison of the configuration of dental arches, paranasal sinuses, mastoids, sella tursica, costal cartilages, calcification of lungs in the premortem and postmortem X-rays are conducted for identification. If a premortem X-ray of a single long bone is available, X-ray of the same bone of the dead body can be taken and compared. Diseases, trauma, tumours, degeneration, vascular grooves and trabecular patterns can be compared. Spine, pelvis and patella will provide comparable features.

## Suspicious Death/Murder

Radiography of the dead body prior to autopsy will help the forensic pathologist in determining the potential cause of death. It will also alert the doctor to focus his attention to specific areas in the dead body. Bony injuries are best detected and studied by X-ray examination prior to autopsy. Fracture of the hyoid bone or cornua of thyroid cartilage in manual strangulation can be best detected in a pre-autopsy radiograph.

Pre-autopsy X-rays of the skull, in the case of fractures of skull and brain trauma will be helpful in determining the direction of impact, nature of the object which caused the fracture and resultant damage to the brain. CT scan will give detailed information about intracranial bleeding and damage to brain. X-ray/CT scan should be invariably taken in all cases of injuries caused by projectiles and sharpnels. This will help the pathologist to recover the foreign bodies without difficulty. CT scan will show the track of the missile and the extent of the damage in the brain.

Radiological findings will provide positive evidence in battered children, battered women and abuse of old people. Classic radiological findings include fractures of various stages of healing, rib fractures, periostitis, etc. CT scan may reveal skull fractures, intracranial bleeding and cerebral edema. Bone scan or scintigraphy will detect trauma to bones and soft tissues, periostitis and osteomyelitis. This method is more sensitive than radiological examination to detect old trauma. There is increased uptake of the isotope in the growing ends of the bones where acute lesions are seen. But the radiation is 2.5 times higher than X-ray examination. Ultrasound scanning of the abdomen and infant brain will reveal hematomas and soft tissue injuries. Three-dimensional ultrasonography methods are of more value in assessing the extent of the lesions.

## Drug Trafficking

To avoid detection, drug traffickers use sophisticated methods for smuggling drugs. Drugs like heroin, cocaine, hashish, marijuana are packed in protective wrappings and swallowed or inserted in the rectum and vagina of the smuggler. Condoms, gloves and balloons are used as wrappings. The packets are in the shape of cocktail sausages having a diameter of 1–2 cm. The carriers are called **body packers** or mules. More than 200 packets have been detected in a single person. One packet may contain 3–7 gm of the narcotic. Majority of the body packers are drug addicts. The packages hidden in the rectum and vagina can be easily detected in physical examination. But the ingested drugs cannot be detected. After reaching the destination, these carriers take a cathartic or enema and pass the wrappings of drug in the faeces. Radiological examination of the abdomen will reveal the presence of the packages as regular- shaped round or oval hyperdense or hypodense shadows. Sometimes hard faecal masses can be mistaken for drug packages. CT scan will be helpful in evaluating doubtful cases.

## Virtual Autopsy

Virtual autopsy or **virtopsy** is a non-invasive technique of examining dead bodies to find out the cause of death in accidental and homicidal deaths. Virtual autopsy does not destroy some of the key forensic evidences which may be destroyed in a classic autopsy. It can also be used in situations where autopsy is not tolerated by certain communities like the Jews. Virtual autopsy combines CT and MR imaging. The CT images provide information about morbid anatomical findings of the body (Figs 32. 11A to C). MR imaging is used to focus on specific areas like soft tissues, muscles and organs of the body. To estimate the time of death, virtopsy uses MR spectroscopy to measure the metabolites formed due to decomposition.

In virtopsy, new generation multislice CT known as MSCT is used. Two dimensional and three D imaging is possible with MSCT. Air embolism, pneumothorax, emphysema, hyperbaric truama, and decomposition effects can be better appreciated in virtopsy. The CT/MRI findings can be correlated with the autopsy findings. In cases where a weapon is used, 3D surface scanning will document the surface of the body. With the help of a computer software, virtual model of an injury with the 3D image of a simulation can be created by using a similar weapon. It will provide a good visual evidence for presenting before the court. In a gun shot injury case, it is possible to determine entrance and exit wounds based on the characteristic fracture pattern with inward and outward bevelling of the bone. CT scanning is an excellent method to view the track of the projectile inside the brain or body organs with associated bleeding and damage to tissues.

## DIRECTIONS TO THE INVESTIGATING OFFICER

## DNA Analysis

DNA typing is an epoch making discovery which has the following several applications in crime investigation:

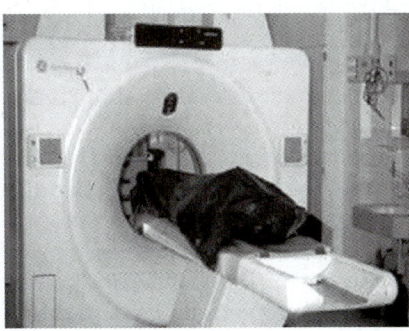 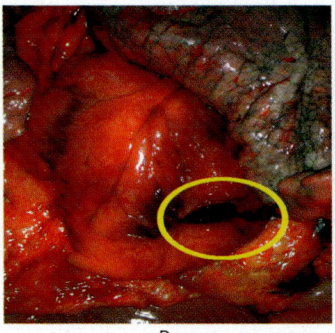 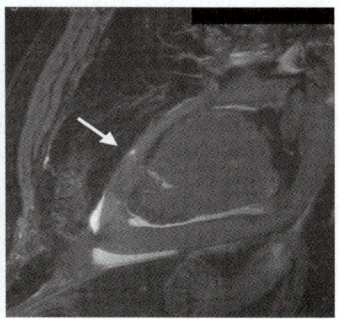

A B C

**Figs 32.11A to C:** Virtopsy: A. MR scanning of dead body, B. Autopsy photograph of stab heart, C. MR scan of heart showing the track of stab wound of heart

1. Personal identity
2. Identification of stains like blood, semen and saliva
3. Sexual offences
4. Disputed paternity

## Collection of Samples for DNA Analysis

Liquid blood, if present in the crime scene can be collected by dipping clean uncontaminated filter papers in it and drying them in air and packed in clean paper or polythene envelopes. These samples need not be refrigerated.

In decomposed dead bodies, it will not be posible to collect unlysed blood for DNA analysis. In that case, request the doctor to collect pieces of skeletal muscle. The muscle tissue should have red tinge. The specimen has to be collected in clean bottles and refrigerated. Skeletal muscle is a good source of DNA.

If the dead body is highly decomposed, teeth, rib, thigh bones and vertebrae are good specimens. Hard cortical bone is better the bone marrow as bone marrow will also undergo changes of putrefaction. Request the doctor to cut pieces of bone using new hack saw blades to prevent contamination. Saw handle should be washed thoroughly before fitting a new blade. Scalp hair with roots can be easily pulled out from a decomposed body. The hairs should be thoroughly dried before packing.

If a bite mark is seen on the dead body, the same may be photographed with a scale placed near the injury. Close up photographs of the injury may be taken. The injury should be swabbed with a clean cotton swab wet with saline or water to collect the salivary stains and buccal epithelial cells for detecting DNA material. The swabs should be dried before packing. The saliva present in the bite mark may contain buccal epithelial cells, a good source for DNA.

Usually the autopsy surgeon collects vaginal swabs/smears and forwards them to chemical examiner for detection of semen and spermatozoa. The chemical examiner discards the specimens after microscopy and chemical analysis. No samples may be available, if the investigator wants to conduct DNA analysis at a later stage. Therefore, it is always better to request the doctor to collect extra samples and preserve them for DNA analysis in such cases. In sensational and controversial cases, the chemical examiner and forensic scienists may be requested to preserve the samples even after analysis or return them along with the report.

Polygraph is not a technique to be used after all other efforts have failed. Routine interrogations prior to polygraph test will not affect the effectiveness of the test. However, third degree methods prior to the test can seriously affect the polygraph diagnosis. Best results are obtained when the test is performed on persons who have been interrogated briefly. It will be very effective when used on a subject who has not been told the important details of the offence.

Polygraph technique is not a substitute for good field investigation. It is only an aid to scientific investigtion. Before subjecting a suspect for polygraph test, some investigation has to be conducted to determine his role in the crime. Information obtained from this investigation will be very helpful for conducting the test. There is a misconception among the investigators that polygraph test can find all about the crime. It can only reveal whether a person is lying or telling the truth with respect to the matter under investigation. But it is possible to obtain a confession from a suspect after the polygraph test detects deception. The polygraph test has a psychological effect in inducing confessions in the guilty. Sometimes a guilty person may confess to the police when he is told that he is going to be subjected to a polygraph test. In order to conduct the polygraph test, all relevant information regarding all the facts of the case should be intimated to the examiner. The circumstances which form the basis for the accusations or suspicions against the suspect should also be provided. A sketch of the crime scene with descriptions may also be provided. Personal information about the subject and his background is also needed. Unless an examiner is well informed about the case, he will not be able to conduct the test well. The investigating officer should meet the polygraph examiner and discuss the case before preparing the test questions. It will be better, if the questions are prepared by them together.

## Narco Analysis

Narco analysis is seldom used by the psychiatrists and investigators in most of the civilized countries as it is a risky procedure which yields unreliable results. But in India, some investigating agencies resort to this method with the help of forensic scientists and doctors. It is quite possible for the subjects to develop fatal or serious adverse effects. Fortunately no fatalities have been reported so far. The courts are not aware of the possible health hazards to which the subjects are exposed to, when they are interrogated under the influence of a narcotic drug. In narco analysis, a narcotic drug is administered for a purpose other than treatment. It can affect the personal safety of the person and can endanger his life. It cannot be considered as a scientific test. It is interrogation of a person in a drugged state and amounts to torture. The method is illegal, unethical, inhuman and gross violation of human rights.

There are scientific methods to detect deception like polygraph and brain fingerprinting. They are non-invasive methods and the subject is not exposed to any kind of physical or mental harm. Polygraph can detect deception and brain fingerprinting can indicate the involvement of the suspect in the crime. The results are also reliable. Coupled with painstaking field investigation, these techniques will help to solve crimes easily.

A three judges bench of the Hon Supreme Court, chaired by Hon.Chief Justice K.G.Balakrishnan , after hearing a number of criminal appeals held that no individual should be forcibly subjected to any of the techniques in question, whether in the context of investigation or otherwise. ( Abstract of the judgement is given as Annexation XV)

Dr. Justice A. R. Lakshmanan, former Chairman of the 18th Law Commission  and a judge of the Supreme Court has opined that it is a welcome verdict ; biut questionable rider. He is of opinion that a wrong cannot become a right when it is done with consent. The rider will affect the common folk who is unaware of the real meaning of consent and its legal implications. ("The Hindu" dated July 9,2010.)

*"The law enforcement agencies should imbibe developments and advances that take place in science as long as they do not violate fundamental legal principles and are for the good of the society"*

# Violation of Human Rights

Human rights refer to basic rights and privileges to which all humans are entitled. Human rights include civil and political rights such as right to life and liberty, freedom of speech and equality before the law. The history of human rights dates back to the ancient times. Proclamations of Emperor Asoka (272–231 BC) contained concepts of human rights. Human rights movements and laws came into existence only by the 20th century. War crimes, atrocities against the prisoners of war and gross abuse of human rights which took place during the world wars lead to the development of modern human rights instruments.

League of nations was established in 1919 after the end of First World War. The goals included prevention of wars, disarmament and settling disputes between nations. The charter of the league of nations led to the Universal Declaration of Human Rights. In 1945, after the Second World War, a new body named United Nations was formed which played a key role in the formulation of International Human Rights Laws. In 1948, United Nations General Assembly adopted the Universal Declaration of Human Rights (UDHR), which is now considered as international customary law. UDHR urges member nations to promote a number of human, civil, economic and social rights which are part of the freedom, justice and peace in the world.

Human rights are primarily governed by the United Nations Security Council and the United Nations Human Rights Council. The latter created at the 2005 World Summit, has a mandate to investigate violations of human rights. Independent experts (rapporteurs) are retained by the council to investigate alleged human rights abuses and to provide the council with reports. The Human Rights Council may request that the Security Council take action when human rights violations occur. This action may be direct actions, may involve sanctions, and the Security Council may also refer cases to the International Criminal Court.

## NATIONAL HUMAN RIGHTS COMMISSION

In India, Human Rights Act came into force in the year 1993 (amended in 2006). It is an Act to provide for the constitution of a National Human Rights Commission (NHRC), State Human Rights Commissions and Human Rights Courts for better protection of human rights and connected or incidental matters thereto. The commission can, inter alia, inquire suo motu or on petition presented to it by a victim or any person on his behalf, into a complaint of violation of human rights or abetment thereof or negligence in the prevention of such violation by a public servant. Commission can summon and examine witnesses under oath. Public records from any court or office can be requisitioned.

It has succeeded in persuading the central government to sign the United Nations convention against 'torture and other forms of cruel, inhuman and degrading punishment or Treatment'. It has brought into sharp focus the problem of custodial deaths and taken steps to see that these are not suppressed by the state agencies and that the guilty persons are made to account for their sins of commission and omission. It has also helped in designing specialised training modules on human rights for introduction in the educational and training institutions.

The National Human Rights Commission soon after its constitution in October 1993, called upon the law and order agencies at the district level throughout the country to report matters relating to custodial death and custodial rape within 24 hours of occurrence.

The Commission found that the postmortem examination in many cases has not been done properly. Usually the reports are drawn up casually and do not at all help in the forming of an opinion as to the cause of death. The Commission has formed an impression that a systematic attempt is being made to suppress the truth and the report is merely the police version of the incident. The postmortem report was intended to be the most valuable record and considerable importance was being placed on this document in drawing conclusions about the death. The Commission was of a prima-facie view that the local doctor succumbs to police pressure which leads to distortion of the facts.

In the year 1995, NHRC has issued directions to all state government to **video film all postmortem examinations done in respect of deaths in police custody and in jails.** The video casettes and the postmortem certificate have to be forwarded to the Commission. The investigating officer has to make necessary arrangement for videography and forwarding the documents to the NHRC.

In 1997, NHRC prepared a model autopsy form taking into consideration the UN **model autopsy protocol.** The commission has also suggested improvements in the conduct of inquests **(additional inquest procedure).** Temperature changes and onset of rigor mortis should be determined to find out the time of death. Accordingly, inquest and autopsy of all custodial deaths and murdered victims of rape, torture, etc. should be conducted as per the NHRC protocol.

The autopsy report and the videograph of the procedure should be sent to the NHRC.

## Torture

The term torture is derived from the Latin word *'torqu-tura'* which means the 'act of twisting'. Since time immemorial, torture has been used as a means of an 'ordeal' or to punish captured enemies. Torture is the infliction of pain, either physical or mental on a person as a means of intimidation, deterrence, revenge, punishment or extortion of information.

Throughout the centuries, all over the world, human beings have been tortured both in body and mind. Torture of the suspects was once considered as a legitimate means for justice to extract confessions or other information about the crime. Often accused persons sentenced to death were tortured prior to execution. Even now torture, cruel, inhuman and degrading treatment of human beings are practiced in two-thirds of the nations of the world. Torture remains a frequent method of repression in dictatorial regimes, terrorist groups and in organised crimes. Even some of the democratic government resort to torture of prisoners of war and detainees under the facade of national security.

Torture is universally considered to be an extreme violation of human rights. Article 5 of the Universal Declaration of Human Rights and Article 7 of the International Convention on Civil and Political Rights provide that 'no one shall be subjected to torture or to cruel, inhuman or degrading treatment or punishment'. In 1984, 128 out of 190 member states of the United Nations have signed an international treaty called the 'UN convention against torture'. The states have accepted their special responsibility to make sure that they must never use torture and must provide support for torture victims.

The World Medical Association's Declaration of Tokyo in 1975 defines torture as " the deliberate, systematic or wanton infliction of physical or mental suffering by one or more persons acting alone or on the orders of any authority to force another person to yield information, to make a confession or for any other reason."

Torture is banned in all circumstances by international law. But in many countries, the law enforcement agencies, the people who should uphold law and protect human rights, often resort to torture. Even in the member states who have acceded and ratified to the UN convention, torture of one kind or another is practiced.

### Methods of Torture

Torture is carried out mainly by criminals, terrorist groups, civil police and other security forces during arrest, detention and interrogation of suspects, accused and prisoners. All types of

physical abuses are practiced on the victims. Sometimes torture may lead to the death of the victim. The signs of torture are not different from those seen in a case of homicide or homicidal attempt. But there may be some characteristic features on the person of a torture victim (Table 33.1). Usually victims are bound and beaten up with hands, fist or blunt weapons. Replication of patterned contusions and abrasions may be seen all over the body. As the victims are detained for long periods after torture, the acute injuries would

| Table 33.1: Instructions to be followed for detection of torture | |
|---|---|
| Torture technique | Physical findings |
| **Beating** | |
| 1. General | Scars, bruises, lacerations, multiple fractures, at different stages of healing, especially in unusual locations which have not been medically treated. |
| 2. To the soles of the feet and ankles | Haemorrhage in the soft tissues of the soles of the feet, fractures of the bones of the feet, aseptic necrosis |
| 3. With palms on both ears simultaneously | Ruptured or scarred tympanic membranes, injuries to external ear. |
| 4. On the abdomen, while lying a table with the upper half of the body unsupported ("Operating table") | Bruises on the abdomen, back injuries, ruptured abdominal viscera |
| 5. To the head | Cerebral cortical atrophy, scars, skull fractures, bruises, haematomas. |
| **Suspension** | |
| 6. By the wrists | Bruises or scars about the wrists, joint injuries. |
| 7. By the arms or neck | Bruises or scars at the site of binding, prominent lividity in the lower extremities. |
| 8. By the ankles | Bruises or scars about the ankles, joint injuries. |
| 9. Head down, from a horizontal pole, forearms placed under the knees with the wrists bound to the "jack" | Bruises or scars on the anterior and backs the knees Marks on wrists and ankles. |
| **Near suffocation** | |
| 10. Forced immersion of head often in contaminated water ("wet submarine") | Faecal material or other debris in the mouth, pharynx, trachea, oesophagus or lungs, intrathoracic petechiae |
| 11. Tying of a plastic bag over the head ("dry submarine") | Intrathoracic petechiae. |
| **Sexual abuse** | |
| 12. Sexual abuse | Sexually transmitted diseases, pregnancy, injuries to breasts, external genitalia, vagina, anus or rectum. |

*Contd...*

*Contd...*

| Torture technique | Physical findings |
|---|---|
| **Forced posture** | |
| 13. Prolonged standing | Dependent edema, petechiae in extremities |
| 14. Forced straddling of a bar | Perineal or scrotal hematomas ("saw horse") |
| **Electric shock** | |
| 15. Cattle prod | Burns: appearance depends on the age of the injury. Immediately: red spots, vesicles, and/or black exudate. Within a few weeks: circular, reddish, macular scars. After several months: small, white, reddish or brown spots resembling telangiectasis. |
| 16. Wires connected to a source of electricity. | - do- |
| 17. Heated metal skewer inserted into the anus | Perianal or rectal burns |
| **Miscellaneous** | |
| 18. Dehydration | Vitreous humour electrolytic abnormalities |
| 19. Animal bites (spiders, insects, rats, mice, dogs) | Bite marks. |

have healed. Then it may be difficult to establish any evidence of torture.

The following types of injuries are usually seen in torture victims:

*Injuries due to restraining:* The wrist and ankles may show linear or patterned abrasions and contusions caused by various types of ligatures like coir, electric wire chain, handcuffs, etc.

*Blunt assault:* Beating is the most common form of torture. The injuries vary according to the type of weapon and the part of the body injured. Blows are inflicted by hand, foot, cane, belt, baton (lathi in Hindi), rifle and gun butt. Many of these produce patterned injuries.

Linear parallel contusions with a central pale area are caused by beating with lathi, cane or a rod (**tram-line bruise**). When the force is more, the bruising will be deep seated and the pattern of the weapon will not be discernible. The skin may be split or lacerated sometimes when a whip or cane is used. Multiple crisscrossing, overlapping linear contusions indicate repeated beating. Usual sites are back, buttocks, thighs, legs and soles of feet. **Rolling** is a peculiar form of torture practiced on suspects to extort confession. The victim is made to lie on a bench with his wrists and ankles tied. Gagging is done to stifle the cries. A round wooden or iron rod 3–4 feet long is rolled over the thighs by two men standing on either side of the victim. Simultaneously beating on the soles with a cane is also carried out (**falanga**). Rolling will result in excruciating pain, rupture of muscle fibres and blood vessels. Rolling has caused death due to damage to the kidneys (lower nephron nephrosis) due to the release of myoglobin, a muscle protein, into blood from damaged muscles.

Blunt assault on the head can cause different types of injuries. On the sides of face, repeated blows with open palms is a common method of torture. Dislocation of teeth, fracture of jaw bones, rupture of tympanic membrane, subluxation of the eye lens, bleeding from the nose and ear are caused. Forcible slapping has resulted in fracture of the temporal bone, intracranial haemorrhage, contusion of brain, cerebral edema and death of the victim in many cases. The victim is suspended from the ceiling by tying the wrists or ankles with a ligature. This method is called **eagle swing.** The suspended victim is beaten on the chest and back with a wooden rod or fists.

## Cut Injuries

It is not uncommon to disfigure or maim the victim by inflicting incised wounds on the face, trunk, nose, ear lobes, fingers or genitals. The victims are later executed by shooting or stabbing.

## Burns

Burning end of a cigarette is pressed on the body of the victim. The temperature of the burning end is around 300 °C. This will scorch the skin and underlying tissues. These are seen as discrete circular areas of reddish yellow parchmented skin. Victim is made to sit naked underneath a burning motor car/cycle tyre suspended above him. Molten rubber drips on the body. Different degrees of burns are sustained. When these heal, there will be severe scarring. Sometimes hot irons are applied to skin.

## Gun Shot Injuries

It is a common practice in foreign countries to shoot the victim through the knee or lower limbs (**knee – capping**) for immobilisation. But generally shooting is not a usual method of torture. But victims are executed after torture by shooting at close range.

## Electrical Torture

High voltage, low amperage direct current (DC) is used for causing painful muscular contractions. This will not cause any injury or death. But DC currents above 50 volts can cause burns and death. Usually, the electrodes are applied to the face, genitals or nipples.

## Suffocation

Victims are suffocated by dipping their head in water or foul liquid such as sewage fluid kept in a bucket **(wet submarining)**. This may sometimes cause sudden death due to drowning or delayed death due to pneumonia.

## Sexual Torture

This includes suspension of weights on the penis and scrotum, application of electricity, chilly powder and other irritants to genitalia, intro-duction of foreign bodies into urethra/vagina, mutilation of sex organs, rape, forced sex with co-victims, forced sex with animals and dead bodies, forced nakedness, verbal sexual abuse, etc.

## Dental Torture

Healthy teeth are extracted using pliers, drilling the teeth using electric drills to expose pulp cavity, etc. are done. These methods will cause intense pain.

## Finger Torture

Finger nails are pulled out using pliers. Pins and pointed objects are introduced underneath the finger and toe nails. These methods will cause excruciating pain.

## Other Forms of Torture

Forcible removal of hair, exposing the eyes to irritant substances, stabbing with pointed objects, exposure to dogs and other wild animals, etc. are practiced. The victims are also tortured mentally. Hooding, prolonged standing, erratic feeding, deprivation of basic needs, forcible administration of faeces, alcohol, cannabis and psychedelic substances, disallowing sleep, exposure to bright lights in a closed cell, etc. are some of the methods of torture.

## ADDITIONAL INQUEST PROCEDURE IN SUSPICIOUS DEATHS

In order to help in proper assessment of 'time since death', determination of temperature changes and development of rigor mortis at the time of first examination at the scene is essential. This can be attained in the present system of inquest by examining the dead body at the scene scientifically for these two parameters either by a medical officer or a trained police officer.

### Essential Requirement for Determining Temperature Changes and Rigor Mortis

The procedure is simple and can be learnt by any police officer, if he is trained properly at the police training institution by a medical officer. This procedure includes:

i. Taking rectal temperature at the first examination of the body at the scene itself conducting the inquest. A simple rectal thermometer can be inserted in the anus of the dead body. After waiting for 3 to 5 minutes, temperature should be read. The temperature so read should be mentioned in the inquest report as also the time of recording.

ii. Similarly for determining rigor mortis, i.e. stiffening of the muscles, the police officer should bend the limbs and see whether there is any stiffness in them. The observations about stiffness be mentioned as also the time in the inquest report. These observations would be helpful to the doctors conducting postmortem examination.

## NHRC GUIDELINES FOR SPEEDY DISPOSAL OF CHILD RAPE CASES

The complaint relating to child rape cases shall be recorded promptly as well as accurately. The complaint can be filed by the victim or an eyewitness or anyone, including a representative of non-governmental organization, who has received information about the offence. The case should be taken as follows:

a. Officer not below the rank of SI and preferably a lady police officer.
b. Recording should be verbatim.
c. Person recording to be in civil dress.
d. Recording should not be insisted in police station, it can be at the residence of the victim.

    i. If the complainant is the child victim, then it is of vital importance that the reporting officer must ensure that the child victim is made comfortable before proceeding to record the complaint. This would help in ensuring accurate narration of the incident covering all relevant aspects of the case. If feasible assistance of a psychiatrist should be taken;

    ii. The investigation officer (IO) shall ensure that medical examination of victim of sexual assault and the accused is done preferably within 24 hours in accordance with CrPC Sec. 164 A. Instruction be issued that the chief medical officer ensures the examination of victim immediately on receiving request from onvestigating officer. The gynecologist, while examining the victim should ensure recording the history of incident;

iii. Immediately after the registration of the case, the investigation team shall visit the scene of crime to secure whatever incriminating evidence is available there. If there are tell-tale signs of resistance by the victim or use of force by the accused those should be photographed;

iv. The investigation officer shall secure the clothes of the victim as well as the clothes of the accused, if arrested, and send them within 10 days for forensic analysis to find out whether there are traces of semen and also obtain report about the matching of blood group and if possible DNA profiling;

v. The forensic laboratory should analyze on priority basis and send report within couple of months;

vi. The investigation of the case shall be taken up by an officer not below the rank of SI. on priority basis and, as far as possible, investigation shall invariably be completed within 90 days of registration of the case. Periodical supervision should be done by senior officers to ensure proper and prompt investigation;

vii. Wherever desirable, the statement of the victim U/S 164 CrPC shall be recorded expeditiously;

viii. Identity of the victim and the family shall be kept secret and they must be ensured of protection. IOs/NGOs to exercise more caution on the issue.

## Trial Court

i. Fast track courts preferably presided over by a lady judge and trial to be held in camera;

ii.   Atmosphere in the court should be child friendly;

iii.  If possible, the recordings be done in video conferencing/in conducive manner so that victim is not subjected to close proximity of the accused;

iv.   Magistrate should commit case to session within 15 days after filing of the charge sheet.

## HUMAN RIGHTS AND POLICING

In a democratic society, it is the responsibility of the state to protect and promote human rights. All state institutions including the police department have a duty to respect human rights, prevent human rights violations, and take active steps for the promotion of human rights. The significant role of the police is to maintain law and order and bring those who break the law including laws which protect human rights. Unfortunately sometimes while discharging this duty, actions of the police conflict with human rights. Police have legal and a moral duty to uphold human rights standards and act strictly in accordance with the constitutional laws.

The Constitution entitles everyone living in India to protection of their human rights. Fundamental rights guarantee basic human rights to all. It assures that the state will safeguard human rights and will protect the liberty, security and privacy of the citizens. Hon: Supreme Court has explained and elaborated the scope of fundamental rights in many decisions. The Court has laid down certain directives for law enforcement. These directives deal with various aspects of police work at the station house or cutting edge level, such as registration of a case; conduct of an investigation; carrying out of an arrest; treatment of an arrested person; grant of bail; questioning of a suspect; and protection of the rights of women, poor and the disadvantaged.

An officer who wilfully or inadvertently ignores Supreme Court directives can be tried in court under relevant provisions of the Indian Penal Code and under the Contempt of Courts Act, 1971. The National Human Rights Commission too has issued guidelines for police officers. The Commission has been established under a special Act of Parliament to protect and promote the human rights of all people living in India. The NHRC addresses violations of human rights by recommending registration of criminal cases against the guilty; disciplinary action against errant officers; and payment of compensation to the victims. Because an overwhelming majority of complaints received by the National Human Rights Commission concern the police, the Commission has made it mandatory to report any case of custodial death or rape within 24 hours and to provide it with a video-film of the post-mortem examination. The Commission has also issued guidelines to the police on encounter deaths; lie detector tests; arrest; and police–public relations.

## DIRECTIVES TO THE POLICE IN RAPE CASES

1.  As soon as a rape victim reports the crime at the police station, she must be informed about her right to get a lawyer before any questions are asked of her. The fact that she was informed of this right must be mentioned in the police report.

2.  The police should make arrangements to provide the victim with a lawyer if she does not have access to one.

3.  Every police station must maintain a list of lawyers capable enough to explain the nature of proceedings to the victim; prepare her for the case; assist her in court and in the police station; and provide guidance on agencies and organizations that help in counselling and rehabilitation of rape victims.

4.  The lawyer so chosen by the police to assist the victim must be approved by the court. However, in order to ensure victims are questioned without undue delay, the lawyer may be authorised to act at the police station before permission of the court is taken.

5.  In all rape trials, anonymity of the victim must be maintained.

6.  Care must be taken to see that the victim is not made to feel small or uncomfortable and her statement is recorded by a woman.

7. Unnecessary references and passing of derogatory remarks that the victim contributed to the crime is not permitted. A rape is a rape, no matter what the reputation or profession of the victim is.

8. The law favours protection of the victim. It lays down that inquiry and trial of rape cases should be held in camera [closed court] and that her identity should not be disclosed to the media.

## DIRECTIVES TO POLICE REGARDING PERSONS UNDER CUSTODY

1. Use of third degree methods or any form of torture to extract information is not permitted.

2. Police personnel carrying out arrest and interrogation must bear accurate, visible and clear identification/name tags with their designations.

3. Particulars of all personnel handling interrogation of an arrested person must be recorded in a register.

4. A memo of arrest stating the time and place of arrest must be prepared by the police officer carrying out an arrest. It should be attested by at least one witness who is either a family member of the arrested person or a respectable person from the locality where the arrest is made. The memo should also be counter-signed by the arrested person.

5. The arrested or detained person is entitled to inform a friend, relative or any other person interested in her/his welfare about the arrest and place of detention as soon as practicable. The arrested person must be made aware of this right as soon as he/she is arrested or detained.

6. The arrested person may be allowed to meet her/his lawyer during interrogation but not throughout the interrogation.

7. The time, place of arrest and venue of custody of the arrested person must be notified by telegraph to next friend or relative of the arrested person within 8–12 hours of arrest in case such person lives outside the district or town. The information should be given through the District Legal Aid Organisation and police station of the area concerned.

8. An entry must be made in the diary at the place of detention in regard to the arrest. The name of the friend/relative of the arrested person who has been informed and the names of the police personnel in whose custody, the arrested person is being kept should be entered in the register.

9. The arrested person should be examined by a medical doctor at the time of arrest if he/she so requests. All bodily injuries on the arrested person should be recorded in the inspection memo which should be signed by both the arrested person and the police officer making the arrest. A copy of the memo should be provided to the arrested person.

10. The arrested person should be subject to a medical examination every 48 hours by a trained doctor who has been approved by the State Health Department.

11. Copies of all documents relating to the arrest including the memo of arrest should be sent to the area Magistrate for her/his record.

12. A police control room should be provided at all district and state headquarters where information regarding arrests should be prominently displayed. The police officer making the arrest must inform the police control room within 12 hours of the arrest.

13. Departmental action and contempt of court proceedings should be initiated against those who fail to follow above-mentioned directives.

Failure to follow proper procedure while arresting and interrogating suspects is a very serious matter. Specific guidelines must be followed while arresting and interrogating suspects. The Supreme Court has said that failure to comply with these guidelines not only renders an officer liable for punishment through departmental action but also amounts to contempt of court.

## NHRC GUIDELINES ON POLYGRAPH (LIE DETECTOR) TESTS

Complaints came to the NHRC that the police, without explaining to people, the full implications of a lie detector test which requires prior injection a drug (?) was making them take it, is violation of their fundamental right against self-incrimination. Since polygraph tests are not regulated by any particular law as such, the NHRC has laid down guidelines for the conduct of these tests. While issuing these guidelines, the NHRC followed the principle: in the absence of a specific law, any intrusion into fundamental rights must be struck down as constitutionally invidious.

Lie detector tests can become an instrument to compel the accused to be a witness against her/himself, in violation of Article 20 (3) of the Constitution. The NHRC said that it was aware that lie detector tests have been held consistent with due process of law by courts in the United States, on grounds that they are a part of everyday life. However, in Indian context, the immunity from invasiveness and from self-incrimination must be read together. General powers of the state cannot intrude upon the liberty or constitutional rights of a person. The invasiveness of a lie detector test overrules the argument of the police that the authority to use lie detector tests comes from their powers under the Code of Criminal Procedure [Cr.PC] to question and interrogate suspects. Holding of such tests is the prerogative of the individual and not an empowerment of the police. It must be regarded as illegal and unconstitutional unless it is voluntarily undertaken under non-coercive circumstances.

### NHRC Guidelines

1. Lie detector tests must not be carried out without the consent of the accused.
2. If the accused volunteers to take a lie detector test, she/he must be given access to a lawyer to explain the physical, emotional and legal implications of the test. The implications must also be explained by the police.
3. Consent to take a lie detector test must be recorded before a judicial magistrate.
4. The magistrate must take into account, the time the accused has been in detention and the nature of her/his interrogation. This should be done to find out whether the accused is being coerced into giving consent.
5. At the time of recording consent, the accused must be represented by a lawyer. The lawyer will explain that the statement (given during the test) does not have the status of a confessional statement given to a magistrate. It will have the status of a statement made to the police.
6. The actual recording of the lie detector test should be done by/in an independent agency such as a hospital and in the presence of a lawyer.
7. A full medical and factual narration of the manner in which information is received must be taken on record.

Forcing a person to take a lie-detector test is illegal. Consent must be taken before subjecting a person to a lie-detector test. Also, there is no scientific evidence to prove that results obtained from polygraph tests are conclusive. Failing a lie-detector test does not mean that the person is guilty. Polygraph tests measure responses on the premise, that a person is being untruthful, if there are sudden changes in her/his breathing, heart and blood pressure rates. A truthful person can fail the test if s/he is nervous, has health problems or is just surprised by the question.

## PROCEDURE IN RESPECT OF INTERROGATION

Methods of interrogation must be consistent with individual rights relating to life,

1. Torture and degrading treatment of suspects is prohibited.
2. Interrogation of an arrested person should be conducted in a clearly identifiable place, which has been notified for the purpose by the government.
3. The place of interrogation must be accessible. Relatives or a friend of the arrested person must be informed where she is being interrogated.

4. An arrested person should be permitted to meet a lawyer at any time during the interrogation.

## NHRC Directions on Mandatory Reporting of Custodial Death/Rape and Video-filming of Post-mortem Examinations

All cases of custodial death and custodial rape whether in police lock-up or in jail must be reported to the NHRC within 24 hours of occurrence by the concerned district magistrate or Superintendent of Police. Failure to report promptly will give rise to the presumption that there is an attempt to suppress the incident. All post-mortem examinations in respect of custodial deaths should be video-filmed and a copy of the recording should be sent to the NHRC along with the postmortem report. Autopsy report forms prescribed by the NHRC should be used to record the findings of the postmortem examination.

# Biological and Chemical Terrorism

Bioterrorism is the deliberate spread of bacteria, viri and their toxins to cause disease in people, animals and agriculture. These agents are propagated through air, water and food. Anthrax, botulism, plague, smallpox, Ebola virus, etc. are used as biological agents. Biological warfare was prevalent even in the ancient times. Romans used to poison the water sources of enemies. They used to dump dead bodies of persons and carcasses of animals who had died of infectious diseases in the wells and ponds. In the year 1710, while waging a war with Sweden, Russians used to throw dead victims of plague into the battle line of the enemy. During the war with Red Indians, the English army used to distribute blankets used by smallpox victims to the enemy barracks. Germans had developed several biological agents like anthrax, plague, cholera and chemical weapons like mustard gas during First World War.

In 1925, 108 countries signed the Geneva treaty banning chemical and biological weapons. But many countries have violated the conditions in the treaty during the Second World War. Several powerful toxins and microbes were developed to annihilate the enemies. America had set up a research wing to develop biological and chemical weapons. The Chemical Corps of USA was concerned with manufacture and deployment of several biological weapons. Great Britain had followed the foot steps of America. A military unit in Japan named 731 division used to sprinkle fleas infected with plague in enemy territories. Israel army used to pollute water sources in Palestine

and Egypt with *Salmonella typhi*, the bacterium which causes typhoid fever. Third World countries like Iraq too had developed several chemical weapons. These weapons were used to kill thousands of Khurds in that country.

In 2001, several members of the American congress and media received letters containing the spores of Anthrax bacilli. Those who handled the letters contracted the disease and five of them died. American President Richard Nixon, prohibited the manufacture and use of chemical and biological weapons by an enactment in 1969. It is rumoured that the human immunodeficiency virus (HIV) was the result of a perversive biological research programme.

## BIOLOGICAL AGENTS

Biological agents and pathogens which are commonly used in bioterrorism are:
- Anthrax (*Bacillus anthraces*)
- Botulism (*Clostridium botulinum toxin*)
- Plague (*Yersinia pestis*)
- Smallpox (variola major)
- Viral haemorrhagic fevers (e.g. ebola, marburg, lassa, machupo)
- Brucellosis (Brucella species)
- Salmonella species
- Typhus fever
- Ricin toxin
- Abrin toxin.

## Anthrax

Anthrax is an infection caused by the spores of a bacterium called Bacillus anthraces. It usually affects animals. Humans who have contact with infected animals or animal products such as wool, hide, etc. can get the disease. There are three types of anthrax infection depending upon the route of entry of the spores.

Infection of the skin is caused by contact with infected animal materials. Blisters and ulcers develop in the skin. Infection of stomach and intestines is caused by consumption of under cooked meat of infected animals. The symptoms are fever, nausea, vomiting of blood and bloody diarrhoea. Infection of the lungs is caused by inhalation of the spores. The symptoms are fever, cough and myalgia. Later serious respiratory symptoms may appear.

Anthrax is propagated by the terrorists in a powder form. Common method is by sending letters smeared with the spores to the target victims. When the letter is handled, the spores will enter the body by inhalation and skin contact. Anthrax spores are highly stable and can be dispersed by enclosing them in bombs and ammunitions. When the bombs explode, anthrax spores are liberated into the atmosphere. Anthrax can be treated with antibiotics. Anthrax vaccination is available as a prophylactic measure against the disease.

## Botulism

Botulism is a disease which causes serious symptoms of the nervous system caused by the toxin generated by the bacterium *Clostridium botulinum*. This toxin is more toxic than cyanide. The toxin is propagated as lyophilised powder enclosed in rockets and bombs. The toxin enters the body through air, contaminated food and water. Symptoms start within 6 hours to 2 days. Double vision, blurred vision, slurred speech, difficulty in swallowing and descending paralysis of muscles are the initial symptoms. Death is due to respiratory paralysis. Antitoxin is effective in reducing the severity of symptoms.

## Plague

Plague is caused by *Yersinia pestis*, a bacterium found in rodents and their fleas. There are two varieties of plague, pneumonic and bubonic. Though both are caused by the same organism, the transmission of the disease is different. Pneumonic plague is transmitted from persons to persons, while bubonic plague is transmitted through the bite of an infected rat flea. One of the methods of propagating plague is by sprinkling infected rat fleas in the enemy country. The fleas kept in porcelain containers are attached to projectiles like rockets and bombs before firing them at the targets.

When the flea bites a person, he develops bubonic plague. The symptoms include swollen and tender lymph nodes called buboes. If it is not treated, the bacteria spread through the bloodstream and infect lungs causing pneumonia. Pneumonic plague develops when the bacteria are released from aerosols during a bioterrorism attack. The infected person will have fever, weakness and rapidly developing pneumonia with difficulty in breathing, chest pain, cough and blood-stained sputum. If not treated, death will occur due to respiratory failure and shock. The condition is treated with broad-spectrum antibiotics. There is no vaccine available to prevent plague. Plague bacteria will be destroyed by sunlight and drying.

## Smallpox

Smallpox is caused by the virus *Variola major*. Symptoms include fever, headache, fatigue, diarrhoea, vomiting and a specific rash. The rash first starts as flat red spots that turn into blisters. Blisters contain a clear fluid first and then pus as the disease progresses. Smallpox is transmitted easily through the atmosphere. As a biological weapon, smallpox is dangerous because of the highly contagious nature. It is spread through aerosols and infected materials. Even though smallpox is eradicated throughout the world, virus samples are available in the laboratories of some countries. There is no specific drug to treat smallpox. Vaccination against smallpox is routinely done in developing countries like India. Vaccine given after the exposure may prevent death.

## Viral Haemorrhagic Fevers

Haemorrhagic fever is caused by *Ebola, Marburg, Lass and Machupo viri. Ebola* infection has a high mortality rate (50–90%). It is believed that some terrorist group possess *Ebola* virus culture. *Ebola* produces multiorgan failure and shock in the victims. *Marburg* virus is equally dangerous with fatality rate of 25–100%. There is no effective treatment and prophylaxis for these viral infections.

## Brucellosis

Brucellosis is an infectious disease caused by the Brucella bacteria. The bacteria first affects cattle, dogs, pigs and other animals. Humans become infected by coming into contact with animals or animal products contaminated with these bacteriae. In humans, a range of symptoms like fever, headache, back pain and weakness are seen. Sometimes endocarditis and encephalitis may develop. Brucellosis can also cause chronic symptoms which include recurrent fever, joint pains and fatigue.

Brucell is also used as a biological weapon. Air, water and food articles are contaminated by the terrorists. The bacteria can also enter through skin wounds. When the cattle are infected their milk will contain the bacteria. If the milk is not pasteurised, bacteria can be transmitted to persons who consume the milk and milk products. The disease is seldom transmitted from person to person. Sexual and breastfeeding transmissions are reported.

## Ricin Toxin

Ricin is a stable toxin easily made from the mash that remains after processing castor seeds (*Ricinus communis*) for oil. Ricin is one of the most poisonous naturally occurring substances known. Poisoning can occur following inhalation, ingestion, or injection of ricin toxin from castor beans. Ricin is toxic by numerous exposure routes and its use by terrorists might involve poisoning of water or foodstuffs, inoculation via ricin-laced projectiles, or aerosolization of liquid ricin or distribution of a powder.

One milligram of ricin can kill an adult. The symptoms of human poisoning begin within a few hours of ingestion. Consuming ricin-contaminated material will cause diarrhea, nausea, vomiting, abdominal cramps, internal bleeding, liver and kidney failure, and circulatory failure. Breathing dust that contains ricin causes cough, weakness, fever, nausea, muscle aches, difficult breathing, chest pain, and cyanosis. Breathing the dust can result in respiratory and circulatory failure. Exposure to concentrated ricin particles in the air is only likely during an act of bioterrorism where large numbers of people would likely experience the signs and symptoms in one place and time. All routes of exposure are very dangerous and can result in death.

## Salmonella Species

The first bioterrorist attack using *Salmonella typhi* bacteria occurred in USA in 1984. This was done by contaminating foodstuffs in restaurants, bars and grocery stores in the city of Dalles in the state of Oregon. Hundreds of persons were infected and developed severe food poisoning. Salmonella infection can cause vomiting, nausea, diarrhea and abdominal pain. It is sometimes associated with very high fever. This condition can last for up to a week. Most severely affected are infants, elderly and those with poor immunity. The poisoning can cause severe symptoms and it can be fatal if not properly treated.

## CHEMICAL WARFARE/TERRORISM AGENTS

Chemical warfare agents are chemical substances used to injure or kill enemies during war. Chemical weapons produce physiological changes on the human body. Some of the substances are lethal, but some injure or incapacitate people. Chemical agents are dispersed as tiny droplets through bombs, chemical shells, spray tanks and missiles. Harmful effects are caused when the chemical is inhaled, ingested or when it comes in contact with skin or mucus membrane. Modern chemical warfare began during World War I. Germans employed chemical agents for the first time.

Chlorine gas was used as a chemical weapon by the Germans against the French. Inhalation of chlorine gas was harmful to the lungs. But it was difficult to transport huge quantities of chlorine gas to the war front. Moreover dispersion of the gas was dependant on the strength and direction of wind flow. Later French attacked Germans with artillery ammunition containing phosgene, another toxic gas. It is estimated that during World War I, 90000 people have died due to the effects of chemical agents. Nazis also developed hydrocyanic acid gas chambers for murdering large number of prisoners of war. Germans also developed mustard gas and various nerve gases.

Iraq was one of the third world countries which stockpiled chemical weapons and used them against Iran in 1983. Several thousand persons have died due to the effect of these chemical agents. It is believed that Russia possesses approximately 40,000 tones of chemical warfare agents. US stockpile consists of 30,000 tones of different agents. In 1992, the chemical weapons convention was adopted by the UN General Assembly. More than 170 countries have signed the treaty. According to the treaty, the countries which ratified the convention should declare the chemical weapons facility immediately and destroy all the chemical weapons in their possession. Organisation for the prohibition of chemical weapons came into existence in 1997 with its headquarters at Hague, Netherlands. This organisation monitors the destruction of chemical weapons and their production facilities all over the world. More than 70 chemical substances are classified as weapons of mass destruction. These agents may be liquid, solid or gas form. Chemical warfare agents are classified into lethal and incapacitating. They are also categorised according to their persistency. Persistency is the length of time a chemical agent remains active after dissemination. Non-persistent agents are purely gaseous and volatile chemicals which lose their effectiveness after a few minutes or hours. Persistent agents remain in the environment for weeks. Chemical agents are generally classified into several categories according to the manner in which they affect human body (Box 34.1).

## Nerve Agents

The first nerve agent **Tabun** was discovered in 1937 by a German chemist. Later **Sarin** and **Soman**, more powerful nerve gases were developed. At present more toxic agents known as **VE, VM, VR and VX** are possessed by certain countries. Among these, **VX** is a persistent poison. Other agents are non-persistent and hazardous on inhalation. These agents are disseminated as vapours and liquids. The action starts within minutes. They are absorbed through skin also.

| **Box 34.1:** Common chemical warfare/terrorism agents and their mode of action | | |
|---|---|---|
| *Nature of chemical* | *Name* | *Mode of action* |
| Nerve agent | Sarin, cyclosarin, soman, tabun, VE, VG, VM, VX | Inactivates the enzyme acetyl cholinesterase accumulation of acetyl choline causing muscarinic and nicotinic effects |
| Asphyxiants | Arsines, hydrogen cyanide, cyanogen chloride | Intravascular hemolysis Prevents cell respiration |
| Vesicants | Sulphur mustard, nitrogen mustard, lewisite | Acid forming—damages skin and respiratory system |
| Choking agents | Chlorine, hydrogen chloride, Phosgene, nitrogen oxide | Acid forming—action more pronounced in respiratory system |
| Lachrymators | tear gas, pepper spray | Irritation of eyes, lachrymation, temporary blindness |
| Incapacitators | Agent 15 quinuclidinyl benzilate | Atropine like inhibition of acetyl choline |
| Cytotoxic proteins | Ricin, abrin | Inhibit protein synthesis |

The symptoms are constriction of pupils, blurred vision, headache, nausea, vomiting, diarrhoea, copious secretions, sweating, muscle twitching, difficulty in breathing, convulsions and unconsciousness.

There are three steps of protection against chemical warfare namely detection of chemical attack, collective protection and decontamination. Civilian organisations must also be prepared to carry out these procedures. Chemical agents are heavier than air and hence they sink to low lying areas. Therefore seeking shelter on high rise buildings and high ground will be helpful. Gas mask and chemical resistant clothing will give protection from inhalation and contact with skin. Special equipments and materials are needed for mass decontamination. Administration of antidotes like atropine may be necessary in the case of nerve agents.

## Asphyxiants (Choking Gases)

Asphyxiants are gases which will damage the respiratory epithelium and lung tissue. Some of the asphyxiants produce systemic toxicity. **Chlorine, arsine, phosgene, cyanogen chloride and hydrogen cyanide** are some of the agents used as asphyxiants.

Inhalation of chlorine gas produces suffocation and laryngeal spasm. There will be increased secretions in the respiratory passage. In severe cases, pulmonary edema will develop leading to difficulty in breathing and cyanosis. Arsine (arseniuretted hydrogen) will cause lysis of blood inside the blood vessels, hemoglobinuria and jaundice which may lead to failure of kidneys. Phosgene ($COCl_2$) or carbonyl chloride is ten times toxic than chlorine. The gas damages the respiratory epithelium and capillaries of lungs producing severe lung edema. The symptoms are lachrymation, choking and a feeling of tightness in the chest.

Hydrocyanic acid at ordinary temperature and pressure is a highly lethal gas. Because of its low density and rapid dispersion, it is seldom used in chemical warfare. It is used in gas chambers for executing prisoners. The gas is absorbed through the respiratory tract. It inhibits the respiratory enzyme cytochrome oxidase and paralyse the oxygen transport system. The cells will not be able to utilise oxygen resulting in tissue anoxia. The blood and skin will be cherry red in colour. The victim will experience nausea, confusion, dyspnoea and seizures prior to death.

## Vesicants (Blistering Agents)

Vesicants are chemicals which produce painful blisters on the skin. The eyes will be affected producing irritation and lachrymation (secretion of tears). The commonly used chemicals are nitrogen mustard, sulphur mustard and lewisite. Nitrogen mustard is an oily liquid having a garlicky smell. It produces vapours at ordinary temperature. It is not soluble in water and persists for a longer time. Sulphur mustard is more toxic than nitrogen mustard. It can cause disruption of the DNA resulting in bone marrow depression. Azoospermia and hair loss are also seen.

Apart from causing respiratory symptoms, the chemical affects the skin producing erythema, blisters and ulcers. The blisters will contain a yellowish serous fluid. The blisters heal very slowly. The chemical can penetrate the clothing and affect the skin. The first step in the treatment is the removal of contaminated clothing. The affected areas should be washed in normal saline. Topical application of cortisone will be helpful to reduce the inflammation. Hemodialysis may be necessary in nitrogen mustard poisoning.

**Lewisite** produces more serious effects than mustard gas. Lewisite is sometimes mixed with sulphur mustard gas to reduce the freezing point. Chemically, lewisite is a lipid soluble arsenic. It is absorbed through skin and mucus membrane. Action of lewisite starts immediately. Blisters which contain a cloudy fluid are produced. Like arsenic it is deposited in the internal organs.

## Lachrymators (Tear Gases)

Lachrymators are chemicals which produce irritation of eyes, large quantity of tears and temporary blindness. These are generally used by the law enforcement agencies to disperse riotous mobs. The commonly used chemicals are *xylyl bromide, enzyl bromide, bromobenzyl cyanide (BBC), bethyl* iodoacetate (KSK), 2 chloroacetophenone (CAP/ CN), orthochlorobenzylidine malononitrile (CS) and dibenzoxazepine (CR), Majority of these agents are liquids which become gases at normal temperature and pressure. The liquid can cause blisters on the skin. Apart from the eye symptoms, respiratory tract is also affected. These are non-persistent in character and the effects last only for a short period. The first line of treatment is to remove the victim from the scene and expose to fresh air. The eyes and contaminated areas should be washed with water.

## Sternutators (Nasal Irritants)

These are chemicals which produce nasal irritation. Common agents are *diphenyl chlorarsine (DA), chlorodiphydro phenarsazine (DM) and Disphenyl cynarsine (DC).* These are solids, which on detonation release huge quantity of smoke. These are used in warfare and riot control. On inhalation, severe pain and irritation of the nose and respiratory passage will develop. There will be incessant sneezing, nausea, vomiting, tightness in the chest and malaise. The first aid is to remove the victim from the scene to prevent further exposure. The eyes should be washed with normal saline. Nose and throat can be irrigated with a 5% solution of sodium carbonate.

## Incapacitating Agents

Incapacitating agents are chemicals which will affect the central nervous system of a person and incapacitate him temporarily. Even though many drugs affect the nervous system and cause various symptoms, anticholinergic drugs are considered as the best to incapacitate the enemy during a conflict. Many nations have developed anticholinergic agents known by different code names. The one developed by the US army is 3-quinuclidinyl benzilate (**BZ**).

A similar chemical in the possession of Iraq is termed 'Agent 15". BZ is dispersed as an aerosol. It may be micropulverised for dispersion or mixed with pyrotechnic burning mixture for dissemination in burning munitions. These chemicals are very stable and persist for 1–2 months in moist air and soil. BZ is odourless and non-irritating and its clinical effects are not seen after 30 minutes to 24 hours. Therefore, exposure can occur without the knowledge of the victim.

BZ is also known as 3 QNB. This chemical affects the smooth muscles, exocrine glands and autonomic ganglia. The symptoms are opposite to those seen in nerve gas poisoning. The skin and mouth become dry. There will be decreased lachrymal, nasal, bronchial and gastrointestinal secretions. Disorientation to time and space is a characteristic feature. There will be hyper-thermia and urinary retention. Poor muscular coordination will lead to ataxia. Speech becomes slurred. The drug can cross the blood–brain barrier and cause mental symptoms like hallucinations, illusions, stupor and delirium. Sometimes the victim may become drowsy, stuporous and comatosed.

The first step in the treatment is decontamination of clothing and skin. Immediate medical attention should be given.

## Accidental Chemical Spill

Apart from exposure from chemical warfare, public are exposed to accidental chemical spill from factories and establishments whcih stockpile dangerous chemicals. In 1984, a worst gas disaster occurred in Bhopal, India. A highly poisonous gas leaked from the Union Carbide factory killing 3800 people and injuring more than 200,000. The gas is believed to be methyl isocyanate, an intermediate chemical in the production of carbamate pesticides. It is a clear, colourless, sharp smelling volatile liquid which is extremely toxic.

On inhalation, severe cough, chest pain, dyspnoea, lachrymation and damage to cornea develop immediately. Due to corneal ulceration and subsequent development of corneal opacities,visual impairment can occur. The gas causes severe pulmonary edema, emphysema, bronchopneumonia, pulmonary haemorrhage and death. Immediate treatment is to decontaminate the skin by removing clothing and washing the eyes and skin with normal saline. Oxygen inhalation, artificial ventilation are needed in pulmonary complications.

## DIRECTIONS TO THE INVESTIGATING OFFICER

Bioterrorism could be a real threat to the community in future. Law enforcement agencies should be able to detect the hazard early and take preventive and curative meaures to save the victims. The significance of bioterrorism is that small amounts of biological agents and toxins can cause mass casualties.

### Recognising a Bioterrorism Event

Reports of an explosion that causes little damage to surroundings.

Detection of devices that disperse a mist or powder with no immediate effects.

Discovery of abandoned spraying equipment or discarded protective suit or laboratory equipment

Presence of unusual swarms of biting insects as they may be used for dissemination of the biological agent.

Observation of large numbers of sick or dying animals (animals and birds are more susceptible and affected before humans).

### Action

Report the event to authorities immediately and alert public health authorities.

Ask the people to remain inside their houses until emergency management teams order to evacuate them.

Wear protective gowns, masks, goggles and gloves.

Wash hands before and after contact with an affected person.

Drink water boiled for half an hour.

Remove all contaminated clothing by cutting them at seams (never pull it over head) and put them in airtight plastic bags for disposal.

### Recognising a Chemical Terrorism Event

Unusual increase in the number of people seeking medical care for respiratory, neurological or dermatological symptoms.

Affecting humans, animals and plants simultaneously.

Birds and insects will die quicly.

Characteristic smell in the affected locality (some of the chemicals may not have any specific smell).

People exposed to the chemical may develop vomiting, difficulty in breathing and fainting.

### Action

Remove people from affected area. If the attack was outside, get inside a building. If the attack was inside a building.

Chemical agents are heavier than air and hence they sink to low lying areas. Therefore seeking shelter on high rise buildings and high ground will be helpful.

Remove the contaminated clothing by cutting them and put them in an airtight plastic bag or container.

Wash the affected areas of the body thoroughly with water.

Provide medical attention to the affected people immediately

# Annexations

## I. ANATOMICAL PLANES AND TERMS

The description of the location of injuries and other morbid anatomical findings on the body are based on the anatomical position and four imaginary planes of the body. The position of a human body standing erect with upper limbs by the side of the body, palms facing forwards, legs together with feet pointing forwards is called **anatomical position** (Annex Fig. 1). The anatomical planes are based on this posture. There are four imaginary planes: median, sagittal, coronal and horizontal. The median plane divides the body into right and left. Sagittal plane is parallel to median plane. Coronal plane divides the body into anterior (front) and posterior (back).

Structures near the median plane are called medial (inner) and those away from midline are called lateral (outer). Structures nearer to the head are called superior, while those close to the feet are called inferior. Distal and proximal are used to describe structures in the limbs. Those nearer to the attachment of a limb are termed proximal and those away are called distal. External and internal refer to the distance from the centre of an organ or cavity. When trunk, feet and palms are referred, ventral and dorsal are synonymously used for anterior and posterior (Annex. Fig. 1).

When injuries are described in autopsy reports or wound certificates, anatomical/technical terms should be avoided as far as possible. When the location of the injury is noted, substitute the anatomical terms with common terms. Few examples are given in the Annex Box 1.

**Annexation Box 1:** Anatomical terms and corresponding common terms

| | | | |
|---|---|---|---|
| Anterior | : Front | Mucosa | : Lining membrane |
| Bronchioles | : Air passage | Patella | : Knee cap |
| Calcaneum | : Heel bone | Pelvis | : Hip bone |
| Calvarium | : Skull cap | Pericardium | : Covering of heart |
| Carpal bones | : Wrist bones | Peritoneal | : Abdominal cavity |
| Clavicle | : Collar bone | Pinna | : Ear lobe |
| Distal | : Away from | Pleural cavity | : Chest cavity |
| Dorsal | : Back | Posterior | : Back |
| Femur | : Thigh bone | Proximal | : Near to |
| Gastric | : Stomach | Scapula | : Shoulder blade |
| Haemorrhage | : Bleeding | Sternum | : Breast bone |
| Homicide | : Murder | Superior | : Above/upper |
| Humerus | : Upper arm bone | Tarsal bones | : Foot bones |
| Inferior | : Below/lower | Thyroid cartilage | : Adam's apple |
| Lateral | : Outer | | |
| Mandible | : Jaw bone | Trachea | : Windpipe |
| Medial | : Inner | Tragus | : Ear lobule |
| Median | : Midline | Ventral | : Front |
| Meninges | : Coverings of brain | | |

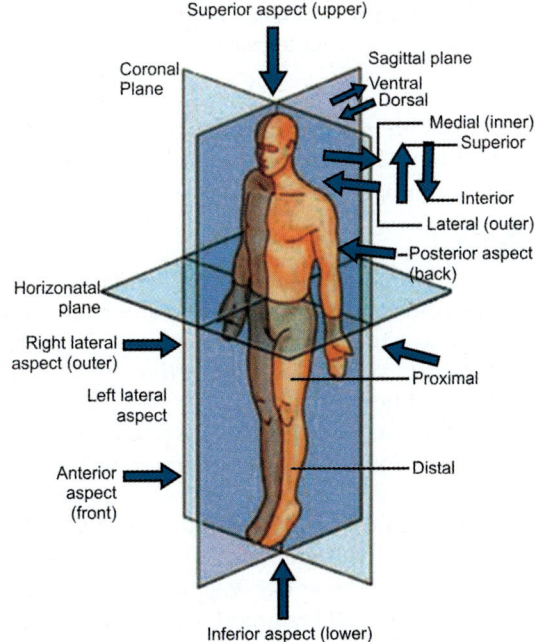

Annexation **Fig. 1:** A natomical planes

## II. BASIC HUMAN ANATOMY AND PHYSIOLOGY

Anatomy is the branch of biology that deals with the structure of living things. Physiology is the study of the functions of living matter. It is concerned with how an organism performs its varied activities: how it feeds, how it moves, how it adapts to changing circumstances, how it spawns new generations, etc. Anatomy and physiology are closely related fields of study. All living things are composed of cells. A single cell is the smallest unit that has all the characteristics of life. Some organisms have only one cell while some have many cells.

In single-celled (unicellular) organisms, the single cell performs all life functions. However, many-celled (multicellular) organisms have various levels of organization within them. Individual cells may perform specific functions and also work together for the good of the entire organism. Multicellular organisms have the following five levels of organization ranging from simplest to most complex.

The levels of organization in the correct order are:

cells → tissues → organs → organ systems → organisms

### Level 1

*Cells:* Cells are the basic structural and functional units of life. May serve a specific function within the organism, e.g. blood cells, nerve cells, bone cells.

### Level 2

*Tissues:* Tissues are made up of cells that are similar in structure and function and which work together to perform a specific activity. Humans have four basic tissues: connective, epithelial, muscle, and nerve.

1. *Epithelial tissue:* The cells of epithelial tissue pack tightly together and form continuous sheets that serve as protective linings in different parts of the body, e.g. the outer layer of the skin.
2. *Connective tissue:* Generally speaking, connective tissue adds support and structure to the body. Some examples of connective tissue include the inner layers of skin, tendons, ligaments, cartilage, bone and fat tissue.
3. *Muscle tissue:* Muscle tissue is a specialized tissue that can contract, e.g. skeletal, smooth and cardiac muscles.
4. *Nerve tissue:* Nerve tissue has the ability to generate and conduct electrical signals in the body. These electrical messages are managed in the brain and transmitted down the spinal cord to the body.

### Level 3

*Organs:* An organ is a structure that contains at least two different types of tissue functioning together for a common function, e.g. liver, kidneys, heart, skin. (Annex. Fig. 2). In fact, the skin is the largest organ in the human body.

### Level 4

*Organ systems:* Organ system is a group of two or more organs that work together to perform a specific function for the organism, e.g. circulatory system, nervous system, skeletal system, ali-

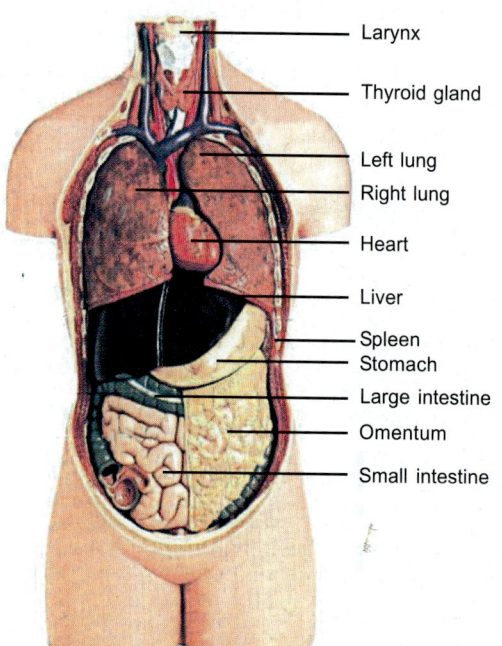

**Annexation** **Fig. 2:** Internal organs

Larynx

Thyroid gland

Left lung

Right lung

Heart

Liver

Spleen

Stomach

Large intestine

Omentum

Small intestine

mentary system, excretory system, reproductive system.

The human body has eleven organ systems. They are skeletal, muscular, integumentary, respiratory, circulatory, digestive, endocrine, excretory, nervous, reproductive, and immune (lymphatic) systems.

## III. SKELETAL SYSTEM

This consists of the skeleton which includes bones, ligaments, tendons, cartilage and attached skeletal muscles. It gives the body basic structure and the ability for movement. In addition to their structural role, the larger bones in the body contain bone marrow, the site of production of blood cells. Moreover, all the bones are major storage sites for calcium and phosphate. Joints are the places where two or more bones meet. Most bones are tied together at joints by tough bands called ligaments. Bones are known by different names (Annex. Figs 3 and 4).

There are 206 bones in the human body. These bones form a rigid framework to which muscles and soft tissues are attached. Vital organs are protected by the bones. For example, the brain is protected by the skull. The heart and lungs are protected by the breast bone (sternum) and the rib cage.

The skeleton is divided into two parts: axial and appendicular. Axial skeleton consists of bones that form the axis of the body. They are: skull, sternum, ribs and the vertebral column. The appendicular skeleton is composed of bones that anchor the appendages to the axial skeleton. It is composed of bones of upper and lower extremities, shoulder girdle and the pelvic girdle.

## Types of Bones

The bones of the body fall into four general categories: long bones, short bones, flat bones and irregular bones. Bones of extremities like femur, humerus, tibia, fibula ulna and radius are long bones. Bones of wrists and ankles are short bones. Flat bones have broad surfaces; examples are skull bones, ribs, shoulder blade (scapula). Irregular bones are of varied size and shape. Vertebrae belong to this group.

## Composition of Bones

Bones are composed of two types of tissues: compact and spongy. Compact bone is dense and hard. The outer aspect of all the bones are compact in nature. Spongy bone, as the name suggests is cancellous and porous in nature. In most of the bones, spongy bone is found inside. Bone tissue is composed of several types of bone cells in a matrix of minerals calcium and phosphate. These give strength to the bone.

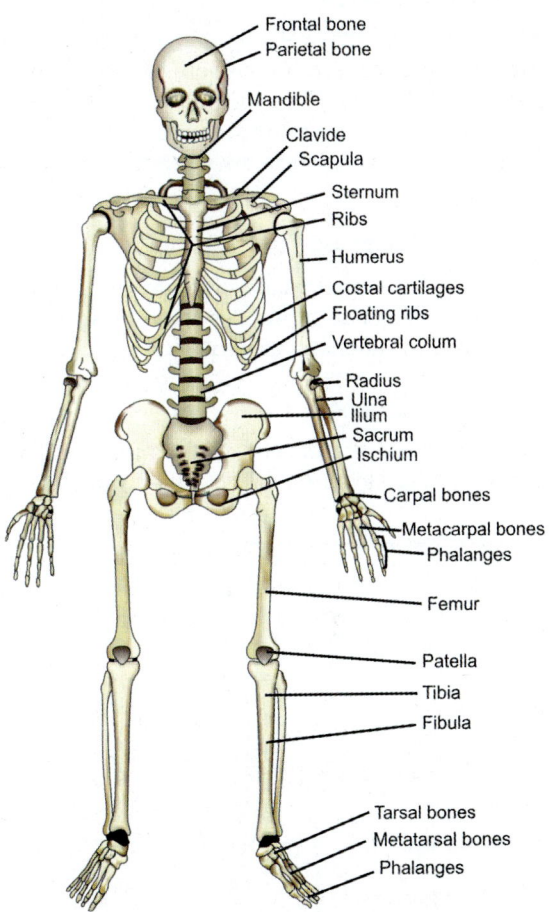

**Annexation Fig. 3:** Human skeleton (frontal view)

## IV. MUSCLE SYSTEM

There are 600 muscles in the human body (Annex. Figs 5 and 6). All the muscles are served by nerves which link them to the brain or spinal cord. Muscles in the human body fall into three types.

### 1. Skeletal Muscles (Voluntary/Striated)

These muscles have the ability to contract producing movement of the body. The muscles are made up of muscle fibres. Each muscle fiber is cylindrical and has striations of alternating dark and light bands. Muscle fibres join together to form bundles and bundles form muscles. Skeletal muscles are controlled by somatic nerves.

### 2. Smooth Muscles

The muscles of the walls of stomach, intestines, bladder, arteries, etc. are smooth muscles. They have no striations. They cannot contract voluntarily. They interlace to form sheets and not bundles. They are controlled by autonomic nervous system.

### 3. Cardiac Muscles

Heart muscle is a combination of striated and smooth muscles. Like smooth muscles these muscles are innervated by autonomous nervous system.

### Muscle Contraction

Motor nerves are attached to the muscles. The nerve ending at the muscle is called motor end plate. When electrical impulse reaches through the nerves, acetylcholine, a compound liberated at the motor end plate facilitates the electrical impulse to pass along the muscle fibers. The muscle fibres are made up of two proteins; actin and myosin. During muscle contraction, these slides past each other to shorten the fiber, thus producing contraction. When muscles attached to both the bones contract or relax, the joint bends or extends.

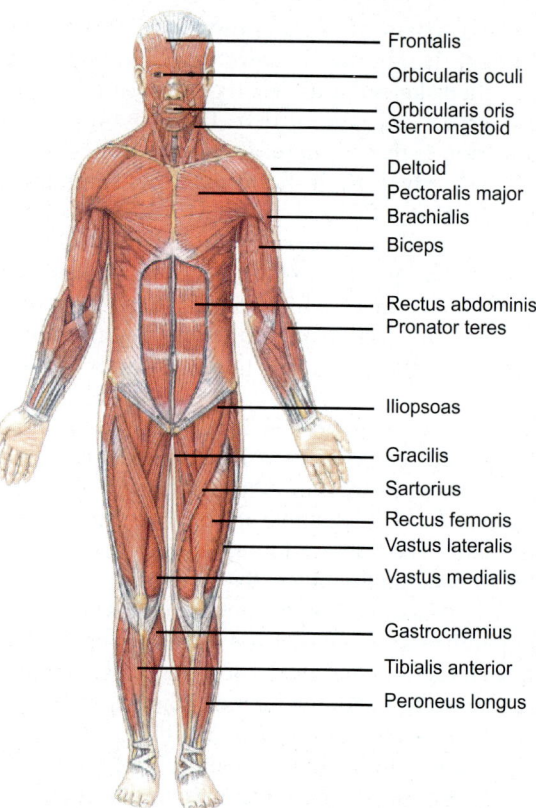

**Annexation Fig. 5:** Major muscles of human body (front aspect)

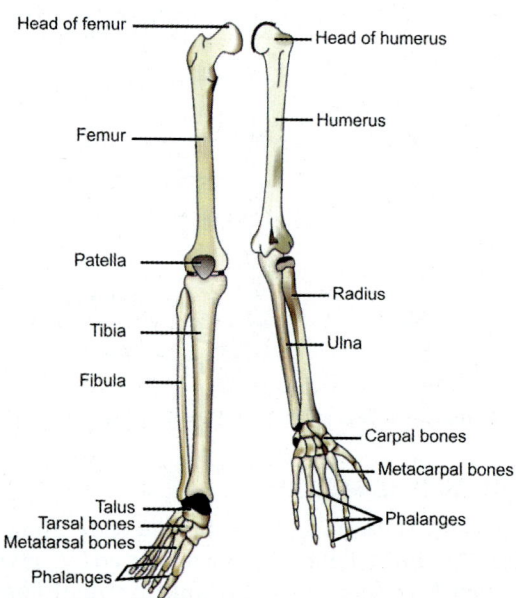

**Annexation Fig. 4:** Bones of the upper and lower limbs

### V. RESPIRATORY SYSTEM

The respiratory system consists of the nose, nasopharynx, trachea, and lungs. The main functions of the respiratory system include:

1. Exchange of oxygen and carbon dioxide,
2. Voice production,
3. Regulation of plasma pH and
4. Olfaction (sensation of smell).

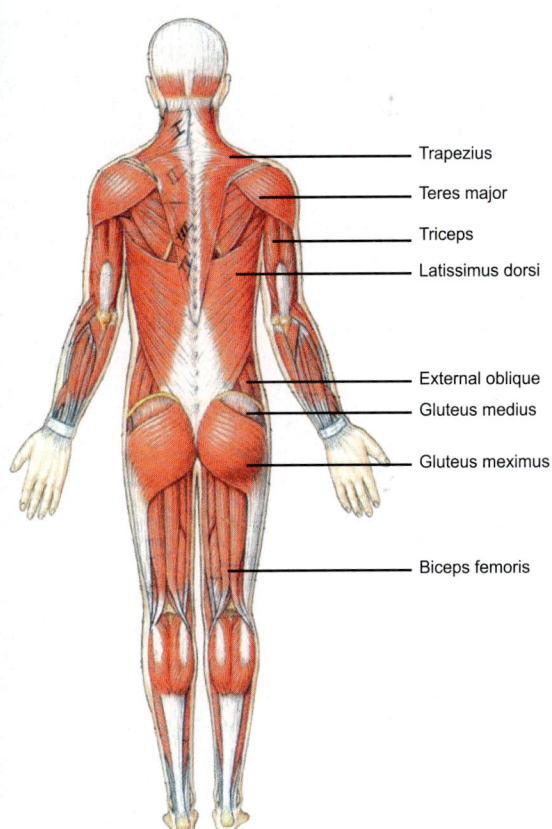

**Annexation Fig. 6:** Muscles of human body (back aspect)

Trapezius
Teres major
Triceps
Latissimus dorsi

External oblique
Gluteus medius

Gluteus meximus

Biceps femoris

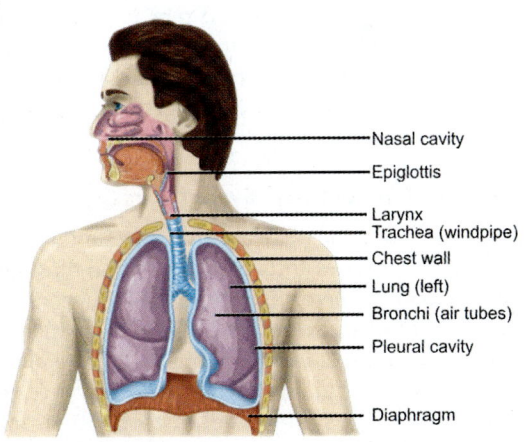

Nasal cavity
Epiglottis
Larynx
Trachea (windpipe)
Chest wall
Lung (left)
Bronchi (air tubes)
Pleural cavity

Diaphragm

**Annexation Fig. 7:** Respiratory system

The main role of the respiratory system (Annex. Fig. 7) is gas exchange between the blood and the environment. Primarily, oxygen is absorbed from the atmosphere into the body and carbon dioxide is expelled from the body. Ventilation occurs under the control of the respiration regulatory center in the brain. Ventilation of the lungs is carried out by the muscles of respiration. Inhalation is initiated by the diaphragm and supported by the external intercostal muscles. Normal resting respirations are 10 to 18 breaths per minute.

Inhalation is driven primarily by the diaphragm. When the diaphragm contracts, the rib cage expands and the contents of the abdomen are moved downward. This results in a larger thoracic volume, which in turn causes a decrease in intrathoracic pressure. As the pressure in the chest falls, air moves into the lungs. Exhalation is generally a passive process; however, active or forced exhalation is achieved by the abdominal and the internal intercostal muscles. During this process, air is forced or exhaled out. The lungs have a natural elasticity; as they recoil from the stretch of inhalation, air flows back out until the pressures in the chest and the atmosphere reach equilibrium.

The right side of the heart pumps blood from the right ventricle to the lungs through the pulmonary artery. The pulmonary arteries have numerous branches which accompany the airways. Upon inhalation, gas exchange occurs at the alveoli, the tiny sacs which are the basic functional component of the lungs. The alveolar walls are extremely thin and permeable to gases. The alveoli are lined with pulmonary capillaries, the walls of which are also thin enough to permit gas exchange. Oxygen in the alveolar air diffuses into the blood in the pulmonary capillaries.

## VI. CIRCULATORY (CARDIOVASCULAR) SYSTEM

The cardiovascular system is composed of the heart, blood vessels and the circulating blood.

### Heart

The heart located in the chest, is a four chambered organ (Annex. Fig. 8) with two upper chambers (left and right atria) and two lower chambers (left and right ventricles). It is composed of muscle called myocardium. The myocardium (cardiac muscle) is a specialised form of muscle, consisting of individual cells joined by electrical connections. The contraction of each cell is produced by a rise in intracellular calcium concentration. Contraction of one cell leads to a wave of depolarisation and contraction across the myocardium. This depolarisation and contraction of the heart is controlled by a specialised group of cells called sinoatrial node (**SA node**) in the right atrium (pacemaker cells). These cells generate a rhythmical depolarisation, which then spreads out over the atria to the atrioventricular node. The atria then contract, pushing blood into the ventricles. The electrical conduction passes via the atrioventricular node to the bundle of His, which divides into right and left branches and then spreads out from the base of the ventricles across the myocardium. This leads to contraction of the ventricles, forcing blood up and out into the pulmonary artery (right) and aorta (left). The atria then refill as the myocardium relaxes. The contraction phase is called systole. The relaxation period, when the atria and ventricles refill, is called diastole.

The heart is the pump responsible for maintaining adequate circulation of oxygenated blood around the vascular network of the body. The right side receives deoxygenated blood from the body at low pressure and pumps it to the lungs (the pulmonary circulation). The left side receives oxygenated blood from the lungs and pumps it at high pressure around the body (the systemic circulation).

The heart needs its own blood supply for its functioning. There are two main coronary arteries, the left and right originating from the aorta (Annex. Fig. 9). These branch further to form several major branches. These branches terminate in arterioles supplying the vast capillary network of the myocardium. Obstruction to one or other of the main branches will lead to death of the heart muscle (myocardial infarction). Sometimes sudden death can also occur.

Heart is responsible for generating the blood pressure that propels blood through blood vessels. The pulsation of the heart is felt at any artery. The pulse rate is equal to the heart rate. Normal rate is 70–80 per minute. The principal function of the heart is to continuously pump blood throughout the body and supply the tissues with oxygen and nutrients and also remove metabolic waste products.

## Vascular (Circulatory) System (Annex. Fig. 10)

The system is made up of arteries, veins and lymph vessels. The arteries and veins carry blood throughout the body, delivering oxygen and nutrients to the body tissues and remove tissue waste matter. The lymph vessels carry lymphatic fluid (a clear, colorless fluid containing water and blood cells). The lymphatic system helps to protect and maintain the fluid environment of the body by

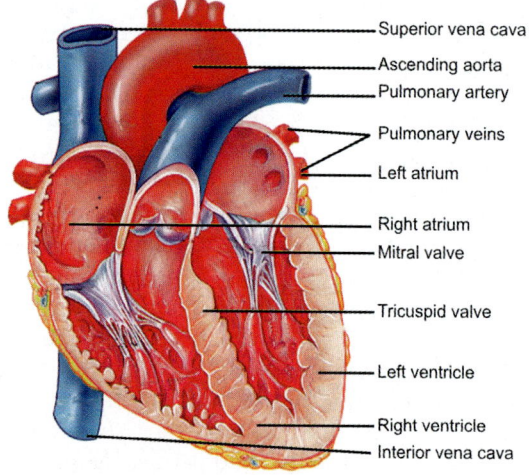

**Annexation Fig. 8:** Anatomy of heart

- Superior vena cava
- Ascending aorta
- Pulmonary artery
- Pulmonary veins
- Left atrium
- Right atrium
- Mitral valve
- Tricuspid valve
- Left ventricle
- Right ventricle
- Interior vena cava

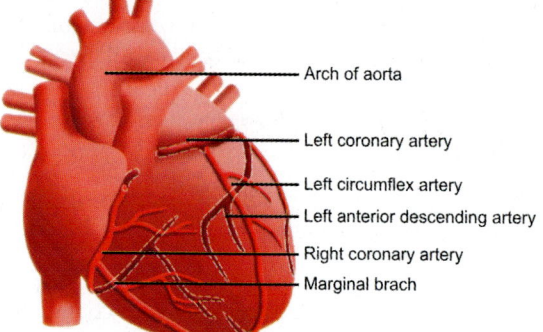

**Annexation Fig. 9:** Blood supply of heart

- Arch of aorta
- Left coronary artery
- Left circumflex artery
- Left anterior descending artery
- Right coronary artery
- Marginal brach

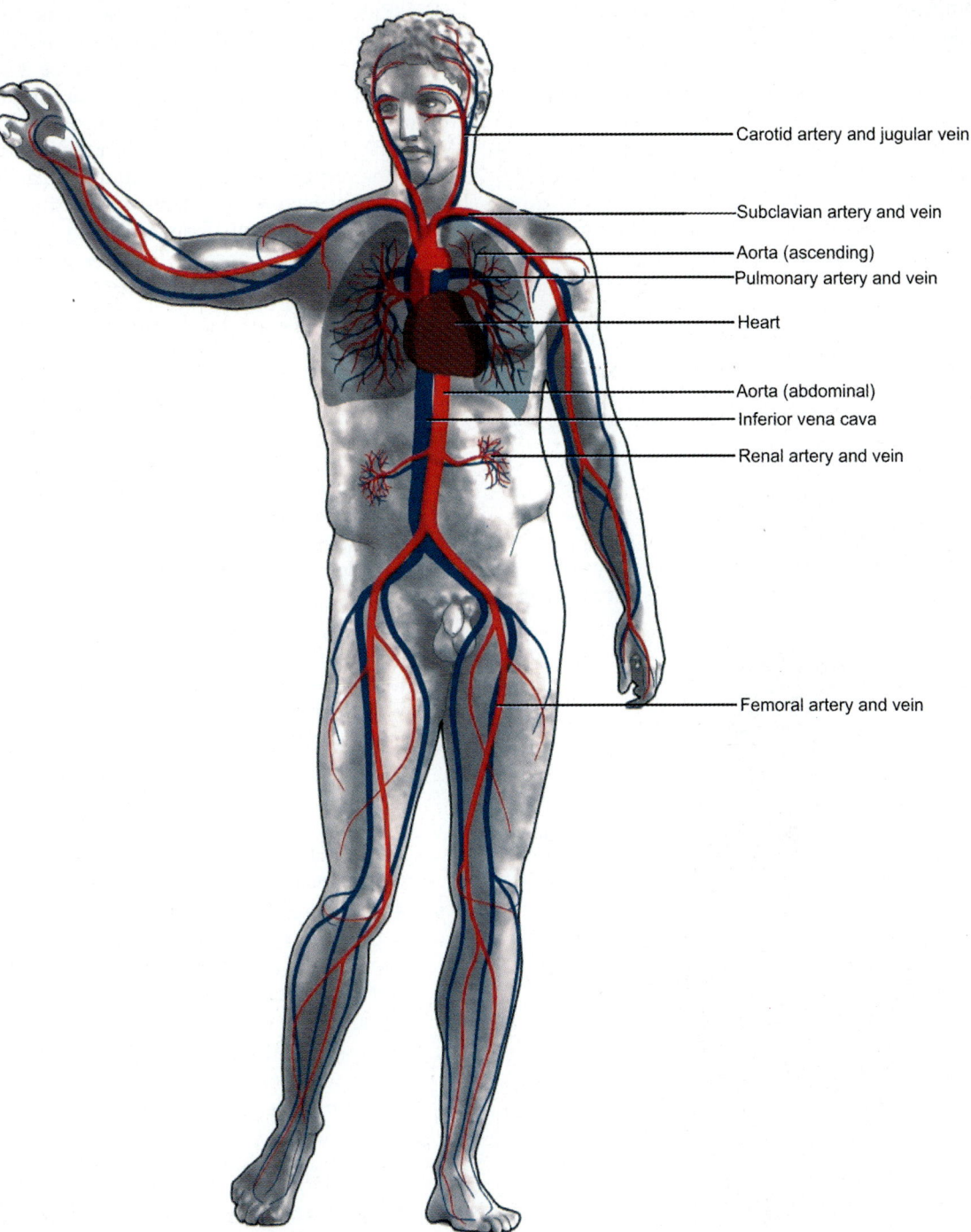

Carotid artery and jugular vein

Subclavian artery and vein

Aorta (ascending)

Pulmonary artery and vein

Heart

Aorta (abdominal)

Inferior vena cava

Renal artery and vein

Femoral artery and vein

**Annexation  Fig. 10:** Circulatory system—major arteries and veins

filtering and draining lymph away from each region of the body.

Heart pumps blood saturated with oxygen through the arteries. The arteries breakdown into smaller and smaller branches in order to bring oxygen and other nutrients to the cells of the body's tissues and organs. As blood moves through the capillaries, the oxygen and other nutrients move out into the cells, and waste matter from the cells moves into the capillaries. As the blood leaves the capillaries, it moves through the veins, which become larger and larger and reach the right side of the heart from where it reaches the lungs for oxygenation. In addition to circulating and lymph throughout the body, the vascular system plays an important role in temperature regulation also.

## VII. GASTROINTESTINAL (DIGESTIVE/ ALIMENTARY) SYSTEM

The overall function of the digestive system is to take in food, break it down to nutrient molecules,

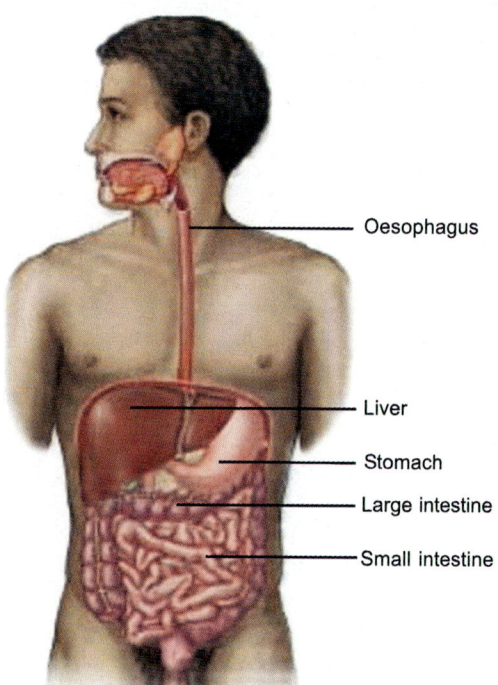

**Annexation Fig. 11:** Alimentary system

Oesophagus

Liver

Stomach

Large intestine

Small intestine

absorb these molecules into the stream, and then rid the body of any indigestible remains. The digestive canal runs from the mouth to the anus and includes the mouth, pharynx, esophagus, stomach, small intestine, and large intestine (Annex. Fig. 11). Accessory digestive organs contribute to the processes of digestion and absorption; but no food or food waste actually passes through them. They include: teeth, tongue, salivary glands, liver, gallbladder and pancreas. The basic processes performed by the digestive system are:

1. *Ingestion:* Food is taken into the alimentary canal.

2. *Propulsion:* Process of moving food through the alimentary canal. Includes deglutition, i.e. swallowing (voluntary) and peristalsis (involuntary). Peristalsis is the primary means by which food is propelled through the GI tract. It involves waves of alternating contraction and relaxation of the smooth muscle in the organ walls.

3. *Mechanical digestion:* Initial breakdown that physically prepares food for further chemical digestion. Includes chewing, mixing of food and saliva by the tongue as well as churning of food in the stomach.

4. *Chemical digestion:* Hydrolytic breakdown of food molecules into their chemical building blocks by enzymes secreted into the alimentary canal. Small amounts occur in the mouth and stomach. Majority occurs in the small intestine.

5. *Absorption:* Passage of nutrients (along with vitamins, minerals, and water) from the lumen of the GI tract across the mucosa and into either or lymph. Primarily occurs in the small intestine.

6. *Defecation:* Elimination of indigestible substances from the body via the anus in the form of faeces

## VIII. ENDOCRINE SYSTEM

The endocrine system is a collection of glands that produce hormones that regulate the body's growth, metabolism and sexual development and function. These glands are ductless (Annex. Fig. 12). The major endocrine glands are:

1. Pineal body,
2. Pituitary gland,
3. Thyroid gland,
4. Thymus,
5. Adrenal glands,
6. Pancreas,
7. Ovaries (females) and
8. Testes (males).

The endocrine system is ban information signal system and uses as the information channel. Glands located in many regions of the body releases into , specific chemical messengers called hormones. The hormones are released directly into the stream and transported to tissues and organs throughout your body. They regulate many functions of the body, viz. mood, growth, develop-

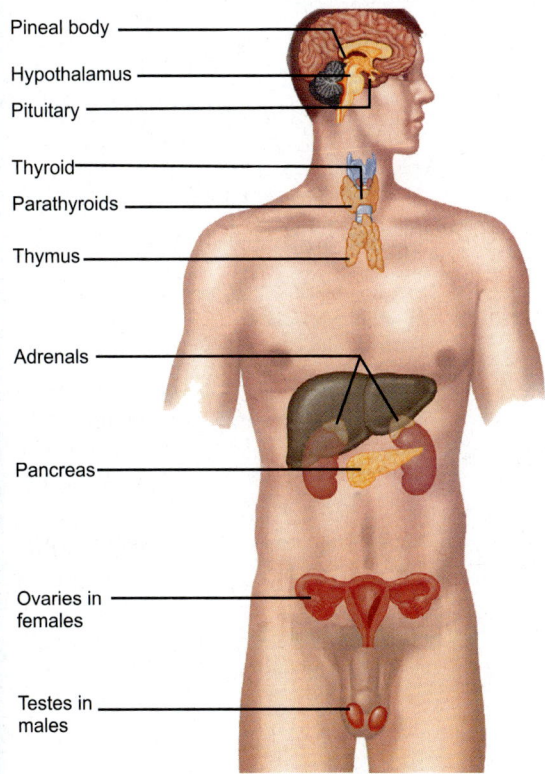

Pineal body

Hypothalamus

Pituitary

Thyroid

Parathyroids

Thymus

Adrenals

Pancreas

Ovaries in females

Testes in males

**Annexation Fig. 12:** Endocrine glands

ment, tissue functions and metabolism, by sending and receiving messages from them.

Dysfunction of the endocrines can produce many disease conditions such as diabetes, hypothyroidism, obesity. The field of medicine which deals with the disorders of the endocrines is called 'endocrinology'. The hormones produced by the endocrines are given in Annex. Table 1.

## IX. NERVOUS SYSTEM

*Major organs:* Brain, spinal cord and peripheral nerves.

### Brain

Human brain is made up of about 100 billion nerve cells which are capable of conducting a great variety of stimuli. It has three main parts called the cerebrum, the cerebellum, and the brainstem (Annex. Fig. 13). The cerebrum is the topmost part of the brain. It is concerned with cognitive, sensory and motor functions. The cerebellum is underneath the back part of the cerebrum. It coordinates the muscular movements and balancing of the body. The brainstem connects with the spinal cord at the bottom of the brain. All the vital centres controlling heart, respiration, etc. are located in the brainstem. Cerebrum and cerebellum are divided into right brain and left brain. The right side controls the left side and the left side controls the right side of the body. Nerves from the right and left side of the body crossover when they enter brain.

Brain is located inside the skull cavity. Brain has three coverings which separate the skull from the brain. This outer covering is the dura mater. The inner coverings are the arachnoid mater and pia mater. Below the arachnoid is the subarachnoid space which contains cerebrospinal fluid, a substance that protects the nervous system. The cerebrospinal fluid (CSF), circulates between layers of the meninges and through cavities in the brain called ventricles. The human brain weighs about 1–1.5 kg. The CSF allows the brain to float, easing the physical stress caused by the brain's mass.

Brain receives signals through nerves from the sense organs. These signals are then processed through out the central nervous system. Reactions

| **Annexation Table 1:** Hormones produced by the endocrines and their function | | |
|---|---|---|
| *Endocrine gland* | *Hormone* | *Function* |
| Hypothalamus | Oxytocin | Contraction of uterus |
| | Vasopressin | Retention of water in kidneys |
| Pituitary | Growth hormone | Stimulates growth |
| | Prolactin | Milk production in breasts |
| | Corticotrophin | Stimulates adrenal cortex |
| | Gonadotrophins | Regulate the function of gonads |
| | Thyroid stimulating hormone | Stimulates thyroid to secrete Thyroid hormone |
| | Follicle stimulating hormone | Sperm production in males and ovum in females. |
| | Luteinising hormone | Stimulates testis to produce male hormone testosterone |
| | Melanocyte stimulating hormone | Stimulates melanin pigment in skin and hair. |
| Pineal body | Melatonin | Antioxidant, causes drowsiness |
| Thyroid | Thyroxin | Affects protein synthesis |
| | Triiodothyronine | Increases basal metabolic rate |
| | Calcitonin | Reduces blood calcium |
| Parathyroid | Parathormone | Increases blood calcium Activate vitamin D |
| Thymus | Thymosin | Development of immune response |
| Pancreas | Insulin | Regulates glucose metabolism |
| | Glucagon | Increases blood glucose level |
| Adrenal cortex | Glucocorticosteroid Immunosuppression | Metabolic hormone, anti-inflammatory |
| | Mineralocorticoids | Increases blood volume by reabsorption of sodium in kidneys |
| | Androgens | Anabolic and virilizing effect |
| Adrenal medulla | Adrenaline | Boosts supply of oxygen to organs and tissues, suppresses non-emergency body processes |
| | Noradrenaline | Constricts blood vessels, Increases blood pressure |
| Ovary | Estrogen | Maturation of female reproductive organs, secondary sex characters |
| | Progesterone | Regulates menstrual cycle |
| Testes | Testosterone | Maturation of male reproductive system and production of sperms |

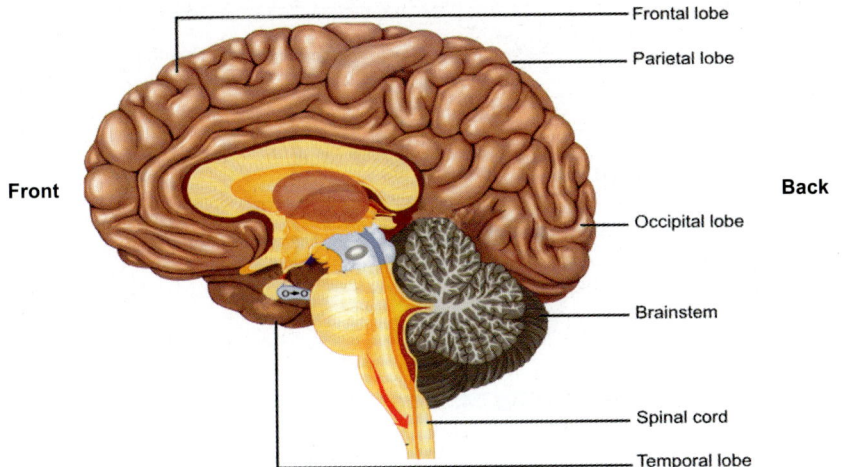

**Annexation Fig. 13:** Human brain

are formulated based upon reflex and learned experiences. An extensive nerve network delivers signals from a brain to control important muscles throughout the body. Anatomically, the majority of incoming and outgoing nerves, are connected to the spinal cord, which then transfers the signals to and from the brain.

Brain has several systems of muscle control. The motor system controls voluntary muscle movement. Nuclei in the brainstem control many involuntary muscle functions such as heart rate and breathing. In addition, many automatic acts (simple reflexes, locomotion) can be controlled by the spinal cord alone.

Brains also produce a portion of the body's hormones that can influence organs and glands elsewhere in the body. Brain also reacts to hormones produced elsewhere in the body. The hormones produced in the pituitary gland in the brain regulate the production of hormones in other endocrine glands.

### Spinal Cord

The spinal cord is a long, thin, tubular bundle of nerves enclosed in the bony vertebral column. It is an extension of the central nervous system from the brain. The main function of the spinal cord is transmission of neural inputs between the periphery and the brain. It is about 45 cm long in

men and 43 cm long in women. The peripheral region contains neuronal white matter tracts containing sensory and motor neurons. Some tracts are ascending (carrying messages to the brain), others are descending (carrying messages from the brain).

Internal to this peripheral region, is the gray, butterfly-shaped central region made up of nerve cell bodies. This central region surrounds the central canal, which is an anatomic extension of the spaces in the brain known as the ventricles and contains cerebrospinal fluid. Coverings of the brain are continuous with spinal cord also.

The human spinal cord is divided into 31 different segments. Motor nerve roots exit from the front and sensory nerve roots enter from the back aspect. These nerve roots later join to form paired spinal nerves, one on each side of the spinal cord (Annex. Fig. 14). There are 31 spinal cord nerve segments in a human spinal cord. The spinal cord is also involved in reflexes that do not immediately involve the brain.

### Peripheral Nerves

The peripheral nervous system extends outside the central nervous system which consists of the brain and spinal cord, to serve the limbs and organs (Annex. Fig. 15). The peripheral nervous system is divided into the somatic nervous system and

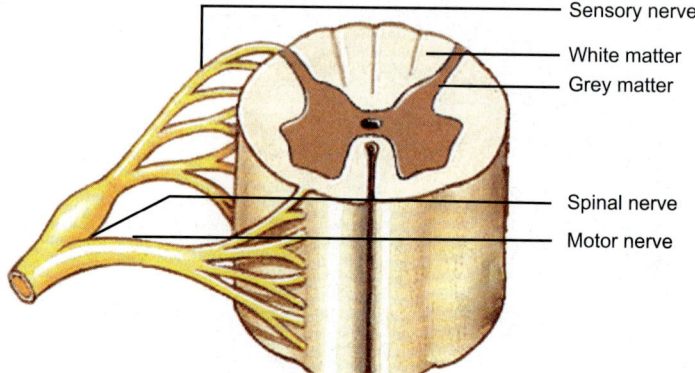

**Annexation Fig. 14:** Cross-section of spinal cord

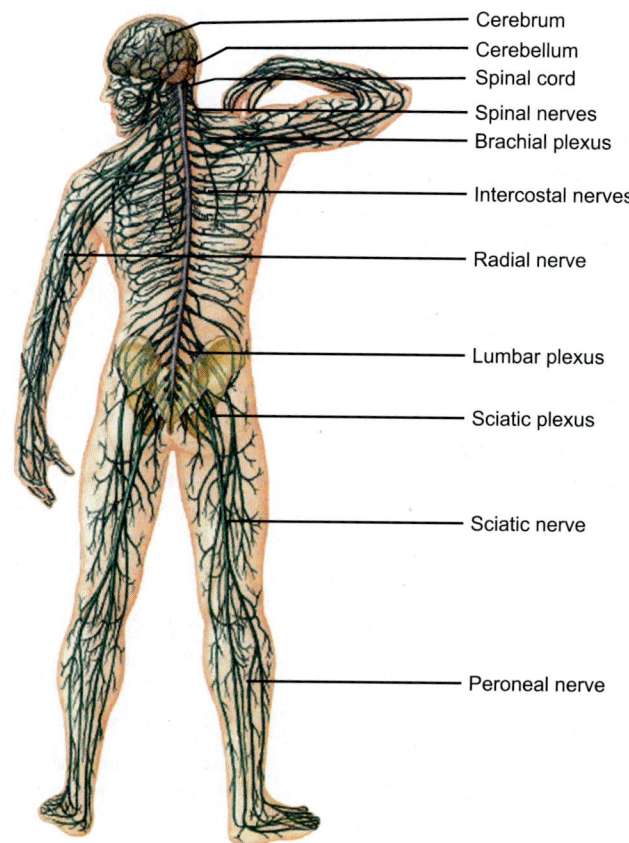

**Annexation Fig. 15:** Peripheral nervous sytem—major nerve plexuses and nerve

the autonomic nervous system. Two main components of the system are sensory (afferent) pathways that provide input from the body into the CNS and motor (efferent) pathways that carry signals to muscles and glands. Most sensory input carried in the PNS remains below the level of conscious awareness. Input that does reach the conscious level contributes to perception of our external environment.

## Somatic Nervous System

This includes all nerves controlling the muscular system and external sensory receptors. External sense organs (including skin) are receptors. Muscle fibers and gland cells are effectors. The reflex action is an automatic, involuntary reaction to a stimulus. Examples of reflex arcs include balance, the blinking reflex, and the stretch reflex. Sensory input from the peripheral nerves is processed by the central nervous system and responses are sent to the organs of the body.

## Autonomic Nervous System

The autonomic nervous system consisting of motor neurons control internal organs. The autonomic nervous system has the sympathetic division, parasympathetic division, and enteric division. The sympathetic nervous system responds to impending danger or stress, and is responsible for the increase of heart-beat and pressure. There will be increased secretion of adrenaline. The parasympathetic nervous system, on the other hand, is evident when a person is resting and feels relaxed, and is responsible for such things as the constriction of the pupil, the slowing of the heart, the dilation of the vessels, and the stimulation of the digestive and genitourinary systems. The role of the enteric nervous system is to manage every aspect of digestion, from the esophagus to the stomach, small intestine and colon. The autonomic system controls muscles in the heart, the smooth muscle in internal organs such as the intestine, bladder, and uterus. Each of these subsystems operates in the reverse of the other (antagonism). Both systems innervate the same organs and act in opposition to maintain homeostasis.

## Special Senses

Input to the nervous system is in the form of our five senses: pain, vision, taste, smell, and hearing. Vision, taste, smell, and hearing input are the special senses. Pain, temperature, and pressure are known as somatic senses.

## X. EXCRETORY SYSTEM

The excretory system is an organ system that performs the function of excretion, the bodily process of discharging wastes. The main components of the excretory system are the urinary system of two kidneys, two tubes that carry urine called ureters, the bladder, and the urethra (Annex. Fig. 16). Other excretory organs are the lungs, skin, sweat glands and liver.

Man has two kidneys. They are bean-shaped organs, located lateral to the spine "behind" the abdominal cavity. At the inner side of the kidney, the pelvis can be found, which forms a small reservoir for urine produced by that kidney. From

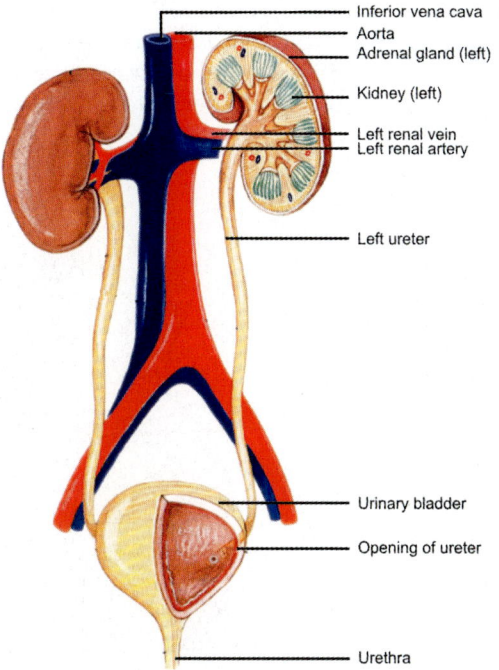

Inferior vena cava
Aorta
Adrenal gland (left)
Kidney (left)
Left renal vein
Left renal artery
Left ureter
Urinary bladder
Opening of ureter
Urethra

**Annexation Fig. 16:** Excretory system

the pelvis, a small tube, the ureter, connects the kidney to the bladder. The urine is squeezed from the kidney towards the bladder (peristalsis) by way of muscle fibers in the wall of the ureters. The kidney is a highly specialized organ that maintains the internal environment of the body by selectively excreting or retaining various substances according to specific body needs. The importance of urine formation and excretion as a life-sustaining function is highlighted in situations in which kidney function is suddenly lost. Without at least one functioning kidney, death can occur within a few days.

## XI. REPRODUCTIVE SYSTEM

The main role of the reproductive system is to produce cells that allow reproduction. In male, sperms are created to inseminate egg cells produced in the female. The reproductive system consists of gonads and internal and external sex organs. The gonads are organs which produce gametes in each sex. They are testes in the male and ovaries in the female. Gametes are cells involved in sexual reproduction. Gamete is a specialized male or female cell with half the normal number of chromosomes that unites with a cell of the opposite sex in the process of sexual reproduction. Ova and spermatozoa are the gametes. The system provides a mechanism for their union and a nurturing environment for the first 9 months of development of the offspring.

## Male Reproductive System

The male reproductive organs are the penis, testes and seminal vesicles (Annex. Fig. 17).

### Penis

Penis is the copulatory organ of the male. It has a long shaft and an enlarged tip called glans penis. The penis is composed of erectile tissue. When the male is sexually stimulated, the spaces in the erectile tissue get filled up with  and the penis become erect and stiff. Urethra passes through the penis and ends in its tip.

### Testes

The testes are situated outside the abdominal cavity within the scrotum. Testes begin their development in the abdominal cavity and descend into the scrotal sacs during the ninth month of fetal development. Testes continuously produce spermatozoa and the male hormone testosterone.

### Spermatozoa

A mature spermatozoan has a head, body and a tail. The head contains a nucleus with 23 chromo-

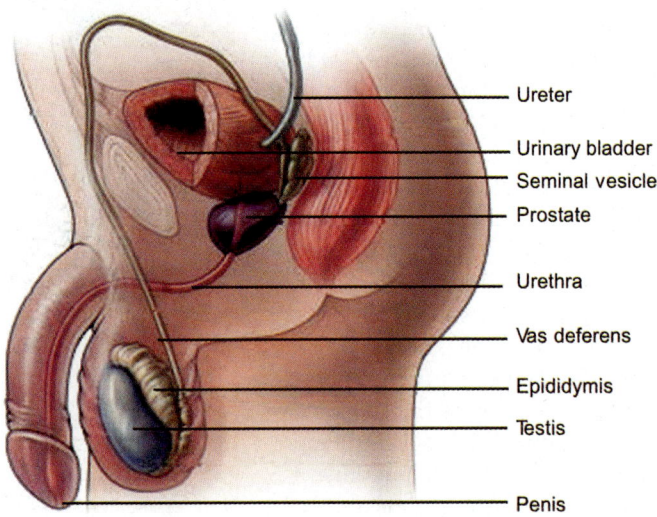

**Annexation Fig. 17:** Male reproductive system

somes. During ejaculation, sperms leave the penis in seminal fluid, produced by the seminal vesicle and prostate glands. During intercourse, semen is deposited in the vagina of the female. Sperms in the seminal fluid enter the uterus and fallopian tubes. If an ovum is present in the fallopian tube, the sperms head penetrates the ovum and unites with it. This process is called fertilisation. The fertilised ovum is called a zygote which may develop into an embryo and later to an offspring.

## Female Reproductive System

This system consists of ovaries, oviducts, uterus, vagina and mammary glands (Annex. Fig. 18). Unlike in males, all these organs are internal. The vaginal orifice opens outside at the vulva which includes labia, clitoris and urethra. Vagina is attached to the mouth (cervix) of the uterus. Uterus is attached to the ovaries by fallopian tubes. In a fertile woman, one ovum matures every month and is released through the fallopian tube into the uterus. During its transit in the tube, a sperm can unite with the ovum and fertilise it. The fertilised ovum implants in the wall of the uterus and develops into a full grown offspring. When the foetus attains full term, the cervix dilates, uterus contracts and expels the foetus outside the uterus through the vagina. If the ovum is not fertilised, it is discarded along with the next menstrual flow.

### Vagina

Vagina is a muscular tube leading from the uterus to the outside of the body in females. The vaginal passage is the receptacle of penis and semen during sexual intercourse. It also acts as the passage of menstrual during menstruation and foetus during parturition. It has a thin membrane called hymen at its outlet, which is usually ruptured during the first intercourse.

### Cervix

Cervix is the lower, narrow portion of the uterus. Top end of the vagina is attached to it. It has an opening which extends to the uterine cavity.

### Uterus

Uterus is a hollow organ composed of muscles. It receives the fertilised ovum from the fallopian tube and implants it in the uterine wall. The foetus derives its nutrition from the vessels specially developed in the placenta. The embryo grows into a foetus till it is delivered after 9 months.

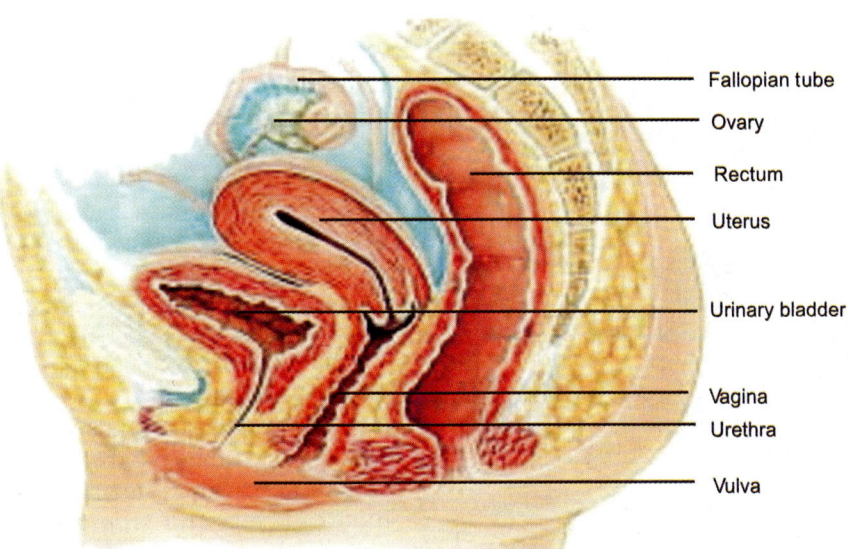

Fallopian tube
Ovary
Rectum
Uterus
Urinary bladder
Vagina
Urethra
Vulva

**Annexation Fig. 18:** Female reproductive system

## Ovaries

There are two ovaries, on either side of the uterus. Ova are produced in the ovaries every month. This process is called ovulation. Ovaries also produce female hormones. The liberated ovum may be fertilised during its transit through the fallopian tube.

## XII. INTEGUMENTARY SYSTEM

This consists of the covering of the body (the skin), including hair and nails as well as other functionally important structures such as the sweat glands and sebaceous glands. The skin is the largest organ in the body and has multiple roles in protection, temperature regulation, sensory reception, etc.

## XIII. LYMPHATIC/IMMUNE SYSTEM

*Major immune systems:* Lymph, lymph nodes, lymph vessels, white cells, t- and b- cells.

Immune system is a group of mechanisms within the human body that protects against diseases. Disorders of the immune system can result in diseases. These diseases are called 'immuno-deficiency diseases'. The immunodeficiency may be congenital or acquired. Acquired immunodefi-ciency is caused by drugs, infections. HIV infection causes acquired immunodeficiency syndrome called AIDS. A hyperactive immune system can damage normal tissues and cause 'autoimmune diseases'. Common autoimmune diseases are rheumatoid arthritis, diabetes mellitus type I, lupus erythematosus, etc.

Hypersensitivity (allergic) reaction is an immune response which damages body's own tissues. Symptoms of hypersensitivity reaction can vary from mild allergic reaction to death. One example is the anaphylactic reaction seen in injection of drugs like penicillin.

## XIV. BLOOD

Blood is a specialised fluid tissue. It consists of formed elements suspended in a liquid matrix, known as plasma. The formed elements consist of erythrocytes (red blood cells), leukocytes (white blood cells), and platelets (Annex. Fig. 19). The average blood volume of an adult is 4.5 to 6 liters in the male and 4 to 5 liters in the females.

*Red blood cells (RBCs):* The red blood cell is a biconcave disc containing hemoglobin, a protein comprising of iron containing 'heme' and a protein 'globin'. Hemoglobin has a unique capacity to transport oxygen to all tissues in the body. The colour of blood depends on the oxygen content. One milliliter of blood contains 4.5 to 6.5 million RBCs.

*White blood cells (leucocytes):* There are four types of white blood cells; neutrophils, Lympho-cytes, eosinophils and monocytes. These cells are mostly defenders of the body against invading organisms. These cells can migrate into tissues and destroy the foreign materials.

One milliliter of blood contains 6000–10000 white blood cells.

*Platelets:* Platelets contain many factors which will enhance their aggregation. Platelets can adhere to the lining membrane of the injured blood vessels and stop bleeding. They are concerned with clotting of blood. One milliliter of blood contains 150,000 to 350,000 platelets.

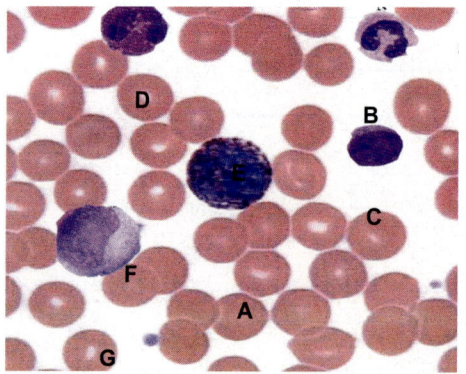

**Annexation Fig. 19:** Elements of blood: A. Red blood cells, B to F – White blood cells, B. Neutrophil, C. Lymphocyte, D. Eosinophil, E. Basophil, F. Monocyte, G. Platelet,

## XV. SUPREME COURT ORDER REGARDING LIE DETECTOR, BRAIN MAPPING AND NARCO ANALYSIS

Criminal Appeal No. 1267 of 2004, Smt. Selvi & Ors. ... Appellants Versus State of Karnataka Criminal Appeal Nos. 54 of 2005, 55 of 2005, 56-57 of 2005, 58-59 of 2005, 1199 of 2006, 1471 of 2007, and Nos.987 & 990 of 2010 [Arising out of SLP (Crl.) Nos. 10 of 2006 and 6711 of 2007]

### Abstract

.......we hold that no individual should be forcibly subjected to any of the techniques in question, whether in the context of investigation in criminal cases or otherwise. Doing so would amount to an unwarranted intrusion into personal liberty. However, we do leave room for the voluntary administration of the impugned techniques in the context of criminal justice, provided that certain safeguards are in place. Even when the subject has given consent to undergo any of these tests, the test results by themselves cannot be admitted as evidence because the subject does not exercise conscious control over the responses during the administration of the test. However, any information or material that is subsequently discovered with the help of voluntary administered test results can be admitted, in accordance with Section 27 of the Evidence Act, 1872. The National Human Rights Commission had published 'Guidelines for the Administration of Polygraph Test (Lie 249 Detector Test) on an Accused' in 2000. These guidelines should be strictly adhered to and similar safeguards should be adopted for conducting the 'Narcoanalysis technique' and the 'Brain Electrical Activation Profile' test. The text of these guidelines has been reproduced below:

(i) No Lie Detector Tests should be administered except on the basis of consent of the accused. An option should be given to the accused whether he wishes to avail such test.

(ii) If the accused volunteers for a Lie Detector Test, he should be given access to a lawyer and the physical, emotional and legal implication of such a test should be explained to him by the police and his lawyer.

(iii) The consent should be recorded before a Judicial Magistrate.

(iv) During the hearing before the Magistrate, the person alleged to have agreed should be duly represented by a lawyer.

(v) At the hearing, the person in question should also be told in clear terms that the statement that is made shall not be a 'confessional' statement to the Magistrate but will have the status of a statement made to the police.

(vi) The Magistrate shall consider all factors relating to the detention including the length of detention and the nature of the interrogation.

(vii) The actual recording of the Lie Detector Test shall be done by an independent agency (such as a hospital) and conducted in the presence of a lawyer. 250

(viii) A full medical and factual narration of the manner of the information received must be taken on record.

C J I —K.G. Balakrishnan
J.R.V. Raveendran
J.J.M. Panchal

# Index